BLACK GENE LIES
Slave Quarter Cures

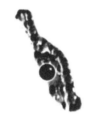

Dr. Joel D. Wallach, BS, DVM, ND

Dr. Ma Lan, MD, MS, LAC

With

Dr. Jennifer Daniels, MD, MBA

BLACK GENE LIES
Slave Quarter Cures

Dr. Joel D. Wallach, BS, DVM, ND
Dr. Ma Lan, MD, MS, LAc
with
Dr. Jennifer Daniels, MD, MBA

Library of Congress Cataloging in Publications Data:

1. History of Physical Bondage
2. History of Political and Financial Bondage
3. History of Health Bondage: Emotional & Physical
4. History of Black Medicine: Slave Quarter Cures
5. High Blood Pressure in Blacks
6. Cardiovascular Disease in Blacks
7. Diabetes in Blacks
8. Obesity in Blacks
9. Arthritis and Osteoporosis in Blacks
10. Cancer in Blacks
11. Slave Quarter Cures: *Materia Medica*
12. The Remedy for the Bondage of Black Gene Lies

Black Gene Lies: Slave Quarter Cures
First Edition, June 2006
Second Edition, October 2014
ISBN No: 0-9748581-3-7

Copyright © June 2006 by Dr. Joel D. Wallach, Dr. Ma Lan and Wellness Publications, LLC. All Rights Reserved

No part of this book may be copied or published in any form without written consent of the authors and publisher.

Printed and published by Wellness Publications LLC
P.O. Box 1222, Bonita, CA 91908
www.drjwallach.com
wellness624@gmail.com

1-800-755-4656 USA and Canada
1-619-420-2435 local and international

About the Authors

Dr. Joel D. Wallach, BS, DVM, ND

Dr. Wallach has been involved in biomedical research and clinical medicine for more than 47 years. He received his BS degree (agriculture) from the University of Missouri with a major in animal husbandry (nutrition) and a minor in field crops and soils; a DVM (veterinary medicine) from the University of Missouri; a three year post doctoral fellowship (comparative pathology /medicine), Washington University, St. Louis, Missouri - The Center for the Biology of Natural Systems (The St. Louis Zoological Gardens, Shaw's Botanical Gardens, Botany Department, Washington University), Iowa State Veterinary Diagnostic Laboratory, Iowa State University, Ames, Iowa; Natal Parks Board, Umfolozi and Hluhluwe Game Parks, Republic of South Africa; St. Louis Zoological Gardens; The Chicago Zoological Gardens (Brookfield Zoo); Shedd Aquarium, Chicago, Il; Yerkes Regional Primate Research Center, Emory University, Atlanta, GA; ND (naturopathic physician), the National College of Naturopathic Medicine, Portland, OR; Harbin Medical University, Harbin, Hei Long Jiang and the Shanghai Medical University, People's Republic of China.

He was a member of NIH site visit teams for facilities using exotic animal models for the study of human disease for four years and was a member of the 1968 National Science Foundation ad hoc committee that authored the 1968 Animal Welfare Act (humane housing, nutrition and care of laboratory and captive exotic species); assistant professor of pathology, Iowa State Veterinary Diagnostic Laboratory, Ames, Iowa; adjunct professor of veterinary pathology, University of Missouri, Columbia, Missouri; a professor of nutrition at the National College of Naturopathic Medicine, Portland, OR; a Consulting Professor of Medicine, Harbin Medical University, Harbin, Hei Long Jiang, People's Republic of China.

Dr. Wallach has appeared as an expert witness in State and Federal Courts as a comparative pathologist.

Dr. Wallach attained the rank of Lieutenant Colonel in the Missouri Air National Guard (131st Tactical Hospital), known as "Lindberg's own," and the Alaskan Air Reserves with responsibilities in public health and prevention and clean up of nuclear, biological and chemical attacks in North America and Europe.

Dr. Wallach was a recipient of the 1991 Wooster Beach Gold Medal Award (Association of Eclectic Physicians) for a significant breakthrough in the basic understanding of the cause and pathophysiology of Cystic Fibrosis. Dr. Wallach was nominated for the 1991 Nobel Prize in Medicine (Association of Eclectic Physicians) for his work in the understanding of the genesis and the pathophysiology of Cystic Fibrosis and other birth defects produced by nutritional deficiencies of the embryo during pregnancy.

Dr. Wallach received the 2004 Guardian of the Constitution Award (Emord & Assoc.) for his proactive and successful litigation efforts in obtaining nutrition claims from the FDA for Selenium and Omega-3 essential fatty acids. He also received the 2004 James Lind Scientific Achievement Award (Emord & Assoc.) for "brilliant discoveries that have paved the way for greater health and longevity" for Americans.

Dr. Wallach has appeared frequently on local and national network and public radio and television (including a special on Cystic Fibrosis with ABC's 20/20), regional and national talk radio programs as an expert on trace mineral, rare earth deficiency diseases, and human health and longevity.

Dr. Wallach is the host of his own syndicated talk radio show programs (Dead Doctors Don't Lie and Let's Play Doctor). Because of his free-wheeling style of humor and ability to zero in on the basic truth in health problems and medical politics he is widely known as the "Rush Limbaugh" of alternative health.

Dr. Wallach has given an average of 300 free health lectures per year for more than 15 years, literally reaching millions of enthusiastic fans. His tape, *Dead Doctors Don't Lie* (translated into eight languages) has sold more than 65 million copies world wide.

Dr. Wallach has produced a CD by the title of *Black Gene Lies II* that was so well received and became so popular that he felt obligated to put more details of the subject of the American medical system falsely blaming degenerative diseases in the Black community to "Black genes," into a book by the same name.

Dr. Wallach has more than 70 peer review publications to his credit including a major reference, *The Diseases of Exotic Animals* - published by W. B. Saunders. This 1,000 page illustrated text is listed by the Smithsonian Institute as, "A recommended reference for all professional zoological parks and Aquariums."

Dr. Ma Lan, MD, MS, LAc

Dr. Ma Lan was educated in the People's Republic of China. Dr. Ma Lan received her MD (medical degree) from the Beijing Medical University; took her residency at the People's Hospital, Beijing and was a staff surgeon at the Canton Air Force Hospital, PRC; she received her MS (master of science) in transplantation immunology from Zhongshan Medical University, Canton, People's Republic of China; as with all Chinese doctors, Dr. Ma Lan was trained in Traditional Chinese Medicine (i.e.- acupuncture, herbs, essential oils, manipulation, food as medicine, massage and hydrotherapy) prior to entering the Western-style medical schools.

Dr. Ma Lan's research credits include being an exchange scholar at the Harvard School of Medicine, Boston, MA; a research fellow in laser microsurgery at St. Joseph Hospital, Houston, TX; the Department of Orthopedic Surgery, the Medical College of Wisconsin, Milwaukee, WI; and the Department of Pharmacology, University of California, San Diego, CA.

Dr. Ma Lan has 10 peer review publications to her credit in the fields of transplant immunology and laser vascular surgery.

Dr. Ma Lan attained the rank of Lieutenant in the Chinese Air Force with primary responsibilities as a general surgeon in the Canton Air Force Hospital, PRC.

Dr. Jennifer Daniels, BA, MD, MBA

Dr. Daniels traces her ancestors back to plantation slaves; she obtained her undergraduate B.A. degree in biology (Premed) from Harvard, Boston, Massachusettes; MD (medical degree) from the University of Pennsylvania, Philadelphia, Pennsylvania and her MBA (Masters Business Administration) from the Wharton School of Business, University of Pennsylvania, with a major in health care financing, organization of health care and the legal aspects of health care.

Dr. Daniels practiced as a primary care physician in Syracuse, New York for more than ten years (1991 - 2001), Clinical Director, Fort Totten Indian Health Service Clinic, Fort Totten, North Dakota, was a consultant for the Veterans Administration Medical Center, Philadelphia, PA analyzing reporting procedures in the hospital laboratory system and has become a historian of economical and effective home remedies of the American colonial slave culture and the current day African American.

Dr. Daniels graduated Cum Laude as a Biology major (Harvard University), she was the recipient of the 1983 McGraw Scholarship, the Henry Kaiser Family Foundation Prize, Harvard-Radcliffe College National Scholar, National Merit Achievement Scholar, President, American Medical Women's Association (Branch 18) and the Dean's List.

Dr. Daniels is nationally and internationally known for a CD of one of her lectures entitled *Slave Quarter Cures* that offers self help treatment options that originated from the 17th century home remedies of American slaves.

Acknowledgements

We gratefully acknowledge Pastor Creflo Dollar and the World Changers Church International, Atlanta, Georgia, for their many forms of support, especially encouragement to explore totally the concept of the *Black Gene Lies: Slave Quarter Cures*.

We gratefully acknowledge Phil Oliver, Genetic Councilor for the Sickle Cell Foundation of Georgia, Support Group, Atlanta, Georgia for introducing us to the tragic health problems in the Black community and introducing us to the iconic figures and political leaders of the American Black community and helping us understand what it meant to be sick and Black in America in the 20th and 21st centuries.

We gratefully acknowledge Ambassador (appointed by President Jimmy Carter as Ambassador to the United Nations) Andrew "Andy" Young (also former mayor of Atlanta and former U. S. Representative from the State of Georgia), who spent literally hundreds of hours sitting in his living room with us or on the phone sharing his views on health care in the Black community and Black politics in America.

We gratefully acknowledge Mike "Stinger" Glenn for opening up to us his vast old book collection of Black history; and John Erpelding for his wisdom and experience related to computer technology and the mechanical construction of this book.

Cover Design

We gratefully acknowledge Jen Loper of Excel Productions and Vince Marasigan of ValMar Printing for their contributions to the cover design.

Table of Contents

About the Authors	iii
Acknowledgements	vi
Introduction	viii
Chapter 1 History of Physical Bondage	1
Chapter 2 History of Political and Financial Bondage	23
Chapter 3 History of Black Health Bondage: Emotional and Physical	80
Chapter 4 History of Black Medicine: Slave Quarter Cures	115
Chapter 5 High Blood Pressure in Blacks	135
Chapter 6 Cardiovascular Disease in Blacks	141
Chapter 7 Diabetes in Blacks	149
Chapter 8 Obesity in Blacks	155
Chapter 9 Arthritis & Osteoporosis in Blacks	165
Chapter 10 Cancer in Blacks	173
Chapter 11 Slave Quarter Cures: *Materia Medica*	185
Bibliography	249
Index	254

Introduction

There are many types of bondage including physical, emotional, political, economic, social and medical.

Between the seventh and the nineteenth centuries Arabs transported approximately 14,000,000 Black slaves over the Sahara desert and the Red Sea for trade and sale throughout the world including the New World colonies.

Slaves were the only form of private, revenue-producing property recognized by universal African Law, and so long before the appearance of White Europeans, Black Africans captured, tortured, killed, ate, bought, traded and sold Black slaves.

Native Americans practiced slavery upon each other long before Europeans arrived in the Americas. Many tribes in the Northwest kept slaves amounting to as many as ten to 15 percent of the total tribal population. The Cherokee employed professional "slave catchers." Routinely large numbers of Native American slaves were tortured, killed and eaten by their Native American owners during redistribution feasts just to show how insignificant the slave was and how wealthy the slave owners were.

Whites in the New World kept a rigid segregation between Blacks and themselves for every aspect of life including where they lived, where they ate and where and how they obtained health care. As a result of the exclusion from White health care systems, Blacks in the American colonies created their own "system" of "slave quarter cures" that were a mixture of African, Native American, Arab and European home remedies, conjure men, healers, root doctors, midwives and in some cases, unique new remedies that had their genesis based on available materials.

The Black people in the Americas have historically suffered from all forms of bondage and have, since the Civil War, been freed from or have in varying degrees extricated themselves from all forms of bondage (including physical, political and financial) except for the last form of human bondage - medical bondage; because of the seamless perpetuation of what we have come to call "the Black gene lies," the Black community in America has in past and even recent history, been denied equal access to government health programs - as it turns out, this situation is not totally bad for those who have embraced, reintroduced and accepted the use of "slave quarter cures."

The medical establishment in industrialized nations, led by the medical establishment in America, continues to perpetuate the false dogma that Black individuals are lesser than White individuals as patients and as care givers - and of course during the 19th and 20th centuries, the American medical system supported this dogma through the pseudoscience of eugenics and later in the 20th and 21st centuries through the false dogmas of genetics.

Yes, there are many diseases that appear in the Black community at a greater rate than in the white community (i.e. - hypertension, type II diabetes, arthritis, osteoporosis, cancer, cardiovascular disease, obesity, etc.), however, the underlying causes are simply cultural dietary choices and nutritional deficiencies and they are absolutely not genetic.

The book, *Black Gene Lies: Slave Quarter Cures*, is a landmark expose that shows that the diseases of the Black population in America, that the medical community attributes to a terrible "Black gene," are in fact caused by regional and cultural eating habits and nutritional deficiencies of trace elements that are easily, safely and economically overcome by the use of simple nutritional supplement programs and herbal remedies.

The medical community in America, by proactively employing the "Big Lie" and the "Stockholm syndrome" in combination, and in a methodical conscious manner, has griped the Black community in America in the most inhumane form of fear, self-recrimination and bondage for the purposes of building an unending income stream for themselves - in effect the Black community is the White doctor's (and some Black doctor's) private hunting grounds and larder.

To understand how the White and Black medical systems and establishment have been able to enslave and milk the assets of the Black community, and the White community for that matter, with chains of DNA, we will look at all forms of bondage and illustrate their similarities.

If every Black (and White) person in America were to follow the guidelines in this book, we would be able to eliminate high blood pressure, diabetes, obesity (10 to 30 pounds per month), arthritis and osteoporosis in the Black community (and White communities) in America in just 90 days and reduce the rate of cancer and cardiovascular disease to almost zero and then they could sing out that old gospel song popularized during the Civil Rights Movement, by Martin Luther King, Jr., "Free at last, free at last. Thank God Almighty, we are free at last."

Dr. Joel D. Wallach & Dr. Ma Lan

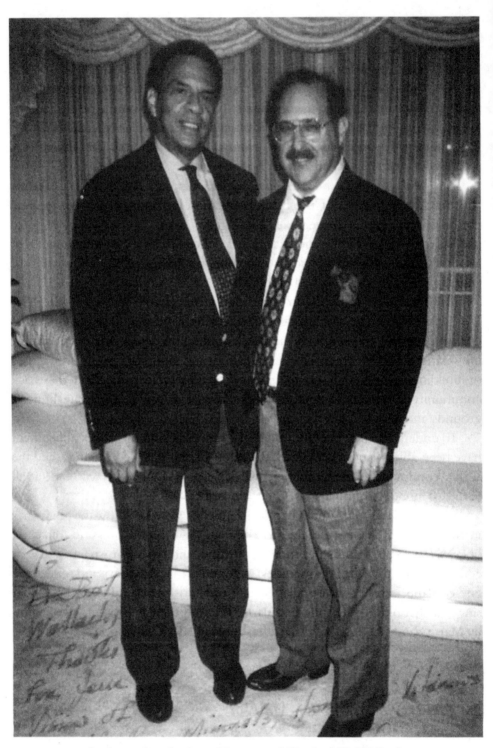

Ambassador Andrew Young and Dr. Joel D. Wallach.

Chapter 1

"History followed different courses for different peoples because of differences among peoples' environments, not because of biological differences among peoples themselves."

*- **Jared Diamond***
Guns, Germs, and Steel

"At some future period, the civilized races of man will almost certainly exterminate and replace the savage races throughout the world."

*- **Charles Darwin***

"Take up the White man's burden -
In patience to abide,
To veil the threat of terror
And check the show of pride;
By open speech and simple,
An hundred times made plain,
To seek another's profit
And work another's gain.

Take up the White man's burden -
The savage wars of peace -
Fill full the mouth of Famine,
And bid the sickness cease."

*- **Rudyard Kipling***
"The White Man's Burden," 1899

"The Negro race has perfect contempt for humanity. Tyranny is regarded as no wrong, and cannibalism is looked upon as desiree quite customary and proper...The polygamy of the Negroes has frequently for its object the having of many children, to be sold, every one of them, into slavery...The essence of humanity is freedom.....At this point we leave Africa, not to mention it again."

- Georg Hegel, 1837

History of Physical Bondage

The beginnings of slavery go back to the earliest of men. Before written history bands of early humans battled between themselves (and took captives) over seasonal food supplies, wild game, territory, water, clay beds, lack of the ability to communicate, fear and just because they didn't know each other.

After the battles, the killed were often eaten. The survivors of the fight were separated into those to be summarily killed and eaten and those to be enslaved as laborers or adopted as members into the band - the latter were usually passive women and little girls.

These early summary killings and cannibalism of the captured weaker individual and groups were the way it was before the appearance of modern cultures, laws and modern religions.

Only crude stone tools and partial skeletal remains give us a hint of who early *Homo sapiens* were - no art, sophisticated weapon or bone tool are to be found. By contrast, the human population of Europe and western Asia between 130,000 and 40,000 years ago is identified by ubiquitous and numerous complete skeletal remains of Neanderthals. They were the first human culture to bury their dead and leave evidence that they treated the sick and infirm.

Archeological evidence of human history passes a crossroad at about 50,000 years ago - this time is called the Great Leap Forward by Jared Diamond. This time was identified in East Africa and is characterized by standardized stone tools and the first preserved jewelry in the form of ostrich-shell beads. Similar evidence of the Great Leap appears in the Near East and in southeastern Europe about 40,000 years ago associated with an innovative, creative and prolific human known as the Cro-Magnons.

Garbage dumps of the Cro-Magnons reveal stone tools, bone tools, fish hooks, needles, awls, engraving tools and multi-piece tools and weapons (harpoons, spear-throwers, and bows and arrows). These tools and weapons allowed for killing dangerous prey and humans from a safe distance that reduced the risk of a disabling injury or death to a hunter or warrior.

The Cro-Magnons are best known for their art, cave paintings, statues and musical instruments. About 40,000 years ago they moved from Africa and Asia into Europe with their modern skeletons, advanced weapons, cultural practices and art.

In just a few thousand years after the appearance of the Cro-Magnon in Europe, the Neanderthal completely disappeared. This fact forces one to come to the conclusion that the modern Cro-Magnon employed their advanced technology and language proficiency to infect, kill, eat, enslave and displace the Neanderthals.

There is no evidence in the form of art or DNA of hybridization between the Neanderthals and the Cro-Magnon peoples - the Neanderthals were either killed and eaten or failed to learn or employ a technique necessary for survival (the placing of wood ashes or plant minerals into gardens and food).

The Americas were settled with humans by 11,000 B.C. Of the inhabitable continents, North America and South America are the ones with the most "compressed" human prehistory.

The Old Testament describes the 400 years enslavement (1000 -1405 BC) of the Hebrews by the Egyptians.

The enslavement of the Hebrews actually started when Joseph's father, Jacob, sent him to check on the status of his brothers and his father's flock. Joseph's brothers were jealous of him because he was his father's favorite and they conspired to kill him. They threw him into a pit, sat down to eat and decide Joseph's fate. His brothers decided to sell him into slavery to the Ishmaelites for 20 shekels of silver (why not sell Joseph and make a profit, rather than simply kill him at no gain) - and the Ishmaelites took Joseph to Egypt.

"Now Joseph had been taken down to Egypt. And Potiphar, an officer of Pharaoh, captain of the guard, an Egyptian, bought him from the Ishmaelites who had taken him down there." Joseph became a successful man and his Egyptian master saw that in all he did Joseph was prosperous. The Egyptian made Joseph the overseer of his house and all that he had.

Over time the Egyptian's wife tried to seduce Joseph, who refused her out of loyalty to his master and "not wanting to sin." The wife complained to her husband falsely that Joseph attempted to seduce her and the captain of the guard put Joseph into jail.

The Pharaoh had a dream that "as he stood by the river; suddenly there came up out of the river seven cows, fine looking and fat; and they fed in the meadow. Then behold, seven other cows came up after them out of the river, ugly and gaunt, and stood by the other cows on the bank of the river. And the ugly and gaunt cows ate up the seven fine looking and fat cows. So Pharaoh awoke.

He slept and dreamed a second time; and suddenly seven heads of grain came up on one stalk, plump and good. Then behold, seven thin heads, blighted by the east wind, sprang up after them. And the seven thin heads devoured the seven plump and full heads. So Pharaoh awoke, and indeed it was a dream."

When the Pharaoh's magicians and wise men of Egypt could not interpret his dreams, the Pharaoh's chief butler, who had been in prison with Joseph, told how Joseph had very accurately interpreted his own dream. As a result the Pharaoh sent for Joseph to interpret his own dreams.

Then Joseph said to Pharaoh, "The dreams of Pharaoh are one; God has shown Pharaoh what He is about to do: The seven good cows are seven years, and the seven good wheat heads are seven years; the dreams are one. And the seven thin and ugly cows which came up after them are seven years, and the seven empty wheat heads blighted by the east wind are seven years of famine.

Indeed seven years of great plenty will come throughout all the land of Egypt. But after them seven years of famine will arise, and all the plenty will be forgotten in the land of Egypt; and famine will deplete the land.

Now therefore, let Pharaoh select a discerning and wise man, and set him over the land over Egypt. Let Pharaoh do this, and him appoint officers over the land, to collect one-forth of the produce of the land of Egypt in the seven plentiful years.

And let them gather all the food of those good years that are coming, and store up grain under the authority of the Pharaoh, and let them keep food in the cities. Then that food shall be as a reserve for the land for the seven years of famine which shall be in the land of Egypt that the land may not perish during the famine.

Then Pharaoh said to Joseph, inasmuch as God has shown you all this, there is now one as discerning and wise as you.

You shall be over my house, and all my people shall be ruled according to your word; only in regard to the throne will I be greater than you. And Pharaoh said to Joseph, 'See, I have set you over all the land of Egypt.'

Now in the seven plentiful years the ground brought forth abundantly. So he gathered all the food of seven years which were in the land of Egypt, and laid up the food in the cities; he laid up in every city the food of the fields which surrounded them.

Then the seven years of plenty, which were in the land of Egypt ended. And the seven years of famine began to come, as Joseph had said. The famine was in all lands, but in all the land of Egypt there was bread.

At this time, Joseph's father sent Joseph's brothers to buy grain from Egypt, so Joseph's ten brothers went down to buy grain in Egypt.

Now Joseph was governor over the land; and it was he who sold grain to all the people of the land. So Joseph recognized his brothers but they did not recognize him. Then Joseph said to his brothers, 'Please come near to me.' So they came near. Then he said, 'I am Joseph your brother, whom you sold into Egypt.'

Now the report of it was heard in Pharaoh's house, saying 'Joseph's brothers have come.' So it pleased Pharaoh and his servants well. And Pharaoh said to Joseph, 'Say to your brothers, do this: load your animals and depart; go to the land of Canaan. Bring your father and your households and come to me; I will give you the best of the land of Egypt, and you will eat the fat of the land.'

Joseph died at the age of 110 years. And so Joseph died, so did all his brothers, and all that generation. But the children of Israel were fruitful and increased abundantly, multiplied and grew exceedingly mighty; and the land was filled with them.

Now there arose a new king over Egypt, who did not know Joseph. And he said to his people, 'look, the people of the children of Israel are more and mightier than we; come, let us deal shrewdly with them, lest they multiply, and it happen, in the event of war, that they also join our enemies and fight against us, and so go up out of the land.'

Therefore they set taskmasters over them to afflict them with their burdens. And they built Pharaoh supply cities, Pithom and Raamses. But the more they afflicted them, the more they multiplied and grew. And they were dread of the children of Israel.

So the Egyptians made the children of Israel serve with rigor. And they made their lives bitter with hard bondage - in mortar, in brick, and in all manner of service in the field. All their service in which they made them serve was with rigor."

The Egyptians were heavy-handed taskmasters who would have engendered the desire for escape for the average human, however, the hostile desert environment surrounding the Hebrews prevented them from simply running away - they were dependent upon their slave masters for their very existence and so they gave up hopes of escape and endured 400 years of slavery, physical bondage, hard labor, depression and disgrace.

Two thousand years ago the ancient Romans and Greeks in the Old World captured, bought and sold, used, abused, tortured, dissected live slaves, sacrificed humans to their gods and killed slaves.

Twelve hundred years ago the Incas and Aztecs in the New World captured, sacrificed, bought and sold, used, abused, tortured and killed and ate slaves. The

Incas and Aztecs had designated helpers to the priests who portioned out the flesh of the sacrificed captives - the heart went to the priests, the right foot and thigh to the emperor and the balance went first to the warrior who had captured them and then to other deserving families of those killed or injured in battle.

These warrior-states grew by extension into neighboring chiefdoms or states, they did not have a great navy to carry armies around the world; as a result they were isolated and had no possibility of invading other continents.

By contrast, the largest human population shift in modern times was the colonization of the New World (the Americas) by the armies of Europeans; with the ensuing conquest came population reduction, or complete extermination of most groups of Native Americans.

The Americas were initially colonized by 11,000 B.C. through Alaska, the Bering Straight and Siberia. Large agricultural societies developed and grew farther South than their original entry routes and developed in total isolation far removed from the complex societies of the Old World.

The first interactions between the "advanced" Old World cultures and the New World cultures started suddenly in A.D. 1492 when Christopher Columbus arrived and "discovered" the heavily populated (Native Americans) Caribbean islands.

Perhaps the most dramatic incident recorded between the Old World and the New World cultures and technologies, was the initial encounter between the Inca emperor Atahuallpa and the Spanish conquistador Francisco Pizarro at the Peruvian highland town of Cajamarca on November 16, 1532.

Atahuallpa was the absolute monarch of the largest and most technologically and culturally advanced political state in the New World. Pizarro represented the Holy Roman Emperor Charles V (aka: King Charles 1 of Spain), monarch of the most powerful state in Europe.

Pizarro led a motley band of 168 Spanish soldiers and was in unfamiliar territory, ignorant of the local culture, completely isolated with no hope of support from navel guns or reinforcements.

Atahuallpa by contrast was in the middle of his own empire of millions of subjects surrounded by his loyal army of 80,000 warriors, just returned from winning a civil war with other Indians. Yet, Pizarro captured and enslaved Atahuallpa within the ensuing minutes after they first looked at each other.

Pizarro held Atahuallpa as his prisoner for eight months, as he exacted history's largest ransom in gold in exchange for the promise to free him. After several tons of gold was delivered Pizarro went back on his promise and executed Atahuallpa:

"Atahuallpa was accused of idolatry, polygamy and incest, which was equivalent to condemning him for practicing a different culture." - Eduardo Galeano

Atahuallpa's capture was critical to the European conquest of the Inca Empire. The Spaniard's superior weapons would have resulted in eventual victory over time, however, the capture and enslavement of Atahuallpa guaranteed a quick and economical conquest.

Atahuallpa was revered by the Inca people as the living embodiment of the sun god who had absolute authority over his subjects - they even obeyed his orders from captivity. Even during the months of Atahuallpa's captivity, Pizarro was able to send out scouting parties under the protection of Atahuallpa without interference throughout the Inca Empire and to send riders to Panama to ask for reinforcements. When battles finally erupted following Atahuallpa's execution, the Spanish were ready with large numbers of well equipped troops.

What happened that bright sunny day at Cajamarca is well documented, as it was recorded in writing by numerous Spanish participants. Jared Diamond wove together the eye witness accounts of six of Pizarro's party, including his brothers Hernando and Pedro:

"The prudence, fortitude, military discipline, labors, perilous navigations, and battles of the Spaniards - vassals of the most invincible Emperor of the Roman Catholic Empire, our natural King and Lord - will cause joy to the faithful and terror to the infidels. For this reason, and for the glory of God our Lord and for the service of the Catholic Imperial Majesty, it has seemed good to me to write this narrative, and to send it to Your Majesty, that all may have a knowledge of what is here related. It will be to the glory of God, because they have been conquered and brought to our holy Catholic Faith so vast a number of heathens, aided by His Holy guidance. It will be to the honor of our Emperor because, by reason of his great power and good fortune, such events happened in his time. It will give joy to the faithful that such battles have been won, such provinces discovered and conquered, such riches brought home for the King and for themselves; and that such terror has been spread among the infidels, such admiration excited in all mankind.

For when, either in ancient or modern times, have such great exploits been achieved by so few against so many, over so many climes, across so many seas, over such distances by land, to subdue the unseen and the unknown? Whose deeds can be compared with those of Spain? Our Spaniards, being few in number, never having more than 200 or 300 men together, and sometimes only 100 and even fewer, have, in our times, conquered more territory than has ever been known before, or than all the faithful and infidel princes posses. I will only write, at present, of what befell in the conquest, and I will not write much, in order to avoid prolixity.

Governor Pizarro wished to obtain intelligence from some Indians who had come from

Cajamarca, so he had them tortured. They confessed that they had heard that Atahuallpa was waiting for the Governor at Cajamarca. The Governor then ordered us to advance. On reaching the entrance to Cajamarca, we saw the camp of Atahuallpa at a distance of a league, in the skirts of the mountains. The Indians' camp looked like a very beautiful city. They had so many tents that we were all filled with great apprehension. Until then, we had never seen anything like this in the Indies. It filled all our Spaniards with fear and confusion. But we could not show any fear or turn back, for if the Indians had sensed any weakness in us, even the Indians that we were bringing with us as guides would have killed us. So we made a show of good spirits, and after carefully observing the town and the tents, we descended into the valley and entered Cajamarca.

We talked a lot among ourselves about what to do. All of us were full of fear, because we were so few in number and we had penetrated so far into a land where we could not hope to receive reinforcements. We all met with the Governor to debate what we should undertake the next day. Few of us slept that night, and we kept watch in the square of Cajamarca, looking at the campfires of the Indian army. It was a frightening sight. Most of the campfires were on a hillside and so close to each other that it looked like the sky brightly studded with stars. There was no distinction that night between the mighty and the lowly, or between foot soldier and horsemen. Everyone carried out sentry duty fully armed. So too did the good old Governor, who went about encouraging his men. The Governor's brother Hernando Pizarro estimated the number of Indian soldiers there at 40,000 but he was telling a lie just to encourage us, for there were more than 80,000 Indians.

On the next morning a messenger from Atahuallpa arrived, and the Governor said to him, 'Tell your lord to come when and how he pleases, and that, in what way so ever he may come I will receive him as a friend and brother. I pray that he may come quickly, for I desire to see him. No harm or insult will befall him.'

The Governor concealed his troops around the square at Cajamarca, dividing the cavalry into two portions of which he gave the command of one to his brother Hernando Pizarro and the command of the other one to Hernando de Soto. In like manner he divided the infantry, he himself taking one part and giving the other to his brother Juan Pizarro. At the same time, he ordered Pedro de Candia with two or three infantrymen to station themselves there with a small piece of artillery. When all the Indians, and Atahuallpa with them had entered the Plaza, the Governor would give a signal to Candia and his men, after which they should start firing the gun, and the trumpets should sound, and at the sound of the trumpets the cavalry should dash out of the large court where they were waiting hidden in readiness.

At noon Atahuallpa began to draw up his men and to approach. Soon we saw the entire plain full of Indians, halting periodically to wait for more Indians who kept filing out of the camp behind them. They kept filing out in separate detachments into the afternoon. The front detachments were now close to our camp, and still more troops kept issuing from the camp of the Indians. In front of Atahuallpa went 2,000 Indians who swept the road ahead of *him, and these were followed by the warriors, half of whom were marching in the fields on one side of him and half on the other side.*

First came a squadron of Indians dressed in clothes of different colors, like a chessboard. They advanced, removing the straws from the ground and sweeping the road. Next came three squadrons in different dresses, dancing and singing. Then came a number of men with armor, large metal plates, and crowns of gold and silver. So great was the amount of furniture of gold and silver which they bore, that it was a marvel to observe how the sun glinted upon it. Among them came the figure of Atahuallpa in a very fine litter with the ends of its timbers covered in silver. Eighty lords carried him on their shoulders, all wearing a very rich blue livery. Atahuallpa himself was very richly dressed, with his crown on his head and a collar of large emeralds around his neck. He sat on a small stool with a rich saddle cushion resting on his litter. The litter was lined with parrot feathers of many colors and decorated with plates of gold and silver.

Behind Atahuallpa came two other litters and two hammocks, in which were some high chiefs, then several squadrons of Indians with crowns of gold and silver. These Indian squadrons began to enter the plaza to the accompaniment of great songs, and thus entering they occupied every part of the plaza. In the meantime all of us Spaniards were waiting ready, hidden in a courtyard, full of fear. Many of us urinated without noticing it, out of sheer terror. On reaching the center of the plaza, Atahuallpa remained in his litter on high, while his troops continued to file in behind him.

Governor Pizarro now sent Friar Vicente de Valverde to go speak to Atahuallpa, and to require Atahuallpa in the name of God and of the King of Spain that Atahuallpa subject himself to the law of our Lord Jesus Christ and to the service of His Majesty the King of Spain. Advancing with a cross in one hand and the Bible in the other hand, and going among the Indian troops up to the place where Atahuallpa was, the Friar thus addressed him: 'I am a priest of God, and I teach Christians the things of God, and in like manner I come to teach you. What I teach is that which God says to us in this book. Therefore, on the part of God and of the Christians, I beseech you to be their friend, for such is God's will, and it will be for your good.'

Atahuallpa asked for the Book, that he might look at it, and the Friar gave it to him closed. Atahuallpa did not know how to open the Book, and the Friar was extending an arm to do so, when Atahuallpa, in great anger, gave him a blow on the arm, not wishing that it should be opened. Then he opened it for himself, and without any astonishment at the letters and paper he threw it away from him five or six paces, his face a deep crimson.

The Friar returned to Pizarro, shouting, 'Come out! Come out, Christians! Come at these enemy dogs who reject the things of God. That tyrant has thrown my Book of Holy Law to the ground! Did you not see what happened? Why remain polite and servile toward this over-proud dog when the plains are full of Indians? March out against him, for I absolve you!'

The Governor then gave the signal to Candia, who began to fire off the guns. At the same time the trumpets were sounded, and the armored Spanish troops, both cavalry and infantry, sallied forth out of their hiding places straight into the mass of unarmed Indians crowding the square, giving the Spanish battle cry, 'Santiago!' We had placed rattles on the horses to terrify the Indians. The booming of the guns, the blowing of the trumpets, and the rattles on the horses threw the Indians into panicked confusion. The Spaniards fell upon them and began to cut them to pieces. The Indians were so filled with fear that they climbed on top of one another, formed mounds, and suffocated each other. Since they were unarmed, they were attacked without danger to any Christians. The cavalry rode them down, killing and wounding, and following in pursuit. The infantry made so good an assault on those that remained that in a short time most of them were put to the sword.

The Governor himself took his sword and dagger, entered the thick of the Indians with the Spaniards who were with him, and with great bravery reached Atahuallpa's litter. He fearlessly grabbed Atahuallpa's left arm and shouted 'Santiago,' but he could not pull Atahuallpa out of his litter because it was held up high. Although we killed the Indians who held the litter, others at once took their places and held it aloft, and in this manner we spent a long time in overcoming and killing Indians. Finally seven or eight Spaniards on horseback spurred on their horses, rushed upon the litter from one side, and with great effort they heaved it over on its side. In that way Atahuallpa was captured, and the Governor took Atahuallpa to his lodging. The Indians carrying the litter, and those escorting Atahuallpa, never abandoned him: all died around him.

The panic-stricken Indians remaining in the square, terrified at the firing of the guns and at the horses - something they had never seen - tried to flee from the square by knocking down a stretch of wall and running out onto the plain outside. Our cavalry jumped the broken wall and charged into the plain, shouting, 'Chase those with the fancy clothes! Don't let any escape! Spear them!' All of the other Indian soldiers whom Atahuallpa had brought were a mile from Cajamarca ready for battle, but not one made a move, and during all this not one Indian raised a weapon against a Spaniard. When the squadrons of Indians who had remained in the plain outside the town saw the other Indians fleeing and shouting, most of them panicked too and fled. It was an astonishing sight, for the whole valley for 15 or 20 miles was completely filled with Indians. Night had already fallen, and our cavalry were continuing to spear Indians in the fields, when we heard a trumpet calling for us to reassemble at camp.

If night had not come on, few out of the more than 40,000 Indian troops would have been left alive. Six or seven thousand Indians lay dead, and many more had their arms cut off and other wounds. Atahuallpa himself admitted that we had killed 7,000 of his men in that battle. The man killed in one of the litters was his minister, the Lord of Chincha, of whom he was very fond. All those Indians who bore Atahuallpa's litter appeared to be top high chiefs and councilors. They were all killed, as well as those Indians who were carried *in the other litters and hammocks. The lord of Cajamarca was killed, and others, but their numbers were so great that they could not be counted, for all who came in attendance on Atahuallpa were great lords. It was extraordinary to see so powerful a ruler captured in so short a time, when he had come with such a mighty army. Truly, it was not accomplished by our own forces, for there were so few of us. It was by the Grace of God, which is great.*

Atahuallpa's robes had been torn off when the Spaniards pulled him out of his litter. The Governor ordered Atahuallpa to sit near him and soothed his rage and agitation at finding himself so quickly fallen from his high estate. The Governor said to Atahuallpa, 'Do not take it as an insult that you have been defeated and taken prisoner, for with the Christians who come with me, though so few in number, I have conquered greater Kingdoms than yours, and have defeated other more powerful lords than you, imposing upon them the dominion of the Emperor, whose vassal I am, and who is King of Spain and the universal world. We come to conquer this land by his command, that all may come to a knowledge of God and of His Holy Catholic Faith; and by reason of our good mission, God, the Creator of heaven and earth and of all things in them, permits this, in order that you may know Him and come out from the bestial and diabolical life that you lead. It is for this reason that we, bring so few in number, subjugate that vast host. When you have seen the errors in which you live, you will understand the good that we have done you by coming to your land by order of his Majesty the King of Spain. Our Lord permitted that your pride should be brought low and that no Indian should be able to offend a Christian'"

The reason for Atahuallpa and his armies appearance in Cajamarca was that they had just won important battles in a civil war and palace revolution against his half brother. Even though Atahuallpa had prevailed in the civil war, the war caused the Inca nation to be vulnerable to outside forces.

The reason for the civil war was an epidemic of smallpox that spread through the South American Indians following the Arrival of the Spanish in Panama and Columbia. The smallpox killed the Inca emperor Huayna Capac and a great number of his court in 1526, including his designated heir, Ninan Cuyuchi. A struggle for the throne ensued between Atahuallpa and his half brother Huascar.

In 1519 Cortes arrived on the coast of Mexico with 600 Spanish soldiers to take on the legendary Aztec warrior nation of 20 million people. The smallpox virus arrived in Mexico in 1520 with an Indian slave from Spanish occupied Cuba. The resulting pandemic immediately killed 50 percent of the Aztecs including the emperor, Cuitlahuac. The fact that the Aztecs were susceptible and the Spanish apparently immune totally demoralized the surviving Aztecs.

In January of 2006, a construction crew discovered the ruins of an old church and burial grounds in the Mexican city of Campeche on the Yucatan peninsula. Researchers who were called in, unearthed some 180 human skeletons. Ten skeletons had characteristics of Africans; four of the skeletons examined bore revealing mineral traces in their teeth that were "in effect birth certificates."

The ratios of strontium in the teeth of the four skeletal remains were characteristic of humans who were born and raised in West Africa. The ratios of the isotopes strontium 87 and strontium 86 were consistent with those in the teeth and bones of people who were born and grew up in West Africa. Five of the other skeletal remains, considered to be African, had isotope ratios typical of people born near Campeche - a second generation.

Many of their teeth were filed and chipped into sharp points in a decorative practice typical of tribal people of Africa. Additional evidence (a pre-1550 medallion) in the grave yard indicated that the skeletons were buried in 1550, thus documenting the earliest remains of African slaves imported into the New World. T. Douglas Price of the University of Wisconsin concluded, "Thus these individuals are likely among the earliest representatives of the African Diaspora in the Americas, substantially earlier than the subsequent, intensive slave trade in the 18th century."

It turns out that colonial Campeche was an important Spanish gateway into the Americas and would have had a heavy Black slave population.

POPULATION LOSSES IN CENTRAL MEXICO (Millions)

```
Millions
35
30
25 * Smallpox
20
15         * Smallpox
10
5                   * Smallpox
2                        * Plague * Hanta virus
1                                          *        *      * S.Pox
0_____ Influenza/measles
1518    1532    1545    1568    1585   1595   1605    1623
(25.2)  (16.8)  (6.3)   (2.7)   (1.9)  (1.4)  (1.1)   (0.7)
```

"Berkeley researchers Cook and Borah spent decades reconstructing the population of the former Aztec realm in the wake of the Spanish conquest. By combining colonial-era data from

many sources, the two men estimated that the number of people in the region fell from 25.2 million in 1518, just before Cortes arrived, to less than 700,000 in 1623 - a 97 percent drop in little more than a century. Sixteenth century Spaniards lumped together all epidemics under the rubric "plague." In addition, native populations were repeatedly struck by (waves of) "cocoliztli," a disease the Spanish did not know(the cause of), but that scientists have suggested might be a rat-bourne hantavirus - spread, in part, by the postconquest collapse of Indian sanitation measures."

By 1618, Mexico's Indian population had dropped from 25 million people 100 years earlier, to a mere 1.6 million; and thus, the Indians were made easy prey for Spanish enslavement. The Spanish were legendary for their cruel and heavy handed enslavement of the captured and surviving Indian populations up and down the west coast of North America and South America. Using mission/fort outposts strategically located on deep-water ports, the Spanish used the slave labor of the Native Americans for farming and the mining of gold, silver and other minerals and jewels between 1526 and the Spanish-American War. The ill gotten gain was then shipped back to Spain.

Throughout the New World, epidemics and pandemics brought by Europeans decimated tribe after tribe before the Europeans physically arrived on the scene - these epidemics and pandemics are believed to have killed 95 percent of the pre-Columbian Native Americans.

The Mississippian chiefdoms, the largest and most successful Native Americans in North America were infected with smallpox and exterminated between 1492 and the late 1600s.

On May 30, 1539, Hernando De Soto landed his private army near what is today Tampa Bay, Florida. De Soto was a unique character: half warrior, half venture capitalist. He became wealthy as a young man in Spanish America by becoming a market leader in the budding slave trade. He rolled his slave profits to fund his expedition for the conquest of the Incas, which added considerably to his wealth.

De Soto joined Pizarro in Tawantinsuyu, gaining a reputation for exreme brutality - he personally tortured Challcochima, Atahuallpa's highest ranking general, before his execution - all this was to gain information about new worlds to conquer - De Soto left Peru and returned to Spain.

In Charles V's court, De Soto persuaded the "bored" king to fund an expedition to the New World for himself. De Soto sailed to Florida with six hundred soldiers, two hundred horses, and three hundred pigs.

For four years De Soto's armed band ravaged and pillaged through what today is Florida, Georgia, North and South Carolina, Tennessee, Alabama,

Mississippi, Arkansas, Texas, and Louisiana, searching for gold, silver and destroying all things that he came across.

The first Black slaves arrived in America in Jamestown in late August of 1619. A Dutch slave trader from the West Indies exchanged his cargo of enslaved Africans to the governor and a merchant for food as reported by John Rolfe to John Smith back in London.

In 1624, the Dutch of New Amsterdam (New York), who had entered into the slave trade in 1621, formed the Dutch West Indies Company imported African Blacks to serve as laborers on Hudson Valley farms. According to Dutch law, the children of manumitted (freed) slaves were still bound to slavery.

By 1625, ten slaves were listed in the first census of Jamestown.

In 1638, the one time price tag for an African slave was $27, while the salary of a White European laborer was $0.70 per day.

The first public slave auction of 23 black slaves was held in the Jamestown Square in 1638.

What were to become the parameters and properties of the "peculiar institution" were defined in the Virginia General Assembly from 1640.

Negro indentures appeared to have been no more than a legal fiction of brief duration in Virginia. Black "freedmen" would live in a legal limbo until the general emancipation in 1864, unable to stand witness in their own defense against the testimony of any Euro-American.

Barbados was the first British possession to enact restrictive legislation governing slaves in 1644, and other colonial administrations, especially Virginia and Maryland, quickly adopted similar rules modeled on it. Whipping and branding, taken from the Roman practice via the Iberian-American colonies appeared early on.

Emanuel, a Virginia slave, was convicted of trying to escape in July 1640; he was recaptured and sentenced to 13 stripes, the letter "R" for runaway branded on his cheek and worked in a shackle one year or more as his master shall see cause.

In 1641 the colony of Massachusetts legalized slavery.

In 1642, the Virginia colony enacted laws that required a fine of those who harbored or assisted runaway slaves. The Virginia law penalized people who sheltered runaways, 20 pounds of tobacco for each night of refuge granted and the slave was to be branded after the second escape attempt.

In 1649, Black slave laborers numbered only 300 in Virginia.

By the 1650s the total world population of human beings had reached 500 million; and some of the indentured servants, White and Black, had earned their freedom.

In 1651 Thomas Hobbes, in *Levisthan*, argued from a mechanistic theory "that man is a selfishly individualistic animal at constant war with others. In the state of nature, life is "nasty, brutish and short."

Because replacements for the freed indentured servants, whether Black or White, were in short supply and more costly, the Virginia plantation owners adopted the "perpetual servitude" policy exercised by the Caribbean land owners. Following the lead of Massachusetts and Connecticut, Virginia legalized slavery in 1661.

The General Assembly of Virginia in 1662 passed an act which directly held that Justinian Code prevailed: *Partvs Seqvitvr Ventrum*; whereby a child born of a slave, regardless of its father's legal status was in fact a slave. A few years later, the numbers of Africans in slavery in Virginia reached 2,000.

Another statute adopted in 1667, established compulsory life servitude: *de addictio*, according to Roman Code - for African Blacks, slavery became an official American Institution.

Originally, the Africans were indentured servants, similar in legal position to poor Englishmen who traded several years of labor in exchange for passage to the Americas.

The concept of a racial "Uncle Tom's Cabin" type of slavery system did not develop until the 1680s.

The word slave did not appear in the Virginia records until 1656. Statutes defining the status of Blacks began to appear casually in the 1660s.

Slave owners were encouraged to baptize their Black and Indian slaves; however, laws were enacted to prevent baptized slaves from being freed:

"It is enacted and declared by this grand (Virginia) assembly, and the authority thereof, that the conferring of baptism doth not alter the condition of the person as to his bondage or freedom."

The "Correction Law of 1669" was passed in Virginia:

"If a Negro slave died at the hands of a master who used extremity of correction to overcome the slave's obstenance, it was not murder."

Lawmakers reasoned that no man would deliberately destroy his own property.

In 1670, Virginia revoked voting rights from recently freed slaves and in indentured servants.

In 1672, the King of England started the Royal African Company to bring shiploads of Black slaves into trading centers like Jamestown, Hampton and Yorktown.

White southerners used the word "servant" until 1865. The word "slave" entered into the Southern vocabulary only as a technical word in trade, law and politics.

Jamestown had exported 10 tons of tobacco to Europe and as a result became a "boomtown." The export industry was growing and the colonists were able to afford two imports that would significantly contribute to their productivity and quality of life - 20 Blacks from Africa and 90 White women from England. The Africans were paid for with trade (food and provisions) and the women were traded from a private English company for 120 pounds of tobacco.

The success of tobacco farming caused African slavery to be legalized in Virginia and Maryland, and slavery became the foundation of the Southern agrarian economy.

Benjamin Franklin was born on January 17, 1706. Boston was 76 years old the year that Franklin was born, the town was not a Puritan "beachhead" any longer, but rather a busy commercial center bustling with preachers, merchants, sailors, and prostitutes. Boston boasted more than 1,000 houses, 1,000 ships registered to its port, and a population of more than 7,000 souls, and the numbers would double every 20 years.

At age 10, with only two years of formal schooling, Franklin started his first full time work as a candle maker with his father. At age 12, in 1718, Franklin was apprenticed to his older brother James as a type setter and writer of poetry.

Initially, Franklin resisted signing the indenture papers as his brother demanded a nine year term of apprenticeship instead of the usual seven.

Franklin was treated like an apprentice instead of a younger brother and he complained that he was subject to "occasional beatings which demeaned me too much." Franklin ran away from his indentured apprenticeship to his brother at age 17 years, much in the same manner as a slave running away from an abusive task master.

By 1715 the numbers of Black slaves reached 24% of the entire Virginia population - up from five percent in 1671.

By 1727, the Junto, a benevolent association was founded by Benjamin Franklin.

Slave uprisings and revolts were dramatic and their effects on Colonial life were dramatic, Genovese reminds us that there was a colorful English North American experience:

The most important slave revolts in the English-speaking North American states occurred in New York City in 1712; at Stono, South Carolina in 1739; in southern Louisiana in 1811; and in Southhampton County, Virginia under Nat Turner in 1831. To them might be added the conspiracy at Point Coupee, Louisiana, in 1795...and the conspiracies of Gabriel Prosser in Richmond, Virginia, in 1800 and of Denmark Vesey in Charleston, South Carolina.

The numbers of African slaves grew slowly at first; by the 1860s slaves had become essential to the economy of the Virginian farming methods. During the 17th and 18th centuries, African slaves lived and worked in all of England's North American colonies.

In 1734, the Great Awakening begins in Massachusetts. This movement encourages Blacks to join the Methodist and the Baptist churches.

In 1749 through 1756 Benjamin Franklin was anguished by the institution of slavery. Slaves made up six percent of Philadelphia's population at that time, and Franklin had published ads in his newspaper that had fostered the buying and selling of slaves:

> "A likely Negro woman to be sold. Enquire at the Widow Reads (Franklin's mother-in-law)."

> "For sale: A likely young Negro fellow - enquire of the printer hereof."

Franklin personally owned a slave couple, but in 1751 he decided to sell them because, as he told his mother, he did not like having "Negro servants" and he found them uneconomical. Yet, at times he would own a slave as a personal servant.

In his article entitled, *Observations on the increase of mankind,* Franklin attacked slavery from an economic point of view. Comparing the costs and benefits of owning a slave, he drew the conclusion that slavery as an institution made no sense. "The introduction of slaves was one of the things that would diminish a nation."

Franklin, however, became fixated with the negative effects that slavery perpetrated against the owners rather than the immorality perpetrated against the slave; he said, "The Whites who have slaves, not laboring, are enfeebled." "Slaves also pejorate the families that use them; white children become proud, disgusted with labor." He continued, "Why increase the sons of Africa by planting them in America, where we have so fair an opportunity, by excluding all Blacks and Tawneys, of increasing the lovely White and Red? But perhaps I am partial to the complexion of my country, for such kind of partiality is natural to mankind."

In his first printing of *Observations*, Franklin observed that, "Every slave being by nature a thief." When Franklin reprinted the work 18 years later, he changed it to say that slaves became thieves "from the nature of slavery." He also removed the entire section about his early view, "The desirability of keeping America mainly White."

In 1756 Virginia's population reached 250,000 (40% being slaves).

In the late 1750s, Franklin became active in the Associates of Dr. Bray, for the formation of schools for Black children in Philadelphia and then widely throughout America. After revisiting the original Black school in Philadelphia in 1763, he wrote an introspective letter regarding his original prejudices:

"I was on the whole much pleased, and from what I then saw have conceived a higher opinion of the natural capacities of the Black race than I had ever before entertained. Their apprehension seem as quick, their memory as strong, and their docility in every respect equal to that of White children. You will wonder perhaps that I should ever doubt it, and I will not undertake to justify all my prejudices."

In 1761, the Quakers were the first group in America to speak out against slavery, and in 1775 the Quakers played a dominant role in the formation of the Pennsylvania Society for the Abolition of Slavery.

Before England prohibited its subjects from participating in the slave trade, an estimated 600,000 to 650,000 African slaves had been transported to North America.

Following the arrival of the 20 African slaves in 1619, the "face" of American slavery began to change from the "tawny" Indian to the "blackamoor" African in the years between 1650 and 1750.

Though the institution of slavery in America was complex, the unsuitability of Native Americans for the labor intensive agricultural practices, their susceptibility to European diseases, the proximity to avenues of escape and their knowledge of living off of the land, and the financial bonanza of the African slave trade led to the transition to an African based institution of slavery.

During this period of transition, the colonial "wars" against the Pequots, the Tuscaroras, the Yamasees, and other Indian nations led to the enslavement and relocations of tens of thousands of Native Americans.

In the early years of the 18th century, the numbers of Native American slaves in areas including the colonies probably reached almost half of the

African slave numbers. During this transitional period, Africans and Native Americans shared the common experience of enslavement. In addition to working together as slaves in the fields, they lived together in communal living quarters (slave quarters), shared recipes for food, and herbal remedies, shared myths and legends and ultimately intermarried.

The intermarriage of Africans and Native Americans was indirectly encouraged by the disproportionate numbers of African men to women (3:1) and the decimation of the Native American men's numbers by disease (smallpox), enslavement and prolonged wars with the better armed colonialists.

A second fact that supports the belief that epidemics devastated Native American populations before the Europeans physically arrived in the New World is that epidemics occurred after they arrived. In her 2001 book, *Pox Americana*, the Duke University historian, Elizabeth Fenn collected evidence that the Western Hemisphere was attacked by two smallpox pandemics just before and during the Revolutionary War.

The smaller of the two pandemics is thought to have begun just outside of Boston in early 1774 and smoldered in that location for several years, killing an average of 10 to 30 victims per day. In Boston the Declaration of Independence was relegated to second place as an event of public interest behind a city-wide smallpox vaccination campaign.

The smallpox virus pandemic spread as far South as Georgia. It decimated the Tsalagi (the group of Native Americans often called the Cherokee, which is a slightly insulting term created by their historical enemies, members of the Creek Confederation) and the Haudenosaunee (the indigenous name for the six nations that made up what Europeans named the Iroquois League). Both groups of Native Americans were allies of the British, and after the epidemic, neither recovered sufficiently to fight the colonists successfully. Smallpox also derailed the British plan to raise an army of Black slaves and indentured servants with the promise of freedom after the war ended - the smallpox killed off almost all of the "Ethiopian regiment" as they were being recruited and trained.

Because of their relative isolation from Europe, the colonists were almost as susceptible to smallpox infection and death as the Native Americans. So many soldiers in the Continental Army fell ill during the epidemic that their leaders worried that smallpox would cause their revolt to grind to a halt.

"The small Pox! The small Pox!" John Adams wrote to his wife, Abigail. "What shall we do with it?" His concerns were quite correct; it was the virus, not the British, that had stopped the Continental Army's excursion into Quebec in 1776. Fenn stated, "One of George Washington's most brilliant moves, was to inoculate the army against the smallpox virus, during the Valley Forge winter of 1778. Fenn went on to say, "Without inoculations, the smallpox epidemic could have easily handed the colonies back to the British."

Native American societies were "matrilineal" and Black African men who married Native American women, became members of their wife's clan and citizens of the respective nation.

As the numbers of the Red and Black relationships grew, the lines of distinction began to blur. The evolution and increase in numbers of "Red-Black" people gained a life of its own. Many of the people who became slaves, free people of color, Africans or Native Americans were most often the product of these integrated relationships and cultures.

In areas such as southeastern Virginia, the Low Country of the Carolinas and Silver Bluff, SC, communities of Afro-Indians began to spring up.

The depth and complexity of this cultural mixture is revealed in a 1740 slave code published in South Carolina:

"All negroes and Indians, (free Indians in amity with this government, and Negroes, Mulattos, and Mustezoes who are now free, excepted) Mulattoes or Mastezoes who are now, or shall hereafter be in this province, and all their issue and offspring ...shall be and they are hereby declared to be, and remain hereafter absolute slaves."

Millions of Native Americans were enslaved, particularly in South America. In the American colonies in 1730, nearly 25 percent of the slaves in the Carolinas were Cherokee, Creek or other Native Americans.

From the 1500s through the 1700s, modest numbers of Whites were also enslaved by simple kidnapping or to work off financial debts or to work off punishment for crimes.

The roots of racial slavery were established early. Acts of resistance that combined the efforts of indentured Irish workers, African slaves, and Native Americans did occur, however, over time these alliances crumbled. Although slaves did not consolidate ethnic identifications on the basis of color, it was generally understood that most Blacks were slaves and no slaves were White. This placed the label of inferiority on Black skin, black intelligence and Black genes.

In America, when a slave was freed, he was still a Black African and the taint of inferiority followed him. Not only did White America become convinced of White superiority and Black inferiority, but it worked diligently to impose these racial beliefs on the Africans.

Slave masters gave a great deal of effort to the education and training of the "ideal slave." In general there were five steps in developing the characteristics of a "good slave."

1) Strict discipline

2) Instill a sense of the slave's own inferiority

3) Complete belief in the master's superior power

4) Acceptance of the master's standards

5) A deep sense of his own helplessness and dependence

There were Black, mulatto and American born slave owners in some colonies in the Americas, and many Whites did not own slaves. Chattel slavery was fundamentally different in the Americas from slavery in other parts of the world because of the racial dimensions.

In December 1835, 500 miles east of New Zealand in the Chatham Islands, hundreds of years of independence came to an abrupt end for the Moriori people in what was to be called the "musket wars." On November 19, 1835, a sailing ship loaded with 500 Maori warriors armed with guns, clubs and axes landed, followed on December 5 by a second ship carrying 400 more heavily armed Maori warriors.

Groups of Maori walked through the Moriori villages, announcing that the Moriori were now their slaves, and summarily killed those who objected. An organized defense could have quickly defeated the invaders, who were outnumbered by at least two to one. However, the Moriori had developed a culture that resolved its differences peacefully and without aggression. The Moriori held a council meeting and concluded that to fight back was futile, so they decided to sue for peace by offering peace, friendship and a division of resources.

Before the Moriori could deliver their offer the Maori mounted a vicious attack. Over the terrible hours of the next few days, they killed hundreds of Moriori, cooked and ate many of the bodies, and enslaved the remainder, and later killing and eating many more over the next few days as suited their will.

A Moriori survivor testified that, " The Maori commenced to kill us (and eat us) like sheep ... (we) were terrified, fled to the bush, concealed ourselves in holes underground, and in any place to escape our enemies. It was to no avail, we were discovered and killed - men, women and children indiscriminately."

A Maori victor said, as a matter-of-fact, "We took possession in accordance with our customs and we caught all the people. Not one escaped. Some ran away from us, these we killed, and others we killed - but what of that? It was in acceptance with our custom."

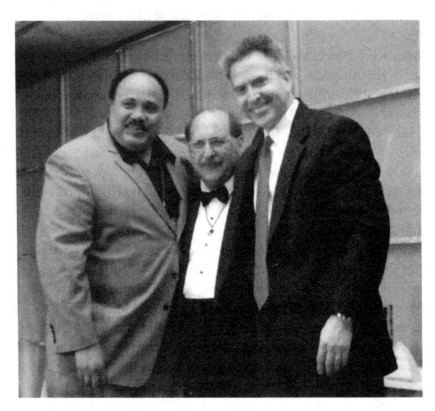

Martin Luther King III   Jonathan Emord, Esq.
Dr. Joel D. Wallach

Chapter 2

"Black is Beautiful."

- John Sweat Rock, March 5, 1858
Crispus Attacks Day, Boston

"To win the war Lincoln must give the Black man the cartridge box, the jury box and the ballot box."

- Frederick Douglass
1862

"The more I consider the subject, the more strongly I am convinced that the most harmful effect of the practice to which people in certain sections of the South have felt themselves compelled to resort, in order to get rid of the force of the Negro ballot, is not wholly in the wrong done to the Negro, but (also) in the permanent injury to the morals of the White man"

- Booker T. Washington
Up From Slavery

"As our commerce spreads, the flag of liberty will circle the globe and the highway of the oceans - carrying trade to all mankind - will be guarded by the guns of the republic. And as their thunders salute the flag, benighted peoples will know that the voice of liberty is speaking, at last, for them .... That civilization is dawning at last, for them."

- Alfred Beverage, 1898
United States Senator

> *"We began with the limited goal of ending racial segregation. But we came to understand segregation as just one aspect of the barrier confronting Black Americans in American Society. The March on Washington became a march for jobs and freedom, because in a nation based on free enterprise, access to jobs and money are an essential component of freedom"*
>
> **- Andrew Young**
> *An Easy Burden* 2004

The History of Financial and Political Bondage

The most primitive of human organizations was the family band. They were hunter gatherers and rarely consisted of more than a dozen people. The successful extended family bands grew in numbers into larger groups known as clans.

Individual members of family bands and clans acquired goods from each other through forms of barter. They often gathered together in larger numbers to raid other non-related family bands or clans for wives, slaves and goods.

Most experts believe that all humans lived in bands until 40,000 years ago and that most still did until 11,000 years ago.

Bands typically do not set up a permanent base of operation such as villages and there is no skill specialization except for age and gender - all are responsible to forage for food. They are typically egalitarian and have no laws, police or agreements to resolve differences between bands. Leadership in bands was not regulated and depended upon individual strength, skills and talents.

Tribes are comprised of hundreds of people often counting many bands and clans, rather than dozens and typically live in villages; however, nomadic herdsmen do often attain the numbers and organizational skills to be called a tribe. The numbers of people in the tribe (measured in the hundreds) are small enough that everyone still knew each other's name and to which band or clan they belonged to. Tribes tended to have an expanded egalitarian leadership system.

Tribes do not have bureaucracies, police forces or taxes and their economies tend to be based on barter. A tribal "Big Man" has no decision making authority, however, they will often take on the role as a chief and redistribute collected goods and food without building or accumulating personal wealth.

On rare occasion, nomads and tribal societies defeated organized states, religions and governments in battle and politics, however, history shows that over the past 13,000 years the nomads and tribesmen more often lost than were victorious.

The historical evidence reveals that tribes evolved into chiefdoms about 5500 B.C. in the Fertile Crescent of Iraq and in 1000 B.C. in Mesoamerica and the Andes.

Chiefdoms characteristically range in size from several thousand to tens of thousands. The majority of people in chiefdoms were not related by blood or marriage and their names were not generally known to each other, which led to many types of conflict and disputes.

The appearance of chiefdoms about 7,500 years ago required that people learn customs and greetings to receive strangers (possibly remote members of their own tribe) without summarily killing, eating or enslaving them.

The chief of the chiefdom was given the right to use force on behalf of the greater community. Different than the tribal Big Man, the chief filled a universally recognized position, which was continued by blood right (of course revolutions and coups did occur to interrupt blood lineage). The chiefdom system resembled certain features of a republic in that he made the important decisions on behalf of his people.

Food surpluses generated in chiefdoms by a few individuals went to feed the chiefs, their relatives, bureaucrats, craftsmen, priests, medicine men and artists.

Chiefdoms continued to obtain goods and services through the barter system; however, they also employed a redistributive economy. The chief would, for example, collect grain during harvest season from all farmers in the chiefdom, then hosting a feast for all members of the chiefdom and providing bread for all or handing it out as needed in the lean months between successful harvests.

Chiefdoms did both good and evil. They tended to provide services that the individual commoner could not afford; however, they also transitioned into "kleptocracies" as they shunted goods and wealth from the general population to the chief, his relatives and appointees.

When a significant amount of the food and goods acquired by the chief was not redistributed to the people as feasts or food in times of drought or famine it was considered tribute - an early form of taxation. A chief could also conscript labor for public works (public buildings, irrigation canals, roads, etc.) and the military. In the absence of sufficient numbers of conscript labor, the chief often turned to raiding neighboring bands, tribes and chiefdoms for sources of slaves.

The chiefs and kleptocrates garnered public support by employing a mix of practices:

1) Disarm the general population and arm the upper classes, nobles, and bureaucrats.

2) Keep the general population satisfied by redistributing a large portion of the collected tribute.

3) Maintain public order and reduce violence and crime.

4) Create a justification for kleptocracy through religion (Egyptians, etc.) and represent the people's voice to their god - the chief often combined the status of chief and priest or god. Chiefdoms usually spent a large portion of the tribute to build statues of gods (Easter Island) and temples.

Political states currently own and rule all earthly land except for Antarctica. Ancient states and modern ones have literate academics and large numbers of literate citizens. The first states as we know them arose first in 3700 B.C. in Mesopotamia and later in 300 B.C. in Mesoamerica, over 2,000 years ago in the Andes, China, and Southeast Asia, and over 1,000 years ago in West Africa.

The populations of chiefdoms ranged from thousands to tens of thousands, while the populations of states were usually greater than one million people.

All ancient states subsidized slavery on a grand scale compared with chiefdoms. Chiefdoms were not more altruistic, but rather early states supported economic specialization, with considerably more specialization of trades, arts, public projects and a full time military. These characteristics of a state required more slave labor than chiefdoms and the greater level of physical and political devastation of state driven wars produced more captives and slaves for the victorious states.

When population densities are low such as in territories populated by hunter-gatherer bands, survivors of the losing faction simply move away from the influence and dominance of the victors.

When populations are made up of tribes and small farming villages, there are rarely areas that the survivors of a war can hide. The winners will usually kill the men and older boys and take the women into their midst as wives. The victors often move some of their own numbers into the village to occupy, direct activities, tax and farm it.

When populations are large in number, the defeated are taken and employed as slaves or they can be left in place to produce food, various goods and services for the victors; but, they will be enslaved politically by installing an occupying governor with a small military force (Romans, Greeks, Spain, England, France, Russia, Japan, Germany, etc.) who was a trusted member of the victorious state; the governor then extracts tribute or taxes to be shipped back to the victorious mother state.

The Spanish conquistadores went to war with the Aztecs specifically to obtain the riches of the New World. Immediately after their victory, the Spanish looked for and obtained the Aztec's tax list. The tax list showed that each year that the Aztec state extracted from subjugated peoples 7,000 tons of corn, 4,000 tons of beans, 4,000 tons of grain amaranth, 2,000,000 cotton garments, large quantities of cacao beans, amber and military equipment.

In 1787, Benjamin Franklin accepted the presidency of the Pennsylvania Society for Promoting the Abolition of Slavery. One of the positions against the immediate abolition of slavery that Franklin had accepted, was that it was not practical or safe to free hundreds of thousands of adult slaves into a society for which they were not prepared (there were 700,000 slaves in the United States out of a total combined population of 4,000,000 in 1790).

Franklin's Abolition Society dedicated itself not only to freeing the slaves, but also to helping them become "good citizens."

"Slavery is such an atrocious debasement of human nature that its very extirpation, if not performed with solicitous care, may sometimes open a source of serious evils," Franklin wrote in a November 1789 address to the public from the society. He went on to say, "The unhappy man, who has long been treated as a brute animal, too frequently sinks beneath the common standard of the human species. The galling chains that bind his body do also fetter his intellectual faculties and impair the social affections of his heart."

Franklin, in his characteristic fashion drew up for his society a meticulous charter and procedures "for improving the condition of free Blacks." He collected a 24 member committee which he then divided into four subcommittees:

A Committee of Inspection, who shall superintend the morals, general conduct, and ordinary situation of the free Negroes, and afford them advice and instruction.

A Committee of Guardians, who shall place out children and young people with suitable persons, that they may (during a moderate time of apprenticeship or servitude) learn some trade or other business.

A Committee of Education, who shall superintend the school instruction of the children and youth of the free Blacks. They may either influence them to attend regularly the schools already established in this city, or from others with this view.

A Committee of Employ, who shall endeavor to procure constant employment for those free Negroes who are able to work; as the want of this would occasion poverty, idleness, and many vicious habits."

In 1790, Franklin presented a formal Abolition Petition to Congress, "Mankind are all formed by the same Almighty being, alike objects of his care, and equally designed for the enjoyment of happiness."

His view was that the duty of Congress was to secure "the blessings of liberty to the People of the United States without distinction of color." He continued, "Congress should grant liberty to those unhappy men who alone in this land of freedom are degraded into perpetual bondage."

Franklin and his abolition petition were angrily attacked by the defenders of slavery; the attack was led by Congressman James Jackson of Georgia, who declared on the House floor that, "the Bible had sanctioned slavery and, without it, there would be no one to do the hard and hot work on plantations." It was the perfect invitation for Franklin's last monumental parody, written less than a month before his death.

Franklin had started his writing career 68 years earlier as a 16 year old apprentice. He had pretended to be a prudish widow by the name of Silence Dogwood, and he continued using these parodies to enlighten his followers ("The Trial of Polly Baker" and "An Edict from the King of Prussia").

Franklin anonymously published in a small local newspaper, with appropriate source citations, a concocted speech said to have been given by a member of the Divan of Algiers one hundred years earlier.

The article was written to mock the speech of Congressman Jackson. It began, "God is Great, and Mahomet is his prophet," They continued to attack a petition by a purist sect asking for an end to the practice of capturing and enslaving European Christians to work in Algeria:

"If we forbear to make slaves of their people, who in this hot climate are to cultivate our lands? Who are to perform the common labors of our city, and in our families? An end to the slavery of infidels would cause land values to fall and rents to sink by half."

"Who is to indemnify their masters for their loss? Will the state do it? Is our Treasury sufficient? …And if we set our slaves free, what is to be done with them? Few of them will return to their countries; they know too well the greater hardships they must there be subject to; they will not embrace our holy religion; they will not adopt our manners; our people will not pollute themselves by intermarrying with them. Must we maintain them as beggars in our streets, or suffer our properties to be prey of their pillage? For men long accustomed to slavery will not work for a livelihood when not compelled.

And what is there so pitiable in their present condition? Here they are brought into a land where the sun of Islamism gives forth its light, and shines in full splendor, and they have an opportunity of making themselves acquainted with the true doctrine, and thereby saving their immortal souls…While serving us, we take care to provide them with every thing, and they are treated with humanity. The laborers in their own countries are, as I am well informed, worse fed, lodged and clothed.

How grossly are they mistaken in imaging slavery to be disallowed by the Koran! Are not the two precepts, to quote no more, "Masters, treat your Slaves with kindness: Slaves, serve your Masters with cheerfulness and Fidelity," clear proofs to the contrary? Let us then hear no more of this detestable proposition, the manumission of Christian slaves, the adoption of which would, by depreciating our lands and houses, and thereby depriving so many good citizens of their properties, create universal discontent, and provoke insurrections."

Like the Algerian divan of Franklin's hoax, the U.S. Congress determined that they did not have the authority to revoke the institution of slavery.

In February 1818, Frederick Bailey (who later changed his name to Frederick Douglass) was born a slave on the Eastern Shore, Talbot County, Maryland.

In August 1824, when he was only six, Douglass' grandmother and he left their home cabin and walked 12 miles to the Wye House - the Great House of the plantation. Frederick was sent to the back yard to play with the other slave children. While he played, Frederick's grandmother left without his knowing and returned to her cabin - Frederick was now on his own as a slave at the age of six.

The Wye House was the classic example of the plantation Great House. Douglass remembered 50 years later:

"Immense wealth and its lavish expenditures filled the Great House with all that could please the eye or tempt the taste. Fish, flesh, and fowl were here in profusion….wild goose, partridges, quails, pheasants, pigeons…..The Teeming riches of the Chesapeake Bay, its rock perch, drums, crocus, trout, oysters, crabs and terrapin….The dairy, too…poured its rich donations of fragrant cheese, golden butter, and delicious cream….The fertile garden….was not behind in its contribution (of) tender asparagus, crispy lettuce,…delicate cauliflower, eggplants, beets, parsnips, peas, and French beans…(There were also) figs, raisins, almonds, and grapes from Spain, wine and brandies from France, teas of various flavor from China, and rich aromatic coffee from Java.

The table of this house groaned under….blood-bought luxuries….Behind the tall-backed...chairs, stood the servants....They resembled the field hands in nothing except their color, and in this they held the advantage of a velvet-like glossiness....The delicately-formed colored maid rustled in the scarcely-worn silk of her young mistress.

Viewed from Col. Lloyd's table, who could have said that his slaves were not well clad and well cared for? Who would have said they did not glory in being the slaves of such a master?"

As a child Douglass was taught to read and write by his master's wife. In his twenties, Douglass declared "that my master was my father; my father was white; and this fact was admitted to...by all."

As to the nature of slavery Douglass wrote:

"The slaveholders, with a craftiness peculiar to themselves, by encouraging the enmity of the poor, laboring White man against the Blacks, succeeds in making the said White man almost as much a slave as the Black slave himself. The difference between the White slave, and the Black slave, is this: the latter belongs to one slaveholder, and the former belongs to all the slaveholders, collectively. The White slave has taken from him, by indirection, what the Black slave has taken from him directly, and without ceremony. Both are plundered, and by the same plunderers. The slave is robbed, by his master, of all his earnings, above what is required for his bare physical necessities; and the White man is robbed by the slave system, of the just results of his labor, because he is flung into competition with a class of laborers who work without wages. The competition, and its injurious consequences, will, one day, array the non-slave-holding White people of the slave states, against the slave system, and make them the most effective workers against the great evil. At present, the slaveholders blind them to this competition, by keeping alive their prejudice against the slaves, as men - not against them as slaves. They appeal to their pride, often denouncing emancipation, as tending to place the White working man, on an equality with Negroes, and, by this means, they succeed in drawing off the minds of the poor Whites from the real fact, that, by the rich slave-master, they are already regarded as but a single remove from equality with the slave. The impression is cunningly made, that slavery is the only power that can prevent the laboring White man from falling to the level of the slave's poverty and degradation. To make this enmity deep and broad, between the slave and the poor White man, the latter is allowed to abuse and whip the former, without hindrance."

Douglass' first marriage was to an illiterate, Black women (five years his senior) by the name of Anna Murray - they were married for 44 years until she proceeded him in death.

In August 1, 1833, slavery was outlawed in the British West Indies, allowing the British antislavery societies to turn their energies to the institution of slavery around the world including the United States.

On Monday, September 3, 1838 Frederick Douglass escaped to New York. He pondered, "Dreams of my childhood and the purposes of my manhood were now fulfilled. A free state around me, and a free earth under my feet! What a moment was this to me! A whole year was pressed into a single day. A new world burst upon my agitated vision."

Frederick Bailey changed his name to Frederick Douglass and became the voice and embodiment of the antislavery movement - who better than an escaped slave, who had the ability to read and write, to speak for the Anti-Slavery Society night after night against the evils of slavery?

With the mix of Black freedmen, slaves and runaway slaves traveling and mixing in public places such as churches, train stations, restaurants and theaters, identification was required by the Black traveler to avoid being arrested and sent back to their owners or "legally" enslaved.

"Jim Crow" was the key figure in a fleet of traveling puppet shows that depicted the Black man as a lazy, ignorant, funny dupe. The federal and local laws that allowed and even fostered the segregation of public places into Negro, Black or "darky" and White facilities were referred to as "Jim Crow Laws."

Douglass entered into the fray of the Jim Crow confrontations in the railroad car - there were Negro cars and White cars. When he first refused to follow the conductor's orders to vacate the White car, the conductor and five other men physically drug him to the Negro Car.

In another incident Douglass entered a first-class car of the Eastern line and was accosted by the ticket conductor; when ordered to remove himself and go to the Negro car, Douglass in a quiet tone retorted, "If you give me one good reason why I should... I'll go willingly." The enraged conductor countered with
"You have asked me that question before," and Douglass came back, "I mean to continue asking the question over and over again...as long as you continue to insult me in this manner," and the conductor returned, "Because you are Black." The conductor asked for help to "snake out the damned nigger." Douglass, a stevedore and marine caulker as a slave, held onto his seat with a tradesman's vice-like grip and dispite the efforts of several large men he was still in his seat when the train arrived at his station.

The railroads refused to stop at stations when Douglass was known to be lecturing in that town. These stories became the grist of the Douglass anti-Jim

Crow lectures; Douglass railed against the Jim Crow Laws with an equal vigor as he did against slavery.

One of Douglass' favorite Jim Crow stories was about a moment when he attended a communion service at the Elm Street Methodist Church in New Bedford and he noticed the "White people gathered round the alter, the Blacks clustered by the door." After the Whites had been given communion, the Reverend Isaac Bonney said (Douglass, when he told the story would mimic the Reverend), "Come up, colored friends, come up! For you know God is no respecter of persons!" Douglass was "willing to be regarded as a curiosity, if I may thereby aid the high and holy cause of the slave's emancipation."

Douglass frequently traveled to Ireland, Scotland and the UK to raise money for the anti-slavery movement by giving lectures against slavery, alcohol and women's suffrage - he had learned to enlist allies. He often declared, "When you tell me there are some Christian slave-holders in the states, I tell you, as well might you talk of sober-drunkards."

In 1839, Lewis Tappan, a Congressional minister, organizes a committee to assist captured and enslaved Black Africans who took command of the slave ship *Amistad*.

In 1841, Cinque, leader of the *Amistad* rebellion, and other Africans represented by John Quincy Adams before the U.S. Supreme Court were allowed to return to Africa.

In the spring of 1845 Frederick Douglass was alerting his audiences to watch for his autobiography. The *Narrative of the Life of Frederick Douglass* (1845) and *My Bondage My Freedom* (1851) would become the universal antislavery text.

In 1846, Lewis Tappan and others founded the antislavery American Missionary Association.

On October 28, 1847, upon returning to the states from one of his speaking tours, Douglass wrote, "I have finally decided on publishing the *North Star* (newspaper) in Rochester and to make that city my future home." Frederick Douglass, former slave, field worker, stevedore, marine caulker and face of the American Anti-Slavery Society became an editor and publisher of a serious newspaper.

William S. McFeely, in his 1991 biography of Douglass, stated that, "From the days of Benjamin Franklin to those of the politically powerful newspaper editors of Andrew Jackson's America, journalism had been a potent calling. Only a rare Black man was a doctor or a lawyer; none was a merchant chief. A Black man who would be heard became a man of the cloth, but Douglass had firmly turned his back on that correct calling. What he would be was an editor."

In 1848, Frederick Douglass met John Brown in Springfield, Massachusetts.

Brown confided to Douglass that he would support a Black insurrection and help to establish a "Black State" in the Appalachian Mountains.

In 1853, Harriet Beecher Stowe, author of *Uncle Tom's Cabin*, recorded in a letter that she had interviewed Douglass and that she had, "enjoyed the pleasure of a personal interview with Mr. Douglass…and I feel bound in justice to say that the impression was far more satisfactory than I had anticipated… …..There did not appear to be any deep stratum of bitterness; he did not seem to me malignant or revengeful. I am satisfied that his change of sentiment was not a mere political one but a genuine growth of his own conviction…..he holds no opinion which he cannot defend, with a variety of richness of thought and expression and an aptness of illustration which shows it to be a growth from the soil of his own mind with a living root, and not a twig broken off other men's thoughts and stuck down to subserve a temporary purpose."

Northern anti-slavery views were agitated by the publication of Stowe's novel, *Uncle Tom's Cabin*. In less than one year after the book's publication in March 1852, more than 300,000 copies of the book were sold in the U.S. alone - a sales record rivaled only by the Bible. Frederick Douglass, "likened it to a flash that lit a million campfires in front of the embattled hosts of slavery."

In 1854, the U.S. Congress passed the Kansas-Nebraska Act which eliminated the federal government's authority to determine which new territories would come into the union as a slave or free state (this had been the federal government's responsibility since the Northwest Ordinance of 1787).

The Northwest Ordinance had kept slavery out of Ohio, Indiana, Illinois, Michigan and Wisconsin. The Kansas-Nebraska Act allowed the post-1854 settlers to make their own determination of slave or free status - Frederick Douglass and his fellow abolitionists were outraged.

Senator Stephan A. Douglas (Illinois), author of the Kansas-Nebraska Act died seven years later, and upon his death Frederick Douglass wrote to Susan B. Anthony, "I rejoice not in the death of any man, but I cannot but feel, that in the death of Stephan A. Douglas, a most dangerous man has been removed. No man of his time has done more than he to intensify hatred of the Negro."

The case of *Dred Scott v. Sanford* finally reached the halls of the U.S. Supreme Court 11 years after the original suit had been filed in Missouri. Scott, a slave, was suing for his freedom on the grounds that his master, an army doctor, had removed him for several years to military bases in both the free state of Illinois and the Wisconsin Territory before returning to the slave state of Missouri. The case wound its way through state and federal courts until it finally reached the Supreme Court in 1856.

The Supreme Court was led by Chief Justice Roger Taney of Maryland, "an uncompromising supporter of the South and slavery and an implacable foe of racial equality, the Republican Party, and the antislavery movement."

On March 6, 1857 the historic decision was read by the 79 year old Taney. The 7-2 decision was complete in its scope and consequences. The Court ruled that, "Blacks are not included, and were not intended to be included, under the word 'citizens' in the Constitution; therefore, Scott had no standing in federal court." He continued, "Blacks were so far inferior that they had no rights which the White man was bound to respect; he went on to say that Congress had exceeded its authority when it forbade slavery in the territories by such legislation as the Missouri Compromise, for slaves were private property protected by the Constitution." Justice Felix Frankfurter later said, the Dred Scott decision was "one of the Court's great self-inflicted wounds."

Shortly after the decision Dred Scott was sold to Mr. Taylor Blow, who promptly freed him - he died a free man within the year.

On October 16, 1859, John Brown commanded an "army" of 22 anti-slavery zealots in an attack on the Federal arsenal at Harper's Ferry. Brown's plan was to seize the weapons and distribute them to the 5,000 slaves in the area and start the Black insurrection. General Robert E. Lee surrounded the arsenal after the attack and either killed or captured all of the rebels. Brown was captured alive, given a trial and later hung for treason.

In March 1861, Abraham Lincoln was sworn in as the President of the United States. The Confederates fired on Fort Sumter in April of 1861 and the Civil War ignited. The new president declared that the war was being fought to preserve the Union - he did not initially design the Civil War to end slavery.

In 1861, an assassination attempt on Lincoln's life was foiled by the famed Pinkerton detective. In the well known "Baltimore Plot" of 1861, local supporters for the secession of the Confederate States planned to assassinate the president-elect as his railroad car passed through Baltimore on his way to Washington D.C. for his inauguration. Detective Allan Pinkerton foiled the plot by talking Lincoln into passing through Baltimore incognito hours ahead of schedule.

In 1862, the state of Massachusetts and its Governor Wendell Phillips, formed the 54th Volunteer Infantry, an "all Black" regiment; their story is documented in the movie *Glory*. Recruits came from many states and Canada; they came at night to prevent the Confederates from detecting them. The recruits were freed slaves and Black men who were born free. Their literacy rate was higher than that of the average Confederate soldier; the youngest man in the regiment was Eli Biddle, a 19 year old, who was a student in a Quaker School - he ran away to join the 54th.

Colonial Robert Gould Shaw, an experienced White officer was appointed by the Department of the Army to command the 54th. White soldiers in the Union Army received $14 dollars per month and their uniform, the Black soldier received only $10 per month and $3 was deducted from their first check to pay for their uniform. The black rank and file grumbled against the inequities until Governor Phillips asked, "If you cannot have a whole loaf, will you not accept a slice?"

The 54th Regiment trained at Camp Megs and all eyes of the nation were upon them. Some troops practiced and polished their skills on their own time and according to Col. Shaw, "The Black man learned faster and better than the Irish I had commanded."

On March 1863, a distinguished crowd, including Frederick Douglass gathered to watch and listen as Governor Andrew spoke to Colonel Shaw while surrounded by the regiment, "Now in the Providence of God, (they have) given to them, an opportunity which, while it is personal to themselves, is still an opportunity for a whole race of men. With arms possessed of might to strike a blow, they have found breathed into their hearts an inspiration of devoted patriotism and regard for their brethren of their own color which has inspired them with a purpose to nerve that arm, that it may strike a blow which, while it shall help to raise aloft their country's flag - their country's flag, now, as well as ours-by striking down the foes which oppose it, strikes also the last shackle which binds the limbs of bondmen in the Rebel States."

On May 28, 1863, at 6:30 a.m. the 54th Regiment, including Frederick Douglass' oldest son, traveled by train from Readville into Boston. Upon disembarking, the 54th Massachusetts formed and lead by Governor Andrew marched down Beacon Street past the reviewing stand to the strains of *"John Brown's Body."* As they arrived at Battery Wharf, they reformed in columns of two and boarded the transport ship *DeMolay*.

Upon arriving at the Union headquarters at Beaufort, South Carolina, the 54th regrouped and was sent south to St. Simons Island off the Coast of Georgia, from which they carried out guerilla raids. These raids by the 54th were led by Colonel James Montgomery, who had earlier led guerilla raids against pro-slavery factions in Missouri. Shortly after their first taste of war the 54th was ordered to attack Fort Wagner, an artillery instillation on Morris Island.

Fort Wagner was designed and placed to guard the Charleston Harbor. On July 18, 1863, Colonel Shaw led the 54th in an attack against the fort. The Confederate defenders of the fort had earlier repelled an attack on July 11 and were inspired by their initial victory and eagerly waiting for their chance to shoot a Black Union soldier.

At a trot the men of the 54th advanced in a frontal attack up the beach - a salt marsh on their left and a flat open beach to their front. The advance was slowed by cannon and small arms fire but the lead ranks of the regiment climbed the parapet to the fort.

Hand to hand combat ensued. The men of the 54th were driven back toward the open, flat beach, however, the regiment did not flee in a route. "This regiment has established its reputation as a fighting regiment - not a man flinched, though it was a trying time," wrote Sergeant Major Lewis Douglass. "Men fell all around me. A shell would explode and clear a space of twenty feet, our men would close up again, but there was no use we had to retreat, which was a very hazardous undertaking. How I got out of that fight alive I cannot tell, but I am here."

During the battle at Fort Wagner, 174 of the Confederate defenders were killed or wounded; 1,515 Union soldiers fell dead. The morning after the battle the men in the fort looked out across the beach and saw "live and dead men strewn in piles and windrows, their bodies horribly mangled….detached arms and legs and heads were splattered all about."

The Confederate defenders buried the dead of the Massachusetts 54th in a common grave and the body of their Colonel Shaw was unceremoniously thrown in with them. Thus the 54th marched into history, won their first battles against the Confederates and went on to distinguish themselves in the island battles off the east coast of the southern states.

There was a total commitment to abolish slavery in the Black communities of the North, however, Frederick Douglass and other Black leaders attempting to recruit Blacks for the Union army, despite the bravery displayed by Black soldiers at the battles of Milliken's Bend and Fort Wagner, the Black soldier was still treated "with scorn" and they were paid less than White soldiers.

According to McFeely, Confederate leaders were "horrified by the prospect of White Southerners being killed by Black men - the ultimate intimacy in their eyes - members of the Confederate Congress on May 1, 1863, put through a formal declaration that Black men bearing arms would be subject to the laws of the state where they were captured; in other words, they would be treated as insurrectionary slaves. The punishment would almost certainly be death."

Douglass was horrified by such a law and protested to President Lincoln and sent a letter resigning from his recruiting responsibilities. On July 30, 1863, President Lincoln signed an order requiring that "for every (Black) soldier of the United States killed in violation of the laws of war a rebel soldier shall be executed."

Douglass, wanting to gain every possible advantage for the abolitionist, visited the president, "I went directly to the White House (and) saw for the first time the President of the United States. Was received cordially and saw at (a) glance the justice of the popular estimate of his qualities expressed in the prefix Honest to the name Abraham Lincoln." Douglass' purpose was to offer a "hint for a discussion from Mr. Lincoln himself. In this I was quite successful for the president instantly…proceeded with…an earnestness and fluency which I had not expected…to vindicate his policy respecting the whole slavery question and especially that in reference to employing colored troops." Douglass left the meeting believing that Lincoln would continue to give support to the Black cause - Lincoln had "charmed his Black visitor totally."

On November 20, 1863, "Lincoln lifted himself up on a chestnut horse and joined a procession to commemorate a military cemetery at Gettysburg. He led an assemblage of nine governors, members of Congress, foreign ministers, military officials and three cabinet officers and an estimated 9,000 citizens."

Lincoln believed, "that the central idea pervading this struggle is the necessity that is upon us, of proving that popular government is not an absurdity; if we fail, it will go far to prove the incapability of the people to govern themselves." At Gettysburg, Lincoln expressed again his conviction:

"Four score and seven years ago, our fathers brought forth upon this continent, a new nation, conceived in liberty, and dedicated to the proposition that all men are created equal.

Now we are engaged in a great Civil War, testing whether that nation, or any nation so conceived, and so dedicated, can long endure. We are met on a great battle-field of that war. We have come to dedicate a portion of that field, as a final resting place for those who here gave their lives, that that nation might live. It is altogether fitting and proper that we should do this.

But in a larger sense, we can not dedicate - we can not consecrate - we can not hallow - this ground. The brave men, living and dead, who struggled here, have consecrated it, far above our poor power to add or detract. The world will little note, nor long remember, what we say here, but it can never forget what they did here. It is for us, the living, rather, to be dedicated here to the unfinished work which they who fought here, have, thus far, so nobly advanced. It is rather for us to be here dedicated to the great task remaining before us - that from these honored dead we take increased devotion to that cause for which they here gave the last full measure of devotion - that we here highly resolve that these dead shall not have died in vain - that this nation, under God, shall have a new birth of freedom - and that, government of the people, by the people, for the people, shall not perish from the earth."

George Gitt, a 15 year old boy who had hidden under the speaker's platform observed, "The extreme brevity of the address together with its abrupt close had so astonished the hearers that they stood transfixed. Had not Lincoln turned and moved toward his chair, the audience would very likely have remained voiceless for several moments more. Finally there came the applause."

On February 1864, Frederick Douglass gave a lecture to the Women's Loyal League entitled *"The Mission of War."* The mission of course was to engender "simply those great moral changes in the fundamental condition of the people…(war) filled our land with mere stumps of men, ridged our soil with 200,000 rudely-formed graves, and mantled it all over with the shadow of death."

Douglass was very aware that in an election year there was a powerful movement afoot for a negotiated peace that would leave slavery in place - "we are in danger of a slaveholding peace… There is but one way to avert this calamity, and that is to destroy slavery and enfranchise the Black man while we have the power. You and I know the mission of this war is National regeneration. I end where I began, no war but an Abolition war; no peace but an Abolition peace; liberty for all, chains for none; the Black man a soldier in war; a laborer in peace; a voter at the South as well as at the North; America his permanent home, and all Americans his fellow countrymen. Such, fellow-citizens, is my idea for the mission of this war."

The South continued to debate whether slavery was their main cause in the war. Senator Stephan A. Douglas, Lincoln's opponent for reelection was willing to allow slavery to continue if the South would negotiate a peace to preserve the Union. Lincoln further interpreted his reelection to be a mandate to pass the 13th Amendment to close the books on slavery in America. On December 6, 1864 he offered an impassioned plea to Congress, "In a great national crisis, like ours, unanimity of action among those seeking a common end is very desirable - almost indispensable."

The Lincoln administration pressed more than a dozen lame duck Democratic Congressmen and promised them to a hailstorm of "political pork" in return for voting with the Republicans to pass the 13th Amendment to the Constitution. The promise of "pork" was rewarded. Sixteen of the Democrats out of 80 voted for the Amendment, allowing the Amendment to pass with two votes to spare 119 to 56. The Republicans broke into a boisterous cheer and "100 cannons thundered a salute in the streets of Washington."

Black citizens were in the Congressional gallery when the final vote was taken - they cheered and wept openly. Lincoln extended a personal invitation to Frederick Douglass to attend the inaugural events at the White House.

On February 1, 1865, Senator Charles Sumner "presented Boston lawyer John Sweat Rock (1825-1866) for admission to practice before the Supreme Court, and Chief Justice Salmon P. Chase swore him in as the first Black man accredited to the highest Court, which eight years earlier had blocked U.S. citizenship to the Negro race (in the Dred Scott Decision)." A year later Rock would be dead of tuberculosis.

Rock was truly a Renaissance man, in addition to law, he apprenticed and was formally trained in dentistry and medicine and at age 27 received his M.D. degree from the American Medical College in Philadelphia in 1852; he was an abolitionist and a journalist who coined the phrase "Black is beautiful."

Lincoln won his reelection bid and on March 4, 1865 was inaugurated. The ceremony was officially photographed by William M. Smith, a patent lawyer and part-time photographer. However, perched on another platform was Alexander Gardner, another photographer who documented the moment with photographs of Lincoln, the vice president, chief justice, and many other dignitaries present for the occasion - a detailed inspection of these photographs also reveals "on a balcony above the stands, standing near an iron railing, a young, black mustached man wearing a top hat gazes down on the president. It is the celebrated actor John Wilkes Booth."

Lincoln's inaugural address was only 701 words but profound:

"Fondly do we hope - fervently do we pray - that this mighty scourge of war may speedily pass away... With malice toward none; with charity for all; with firmness in the right, as God gives us to see the right, let us strive on to finish the work we are in; to bind up the nation's wounds; to care for him who shall have born the battle, and for his widow and orphan - to do all which may achieve and cherish a just and lasting peace, among ourselves, and with all nations."

On April 3, 1865, Richmond, Virginia, capital city of the Confederacy, was captured by the Union forces led by General Ulysses S. Grant.

On April 7, 1865, John Wilkes Booth was having drinks with a friend and fellow actor, Samuel Knapp Chester, at the House of Lords Saloon in New York City. Booth, slamming the bar with his fist shared, "What an excellent chance I had, if I wished, to kill the President on inauguration day! I was on the stand, as close to him nearly as I am to you."

On April 9, 1865, in a small house near the Appomattox Courthouse, General Robert E. Lee, commander of the Army of Northern Virginia, surrendered. The "vanquished commander, six feet tall and erect in bearing, arrived in full-dress uniform with sash and jeweled sword; (Grant), the victor, five foot eight with stooped shoulders, appeared in his usual private's blouse with mud-splattered trousers tucked into muddy boots. There in the parlor of a humble house the son of an Ohio tanner dictated surrender terms to the scion of a First Family of Virginia."

Booth, having returned to Washington, D.C. the day before Lee's surrender, wandered the streets of D.C. in great despair and depression - "his great cause was all but lost."

On the night of April 11, 1865 a crowd of several thousand overjoyed citizens marched up to the front door of the White House and begged for Lincoln to come out and speak, "Speech, speech!" According to Elizabeth Keckley, Mary Lincoln's Black dressmaker and confidante, "Close to the house the faces were plainly discernible, but they faded into mere ghostly outlines on the outskirts of the assembly; and what added to the weird, spectral beauty of the scene, was the confused hum of voices that rose above the sea of forms, sounding like the subdued, sullen roar of an ocean storm."

Lincoln spoke:

"We meet this evening, not in sorrow, but in gladness of heart. The evacuation of Petersburg and Richmond, and the surrender of the principal insurgent army, give hope of a righteous and speedy peace whose joyous expression can not be restrained. In the midst of this, however, He from whom all blessings flow, must not be forgotten...no part of the honor...is mine. To General Grant, his skillful officers, and brave men, all belongs." Lincoln continued with a description of the newly organized state government of Louisiana, "It is also unsatisfactory to some that the elective franchise is not given to the colored man. I would myself prefer that it were now conferred on the very intelligent, and on those who serve our cause as soldiers."

In the otherwise joyous crowd John Wilkes Booth brooded over the speech and commented to his coconspirator, David Herold, "That means nigger citizenship, now by God, I'll put him through." And as he walked away Booth continued, "That is the last speech he will ever give."

Booth's original plan was to take a small band of men and in a bold move kidnap Lincoln and spirit him to Richmond (the capital of the Confederacy and only 100 miles south of Washington, D.C.) and use the captive president to leverage an end to the war in the favor of the Confederacy. The fall of Richmond and the surrender of Lee's army rendered that plot impossible.

On Good Friday, April 14, 1865 Lincoln sent a messenger notifying the Ford theater that he would require the presidential box as he would attend that evening's play - *Our American Cousin,* and would be there at 8:30 p.m. as the curtain went up.

Booth, knew the physical plan of the theater like the back of his hand, the theater was his lair and Lincoln was coming, unknowingly straight to him! Booth also knew the play, "its duration, its scenes, its players, and, most important, as it would turn out, the number of actors onstage at any given moment during the performance." It was perfect!

Booth's checklist was substantial; however, he had already put it together for the kidnapping plot so he did not have to start at the beginning, "horses, weapons, supplies, alerting his fellow conspirators that a plan had been put into place, casing the theater, etc." all needed to be checked and rechecked within an eight hour time frame - it was like a episode of the 2006 TV series "24" - the clock was ticking!

By late afternoon Booth went to his hotel and chose and loaded his primary weapon, a .44-caliber, single-shot, muzzle-loading percussion cap pistol manufactured by Henry Deringer of Philadelphia - it could be fired only once - the first shot must count. Booth's secondary, backup weapon was a Rio Grand Camp Knife.

At 8:00 p.m., thirty minutes before the curtain went up at the Ford Theater, Booth called together his coconspirators, Lewis Powell, David Herold and George Atzerodt. They would not only assassinate Lincoln, but they also planned to kill Vice President Andrew Johnson and Secretary of State William H. Seward. At 10:00 p.m. they were instructed to strike simultaneously and kill Lincoln, Johnson and Seward.

Atzerodt was to shoot or stab to death Vice President Johnson in his unguarded hotel room at the Kirkwood House; Powell, also was to carry a revolver and a knife and assisted by Herold, was to murder Seward; Booth himself would kill Lincoln.

Atzerodt consumed a great deal of liquor, got drunk and did not even make an attempt to kill Johnson.

Powell, carrying a fake "prescription" as a rouse (Seward had been critically injured in a runaway carriage incident earlier that week), gained entry into the Seward home and attacked the Secretary with his knife (his revolver had been damaged in a fight gaining entry into Seward's bedroom) - Seward was severely injured in the face and neck by Powell's attack but lived.

Herold, who was supposed to hold the getaway horse, became frightened, ran away, and left Powell to his own fate as the commotion erupted from the Seward house.

Booth left his horse to be hand held by John Peanut, a snack salesman for the theater; he crossed under the stage via a tunnel to the far side of the stage - he exited the building, entered the next door bar and had a last drink at about 10:00 p.m.

After his drink, Booth returned to the theater lobby, then climbed the stairs and walked slowly to the unguarded door of the vestibule that led immediately to the presidential box. There was no policeman or military officer, only Lincoln's valet, Charles Forbes. Booth showed Forbes a calling card - the famous actor could gain entrée to any event.

As Booth opened the door to the box he would have instantly noticed that there was no hidden guard. James Ferguson, a witness, noted, "I looked back and saw him (Booth) step down one step, put his hands to the door, and his knee against it, and push the door open." There was no one to block his path to Lincoln.

From his rocking chair Lincoln reached out and held his wife's hand. In a playful mood, Mary, goaded Lincoln for being so forward, "What will Miss Harris think of my hanging on to you so?" Lincoln replied, "She won't think anything about it."

Booth closed the outer vestibule door so quietly that the occupants of the box including Lincoln did not hear him. Booth, then retrieved a pine bar from a music stand (he had hidden the piece of lumber along the floor molding under the wallpaper earlier that day), placed one end into a hole he had predrilled in the front wall and wedged the other end of the bar against the door to prevent entry into the box from the outside - still no one heard the stealthy maneuvers.

Lincoln was sitting in a high-backed rocking chair immediately inside the box. Mary Lincoln sat on the president's right, on a wood cane-bottomed chair. On Mrs. Lincoln's right sat their guests, Miss Harris on another similar chair and her fiancee', on the far right of the box was Major Rathbone on a sofa. Booth could enter the box and attack Lincoln without having to confront the Major.

Act 3, scene 2 were just beginning - there were now four scenes left before the end of the play. It was about 10:11 p.m. After a few more moments one of the main characters, one Asa Trenchard, played by the well known comic actor, Harry Hawk would be the only actor on the stage.

Armed with his 44-caliber single shot Deringer pistol in his right hand and his Rio Grande Camp Knife in his left, Booth waited until Hawk, alone on the stage shouted a litany of insults toward the exiting female character, "Don't know the manners of good society, eh? Wal I guess I know enough to turn you inside out, old gal...you sockdologizing old mantrap!"...Then he entered the box as the crowd burst into uproarious laughter.

Booth immediately raised his right arm to the height of his shoulder, pointing the pistol at Lincoln's head. And as the laughter reached a peak, Booth pulled the trigger.

James Ferguson described the scene, "The President at the time he was shot was sitting in this position: he was leaning his hand on the rail, and was looking down at a person in the (theater), not looking at the stage. He had the flag that decorated the box pulled around, and he was looking between the post and the flag." The bullet hit the President in the head just below his left ear and traveled in a diagonal path through Lincoln's brain. The one ounce lead ball ground through his brain and came to a stop behind his right eye.

Lincoln was instantly brain-dead, however, his heart was still beating, but his respiration had briefly stopped. Lincoln appeared to the audience as if he was "bored" with the play and had fallen asleep.

Major Rathbone got up and rushed the assassin - he and Booth grabbed each other; Booth yanked free and yelled, "Freedom!" and drove his right arm up as high as he could reach, and in a wide arc drove the large-bladed knife at Rathbone's chest. Rathbone defended himself by throwing up his arm and took the impact of the blade in his upper arm.

Booth, now devoted his full attention to his own escape, he threw his leg over the box rail as Rathbone caught his coattail. As he attempted to pull free, Booth became tangled in the portrait of George Washington and one of his spurs became tangled in the red, white and blue bunting decorating the box. Booth landed off balance and broke his left leg (the small fibula) near the ankle (his heavy leather riding boot acted as an effective splint).

Booth gathered himself up straight and shouted, "Sic semper tyrannis." The Latin words he shouted were the State Motto of Virginia, "Thus always to tyrants." Booth then screamed, "The South is avenged." And as he fled he yelled, "I have done it!"

Booth ran to the alley and took his horse from Peanut, literally kicked Peanut out of the way with his good leg and rode off on his horse at a gallop.

It took a full 12 days after the assassination of Lincoln for Booth to be cornered by a Union cavalry patrol and killed. The following account by James L. Swanson gives a word picture of Booth's last moments:

"John Garrett (a Confederate sympathizer) asked them (Booth and Herold who had rejoined Booth and was guiding him through the Virginia countryside) where they thought of sleeping. Why, 'in the house,' of course Booth replied. No, gentleman, you can't sleep in my house. Booth was incredulous. Was John Garrett denying him the bed that, only a night before, was his? Booth sensed the weight hanging from his hips. He was still wearing the pistol belt. He had never unbuckled it it since the cavalry rode past that afternoon. And Herold's carbine was close by. With his revolvers and knife within easy reach, Booth considered Garrett's poor manners. Garrett's father had kindly offered Booth shelter one day, and John cruelly robbed it from him the next. The prospect of another night sleeping on the ground was hateful to Booth. He could always threaten the Garretts, just like when he had menaced the cowering Black man, William Lucas. His weapons would certainly get him back upstairs, onto that restful mattress and soft pillow.

John Garrett still did not know the true identity of the man he was throwing out of his house. He was pretty sure that the 'Boyd cousins' were in some kind of trouble, but he failed to imagine its magnitude, and that Lincoln's killer was a guest at his family's dinner table. This was the man that had put a bullet in the brain of the President of the United States, who ordered the murders of the Vice President and Secretary of State, and had threatened to cut the throat of a harmless, Black freedman who dared refuse Booth the accommodations of his humble cabin. John Wilkes Booth fancied himself a paternalistic, courtly man, and in truth he often was. But when pressed he could also become a ruthless, vicious one. What, then, was Booth going to do with the young, poorly mannered Mr. John Garrett?

David Herold intervened: 'We'll sleep under the house then.' Herold had hoped to defuse the situation, but the obstinate Garrett would not budge an inch.

"Impossible," he retorted, "The dogs sleep under there and would bite them," perhaps even attacking them in their sleep.

Persistant, Herold tried again: 'Well, what's in the barn then?' Hay and fodder, John Garrett replied. 'We'll sleep in the barn then,' Herold announced in a voice indicating that the matter was closed. Garrett relented. He could not eject them from Locust Hill by force. There were children in the house. The 'Boyds' were better armed, and any violence might endanger not just him, but the whole family.

Booth and Herold headed toward their new quarters, a modest-sized tobacco barn, 48 by 50 feet, with a pitched roof, that stood 150 to 200 feet from the main house. By 9:00 p.m. Booth and Herold had lain down on the plank floor and settled in for the night. Unbeknownst to them, the Garretts, already guilty of inhospitality, were at that moment conspiring to commit a worse crime, treachery. Lincoln's assassin had just walked into a trap.

John and William Garrett swung the barn door shut behind the fugitives. Neither Booth nor Herold paid heed to the black, iron lock. Perhaps, blinded by the dark, they failed to see the sturdy piece of hardware as they passed through the doorway. As soon as the door closed, John Garrett whispered to his brother, 'We had better lock those men up.' John was sure that the 'Boyds' were scheming to steal their horses in the middle of the night.

What better way to foil a horse theft than by imprisoning the strangers in the tobacco shed until tomorrow morning? John crept around the perimeter of the building until he found a crevice between the boards, close to the ground. Dropping to his belly, he pressed his ear to the crevice and eavesdropped on

Booth and Herold. John wanted to 'see if I could find out anything about them. I thought that maybe they would be talking together and I might learn what their intensions were.' But the strangers frustrated Garrett's primitive effort at intelligence gathering: 'they were talking to each other in a low tone (and) I could not distinguish a word they said.'

While his brother John eavesdropped, William Garrett tiptoed to the front door and, as quietly as he could, inserted the key into the lock. To avoid alerting the barn's occupants he turned the key slowly, so the locking mechanism would softly grind, and not loudly snap into place. It worked, Booth and Herold did not hear the sliding bolt; they did not know that they were prisoners.

The (Garrett) brothers returned to the house in time for nightly family worship conducted by their father. After evening prayers, they retired to their room, each man with a bed to himself again, now that they had thrown Booth and Herold out of the house. Still, John Garrett remained uneasy. What if the 'Boyds' broke out of the barn? Then they would in their anger, steal the horses for sure. John suggested to William that they spend the night outside and keep the barn under surveillance. Both Garretts grabbed the blankets from their beds, William siezed his pistol (from its shelf), and they hustled outside. They chose one of the two corn houses as their guard post: 'We unlocked the corn house between the barn, or tobacco house, and the stables and spread out the blankets and lay down there.' There they watched and waited, observing the barn and listening keenly for suspicious sounds in the night.

The cavalry patrol approached (the town of) Bowling Green at around 11: 00 p.m., April 25. About a half a mile out, Doherty ordered ten of his men to dismount, and, by stealth, to follow Detective Baker into the town. Doherty, Conger, and Rollins rode quietly with the main body into the town and, by midnight, found the Star Hotel. They immediately commanded their men to surround the hotel and allow no one to leave. But their mission was thwarted, albeit temporarily, by an embarrassing incident. Lincoln's assassin might be sleeping inside, but, comically, they could not get in. 'We knocked about fifteen minutes at each door with receiving any reply,' according to Doherty. When no one answered the front door, they tried the side door, but no one answered there, either. Eventually they saw a Black man walking down the street, and they dragooned him for assistance. He took Conger and Doherty around to the back and showed them the entrance to the 'Negro house' at the rear of the Star. Baker was already lurking at the front door. They crept into the building and almost immediately encountered another Black man. 'Where is Willie Jett?' Doherty asked. In bed, the servant replied. Conger demanded to know where the room was.

Mrs. Julia Gouldman, now awake, opened the door between the hotel and the Negro house. Doherty and Conger pushed through without an introduction and asked her a single question: where was her son, Jesse? She led them upstairs to a second-floor bedroom. Prepared for anything, the officer and detectives rushed in and discovered Jesse Gouldman and Willie Jett sharing a mattress. Already awakened by the commotion, Jett tried to get out of bed. 'Is your name Jett?' Conger demanded. 'Yes, sir,' came the meek reply. 'Get up: I want you!' the detective thundered. Jett stood up and yanked on his pants. Then they seized him, hustled him downstairs roughly, and confined him in the parlor. The trio did everything possible to frighten Jett: 'We…informed him of our business,' said Doherty, 'telling him if he did not forthwith inform us where the men were, he should suffer.'

Conger reclined in a chair and studied the captive: 'Where are the two men who came with you across the river at Port Royal?'

Jett, eyeing Baker and Doherty nervously, approached Conger and whispered a plea: 'Can I see you alone?' 'Yes sir: you can,' Conger replied magnanimously. Conger asked his counterparts to leave the parlor. The moment they departed, Jett extended his hand to the detective in supplication and betrayed John Wilkes Booth: 'I know who you want; and I will tell you where they can be found.'

'That's what I want to know,' Conger encouraged him.

All that this Confederate Judas begged in return was privacy: Willie wanted no audience to witness his shame.

'They are on the road to Port Royal,' Jett confided, 'about three miles this side of that.'

But where, exactly, queried Conger: 'At whose house are they?'

'Mr. Garrett's,' Jett said, adding, 'I will go there with you, and show where they are now; and you can get them.' Willie Jett proved not only a Judas, but an enthusiastic one: 'I told them everything from beginning to end. I said I would pilot them to the house where Booth was.'

Conger realized Jett would be an invaluable guide. Without him it might be difficult, if not impossible, to locate the Garrett farmhouse in the middle of the night.

'Have you a horse?' Conger asked.

'Yes, sir.'

'Get it, and get ready to go!'

Conger sped Jett upstairs under guard to finish dressing. Quickly he put on his shirt and coat and pulled on his boots. By the time he returned to the parlor, the detectives had already sent a Black servant to get his horse.

'You say they are on the road to Port Royal?' Conger asked.

'Yes, sir,' Jett verified.

Conger could not believe it: 'I have just come from there.'

The news surprised the young Confederate: 'I thought you came from Richmond: If you have come that way, you have come right past them. I cannot tell you whether they are there now or not.'

Perhaps, when the cavalry thundered past Garrett's farm several hours ago on its way to Bowling Green, it had spooked Booth and Herold and prompted them to flee elsewhere. That was beyond Jett's control, he made clear to Detective Baker. It was not his fault if the cavalry had scared off the assassins. The news stunned Baker. A few hours ago, he and the Sixteenth New York had ridden through Port Royal, and then past the farm. The fugitives, Baker guessed, must have heard the pounding hooves of their horses. Booth and Herold had been within his grasp and he had ridden right past them! Around midnight, Conger, Baker, and Doherty, hoping they were not too late, turned the troops around and galloped back to the farm.

Conger, Baker, Doherty and Jett hurried out of the Star Hotel and mounted their horses. At about 12:30 a.m., Wednesday, April 26, the Sixteenth New York Cavalry headed for Garrett's farm and, they hoped, a rendezvous with Lincoln's assassin. Baker warned Jett not to try any tricks: 'He shook hands with the Colonel, and promised on his honor as an (Confederate) officer and a gentleman that he would be true to us. We told him that if he deceived us, it would be death to him - we thinking that perhaps it might be his design to lead us into an ambuscade.'

After two hours in the saddle, Jett told Conger that he should slow the column: 'We are very near ... now to where we go through: let us stop here, and look around.' In the dark, Jett had trouble finding the gate to the road that led to Garrett's house. Conger ordered the patrol to halt. He and Jett rode on alone. It was just a little way up, Willie reassured him. Conger trotted ahead of Jett. His eyes scanned the dark roadside but detected no opening. All Conger could see was a 'bushy, unbroken fence line skirting the road.' He turned his horse around and retreated. There is no gate he complained to Jett.

Then it is just a little farther up the road, Booth's Judas promised. It is hard to judge these distances in the dark. They rode on three hundred yards more, and Baker spurred ahead from the main body to help Conger search for the gate. This time they found it. After unlatching it, Conger sent Baker ahead to find and open the second gate; Jett had told them that it would block their way. Baker vanished into the black night while Conger backtracked to fetch the cavalry. The detective asked Jett a final question: 'when the cavalry charges down that road, where should they look for the house?'

As before, Jett obliged: 'I took them to Garrett's gate and directed them how to go into the house and they went in, leaving me at the gate.'

Conger ordered Jett and Rollins to remain at the gate, guarded by only one trooper. Soon Baker located the last roadside obstacle that separated them from Booth: 'We found a gate, fastened by a latch, dismounted, opened the gate, and the command came through, and a charge was ordered.' The Sixteenth New York Cavalry raced up the dirt road and toward the farmhouse.

As the Sixteenth New York closed in on Booth and Herold, the nation did not hold its collective breath, awaiting the exciting climax of the manhunt. Nobody - not Stanton, his officers, the other pursuers, or the press - knew that Conger, Baker, and Doherty had tracked Lincoln's assassin to Port Royal, and to the Garrett farm. Elsewhere, all over Virginia and Maryland, other manhunters, ignorant of was happening at Garrett's farm, continued the chase. In Maryland, S. H. Beckwith, the man whose tip had set in motion the sequence of events that led the Sixteenth New York to Booth's hiding place, sent, at 1:30 a.m., April 26, another telegram to Major Eckert. The Major did not receive it until 8:00 a.m. And Booth had escaped Maryland days ago.

The telegram read:

Immediately after reporting to you to-day I proceeded with Major O'Beirne to Bryantown, thence to Turner's house, where Booth and Herold were seen by two servants to enquire about food, then enter pine thicket about twenty rods distant from the house and two miles north from Bryantown. Parties on the ground had been through, losing the track and accomplishing nothing. We at once penetrated the thicket and deployed. After following probable routes I struck the crutch track, and we followed it in a direction circling around toward a piece of timber from which they first issued far enough to justify the belief they are still in same vicinity from which they started, and that while the troops were searching the thicket where they were last seen, they, by taking course above described, gained time to temporarily conceal ourselves again. It appears to us from all we can learn that troops have not been pushed through with much system. The colored troops, while deployed and advancing, upon hearing a shout on one part of line, made rush in that direction, leaving considerable space uncovered. Cavalry has been operating, and tonight have strong line of pickets around timber. I made a map to-day for immediate use, but it would have assisted much if we had a county survey map and a compass. I left Major O'Beirne at Bryantown, where he was preparing to co-operate with others and make an early and systematic scouring.

The Sixteenth New York did not need compasses or survey maps. Only a few hundred yards separated them from Booth now.

The dogs heard it first. Rising from the southwest. Distant sounds, yet inaudible to human ears, of metal touching metal; of a hundred hooves sending vibrations through the earth; of deep, labored breathing from tired horses; of faint human voices. These early warning signs alerted the dogs sleeping under the Garrett's front porch. At the farm, John Garrett, corn-house sentinel, was already awake and became the first one there to hear their approach. William Garrett, lying on a blanket a few feet from his brother, heard them, too.

It was dark and still inside the farmhouse. Old Richard Garrett and the rest of his family had gone to bed hours ago.

All was quiet, too, in the tobacco barn. It was well past midnight, and the Garretts' unwitting prisoners were asleep. As far as John and William could observe from their hiding place, neither Booth (nor) Herold stirred during the night, realized their predicament, and tried to escape their rustic jail. The horses were safe, and the suspicious 'Boyd' cousins were trapped. The barking dogs and the clanking, rumbling sound finally woke up Booth. Recognizing the unique music of cavalry on the move, the assassin knew he had only a minute or two to react before it was too late.

Booth woke up Davy fast. 'The cavalry is here,' Booth hissed in a low whisper. The assassin's groggy companion snapped to attention. They snatched up their weapons and rushed to the front of the barn. 'We went right up to the barn door and tried to get out,' recalled Davey (Herold), 'but found it was locked.' The Garretts had imprisoned them! Booth wasted no time and began trying to pry the lock from its mountings. Every second was precious: they had to flee the barn before Union troops surrounded it. Booth guessed that the riders would move on the farmhouse first. He and Herold had to clear out of the tobacco barn before the cavalrymen turned their attention to the outbuildings. No doubt the treacherous Garrett boys would guide the Yankees to the right one.

Booth wheeled around one hundred and eighty degrees. 'Come on!' he called to Davey. The assassin scampered fifty feet to the back wall. 'We went directly to the back end of the barn, and we tried to kick a board off so we could crawl out,' witnessed Herold. Booth impaired by his injury, and hobbled by his crutches, could not leverage his full weight on his left foot to swing a powerful kick with the right. He struck weakly. The board did not give. Davey fared no better. 'Let's kick together!' Booth proposed. They aimed their kicks to strike one board together. Still the iron nails held tight as though cemented into the framing. David Herold was getting worried: 'Although we did, our kicks did not do the work.'

The Union column raced up the road and threw a cordon around the Garrett farmhouse. Edward Doherty, Luther Baker and Everton Conger dropped from their saddles, leapt up the porch, and pounded on the door. Awakened by the commotion, Richard Garrett climbed from his bed and walked downstairs in his night clothes.

David Herold panicked: 'You had better give up,' He urged Booth.

'No, no,' the actor declared, 'I will suffer death first.'

Doherty, Baker, and Conger waited impatiently on the front porch, and the trio pounced as soon as old man Garrett opened the door.

Conger barked first: 'Where are the two men who stopped here at your house?'

Startled, Richard Garrett replied vaguely: 'They have gone.'

'Gone where?' Conger demanded.

'Gone to the woods,' explained Garrett.

'What!' Luther Baker interrupted mockingly, 'a lame man gone into the woods?'

'Well, he had crutches,' old man Garrett pointed out.

'Will you show me where they are?' Baker continued.

'I will, Garrett promised, 'but I will want my pants and boots.'

Garrett's interrogators refused to let him back into the house to dress, so his family passed his clothes and boots to him through the door. There on the front porch, in full view of the soldiers, he dressed himself.

Conger decided to play the old man's game, at least momentarily; 'Well Sir, whereabouts in the woods have they gone?'

Garrett began a long-winded story of how the men came there without his consent, that he did not want them to stay, and that....'

'Enough,' Conger interrupted: 'I do not want any long story out of you: I just want to know where the men have gone.'

Richard Garrett was afraid, and he babbled his defensive monologue all over again. Conger had heard enough. He turned from the door and spoke gravely to one of his men: 'Bring the lariat rope here, and I will put that man up to the top of one of those locust trees.' Even under the threat of hanging, marveled Conger, Garrett 'did not seem inclined to tell.' A soldier went to get the hemp persuader.

John Garrett emerged from the corn house, walked up to the nearest cavalry man, and asked whom they were pursuing. 'That, I cannot tell you,' the trooper answered mysteriously, telling another soldier to take John to the house. When they got near the house, John saw Doherty, Conger and Baker on the front porch talking to his father. Spotting John Garrett, Conger bellowed to his soldier escort, 'Where did you get this man from?' John Garrett spoke up and came to the rescue of his tongue-tied father.

'Don't hurt the old man: he is scared. I will tell you where the men are you want to find,' he said.

'That is what I want to know,' said an exasperated Conger. 'Where are they?'

Before John had time to answer, Doherty seized him by the collar, pushed him down the steps, put a revolver to his head, and ordered him to tell him where the assassins were.

'In the barn,' John Garrett cried out. 'The two men are in the barn.'

'Not good enough,' warned Conger: 'There are three rooms around here, the tobacco-house and two corn houses; if you don't tell me the exact house he is in, your life will pay the forfeit.'

'They are in the tobacco barn,' divulged Garrett.

'Show me the barn,' Doherty commanded.

Booth and Herold heard the soldiers rush and surround the barn. Maybe stealth could save them just once more, like it had served them in the pine thicket. Booth hushed Herold to remain silent and motionless: 'Don't make any noise,' he whispered, 'maybe they will go off thinking we are not here.' Conger, close to the barn now, heard someone moving around inside, rustling the hay. It was David Herold walking about, failing to heed Booth's orders to take cover and, stupidly, revealing that they were in the barn.

The leaders of the Sixteenth New York expedition were not done with John Garrett. They had a special mission for him. Luther Baker summoned John to his side and pointed to the tobacco house: 'You must go in to the barn, and get the arms from those men.' Garrett objected to the suicidal plan. Ignoring his reaction, Baker went on: 'They know you, and you can get in.' Yes, Booth and Herold did know John Garrett-as the man who ordered them out of his house, refused them the comfort of a bed, and locked them in the barn. That is precisely why he refused Baker's request. He had seen Booth's weapons and knew he would not hesitate to exact vengeance for Garrett's inhospitality and betrayal. No, he would not be the assassin's last victim.

Perhaps Garrett did not understand, Baker explained to him, that this mission was not optional: 'I want you to go into that barn and demand the surrender of the arms that man has and bring them out to me. Unless you do it, I will burn your property.' Baker didn't mean just the tobacco barn. He meant it all-house, barn, corn houses, and stables. Either John went in, or Baker would, 'end this affair with a bonfire and a shooting match.'

By now William Garret had also emerged from the cover of the corn house and joined his brother near the tobacco barn. William, who had imprisoned the fugitives, pulled the key from his pocket and surrendered it to Baker.

Baker stepped forward and shouted to John Wilkes Booth: 'We are going to send this man, on whose premises you are, in to get your arms, and you must come out, and deliver yourselves up.' Booth said nothing. It might be a trick, he considered. He readied himself for a dismounted charge by more than twenty cavalrymen the moment the door opened. Baker, key in hand, strode right up to the barn door. He stood within close range of Booth's pistols now. Baker inserted the key, turned the lock, and, slowly, opened the door a little. Booth remained invisible, hiding just several yards away in the black, inner recesses of the barn. He saw movement. He held his pistols tightly, fingers in the trigger guards, thumbs ready to cock the hammers of the single-action colts. But he held his fire. Baker seized John Garrett and half-guided, half-pushed him through the door and closed it behind him.

John Garrett stood alone, in the dark, at the mercy of Lincoln's killer. He spoke timidly to the unseen fugitives, reporting that, 'the barn was surrounded, that resistance was useless, and that (you) had better come out and deliver (yourself) up.'

A growling, tenor voice, dripping with malice, echoed from the darkness in reply: 'You have implicated me.'

Garrett tried to reason with them: 'Gentlemen, the cavalry are after you. You are the ones. You had better give yourselves up.'

Then, like a ghostly apparition, John Wilkes Booth's pale, haunting visage emerged from the void, like a luminous portrait floating on a black canvas. Then he exploded: 'Damn you! You have betrayed me! If you don't get out of here I will shoot you! Get out of this barn at once!' Garrett glimpsed Booth's right hand in motion. The assassin, while cursing Garrett, slowly reached behind his back for one of his revolvers.

Like Harry Hawk had done on the stage of Ford's Theater after Booth jumped from the president's box, a terrified John Garrett turned and ran, escaped the barn, and nearly leaped into Conger's arms. 'Booth was going to kill him,' Garrett pleaded.

Conger was skeptical: 'How do you know he was going to shoot you?'

'Because,' Garrett claimed in a tremulous voice, 'he reached down to the hay behind him to get his revolver.' 'He had come out of the barn just in time,' he insisted.

Finally, at the climax of a twelve-day manhunt that had gripped the nation, a heavily armed patrol of Sixteenth New York Cavalry had actually cornered Lincoln's assassin. The situation demanded decisive action, but, at the critical moment, Conger and the others hesitated. Instead of ordering their men to rush the barn and take Booth, they decided to talk him out, and then they delegated the job to a solitary, unarmed man, a civilian - and an ex-rebel soldier, no less - to negotiate Booth's surrender. It was a clear abdication of command responsibility. Twenty-six cavalrymen, each armed with a six-shot revolver, not counting other weapons, could pour a fusillade of 156 conical lead pistol bullets into the barn before having to reload. In response, Booth could fire a mere 12 rounds from the revolvers and seven from the Spencer carbine. He wouldn't have time to reload. Or the troops could, without warning, before they fired a shot, charge the barn and try to take Booth by surprise. In the dark, and in the few seconds before they seized him, Booth could not pick off more than a few of them before he was subdued. Stanton wanted Booth alive for questioning.

Even after John Garrett's ill-advised, failed mission, Doherty, Conger, and Baker dithered, pursuing a strategy of talk, not action. The trio deputized Baker as their spokesman. Baker shouted an ultimatum to the occupants: 'I want you to surrender. If you don't, I will burn this barn down in fifteen minutes.' If the fugitives refused to come out voluntarily, he resolved, then, the flames would drive them out. Baker, Conger, and Doherty awaited an answer. It was 2:30 a.m., Wednesday 26. From the time the Sixteenth New York arrived at Garrett's farm until this moment, the fugitives had not spoken one word to their pursuers. Then came the first contact.

A voice speaking from inside the barn bellowed three pointed questions: 'Who are you?' 'What do you want?' 'Whom do you want?'

It was John Wilkes Booth. The assassin stepped to the front of the tobacco barn and peered through a space between two boards, eyeballing his counterpart, whom he took, mistakenly, as an army captain.

'We want you,' Baker replied, 'and we know who you are. Give up your arms and come out.'

Booth stalled to preserve his options: 'Let us have a little time to consider it.'

Surprisingly, Baker agreed to the delay: 'Very well.'

Ten or fifteen minutes elapsed without communication between the parties. But the manhunters maintained a keen vigil on all four of the barn walls to ensure that their prey did not slip out unnoticed through a crevice between the boards.

In the meantime, Booth and David Herold got into a heated argument. Davey had no more fight left in him. 'I am sick and tired of this way of living,' he had complained to his idol on the afternoon of the twenty-fifth, less than twelve hours ago. Herold had convinced himself, naively, that once he talked his way out of trouble the soldiers would send him home. After all, in his mind, he wasn't guilty of anything. Booth killed Lincoln, and Powell stabbed Seward. Davey just came along for the ride. Booth could roast alive in the tobacco barn if he chose, but not him. 'You don't choose to give yourself up, let me go out and give myself up,' Herold proposed.

'No, you shall not do it,' Booth growled in a low voice, so that the soldiers hovering on the other side of the boards could not hear him.

Herold implored Booth to release him from the assassin's service, speaking so loudly that some of the soldiers heard his begging.

Herold started for the door, but Booth menaced him: 'He threatened to shoot me and blow his brains out,' Herold complained. Furious, the actor denounced his hitherto faithful companion: 'You damned coward! Will you leave me now? Go, go! I would not have you with me.'

Baker, counting down the minutes on his pocket watch, shouted to Booth that, 'he was running out of time. Only five minutes more, and he would torch the barn.'

Again, Booth asked: 'Who are you? And what do you want?'

Before Baker could reply, Conger took him aside, out of earshot, and suggested how to continue the negotiations: 'Do not by any remark made to him allow him to know who we are: you need not tell him who we are. If he thinks we are rebels, or thinks we are his friends, we will take advantage of it. We will not lie to him about it; but we need not answer any question that has any reference to that subject, but simply insist on his coming out, if he will.'

Baker agreed with Conger, telling Booth, 'It doesn't matter any difference who we are: we know who you are, and we want you. We want to take you prisoners.'

Booth corrected him. There was no more than one prisoner available for the taking: 'I am alone, there is no one with me.'

Baker rebuked the assassin: 'We know that two men went in there and two must come out.' Conger worked his way around the barn's perimeter to select the best place to light the fire.

'This is a hard case,' Booth confided to Baker, 'it may be I am to be taken by my friends.' That assassin held the forlorn hope that (the) soldiers surrounding the barn were Confederate, not Union.

'I am going,' insisted Davey. 'I don't intend to be burned alive.'

Booth relented. Forcing Davey to share his fate would serve no purpose. And it would be wrong. Herold had had several chances to abandon Booth during the manhunt - in Washington on assassination night, in the pine thicket, or during the night the assassin slept alone at Garrett's farm. But on every occasion, the loyal Herold returned to share Booth's fate. Almost certainly, Booth must have concluded that it would be ungrateful, even ungallant, to deny his young follower the chance to live. When others had betrayed Booth, Herold had stuck by him. It was harsh to call him coward now. This was the last act. It was time to claim center stage alone. The actor called out to Baker: 'Oh Captain -there is a man here who wants to surrender awful bad.'

Too excited to remain silent, Lieutenant Doherty blurted out: 'Hand out your arms.' Yes, chimed Baker almost simultaneously, 'Let him hand out his arms.'

Their demands perplexed Herold. Would they refuse his surrender until he first handed over Booth's firearms? His master might let him go, but Davey knew that Booth would never give up his guns. 'I have none,' Herold pleaded.

Doherty did not believe him: 'Hand out your arms, and you can come out.'

'I have no arms,' Herold whimpered, 'let me out.'

Luther Baker scoffed at Herold's stubborn denials: 'We know exactly what you have got.' The Garrett's, helpfully, had provided Baker and the other officers with a complete inventory of the fugitive's arms and equipment: two revolvers, one Spencer repeating carbine, one Bowie knife, a pistol belt, a couple of blankets, and the clothes on their backs. 'You carried a carbine,' Baker insisted, 'and you must hand it out.'

The back-and-forth bickering over the arms devolved into comedy, with one officer and two detectives proving themselves too incompetent to communicate the peaceful, willing surrender of Lincoln's assassin and his guide. Booth spoke to end the empasse: 'The arms are mine; and I have got them.'

Baker disputed the assassin: 'This man carried a carbine, and he must hand it out.'

Booth argued back: 'Upon the word and honor of a gentleman, he has no arms: the arms are mine, and I have got them.' And he would not give them up. 'I own all the arms and intend to use them on you gentlemen.' As this wore on, Booth reminded the nitpicking officers that 'There is a man in here who wants to come out.'

Yes, Herold affirmed: 'Let me out, quick; I do not know anything about this man, he is a desperate character, and he is going to shoot me.'

Booth supported Herold's charade: 'Let him out; that young man is innocent.'......

'Whoever you are, come out with your hands up,' a voice outside the barn shouted.

Davey turned away from Booth and faced the door, now ajar and ready for his passage from fugitive to captive. Doherty ordered Herold not to walk through the door just yet. First he wanted to see his hands to confirm that he was unarmed. The lieutenant told Davey to thrust only one hand through the doorframe. The frightened youth complied, and in a moment Doherty saw a spot of open-palmed, white flesh protruding through the entryway. The lieutenant signaled Davey to send through the other hand. It too was empty.

Doherty sprung to the door, seized Herold by the wrists, and yanked hard, pulling him forward through the doorway, and throwing him off balance. Davey's captor tucked his revolver under his armpit, ran both his hands down Herold's body to see if he had any hidden arms, and found none. Then he asked Herold, 'Have you got any weapons at all about you?'

'Nothing at all…,' swore Davey. The lieutenant grabbed Herold by the collar……(and) marched him away from the barn.

Conger and Baker wanted to burn the barn…Indeed, the only danger would be to the men who had to get close enough to the barn to lay the kindling against the timbers. Booth might be able to…. shoot them in the head at point-blank range. They (considered) the risk involved and concluded that the (task) didn't have to fall to their own men.

Conger sent for the Garrett sons. He had one more job for them, he explained: 'collect a few armfuls of straw and pile them against the side of the barn. John Garrett roamed the grounds but could not find any fresh straw. 'It was all in the tobacco barn with Booth,' he told Conger. 'Then find something else that will burn,' the detective ordered. John Garrett gathered pine twigs and set them next to the barn. He returned with a second armful and bent low to arrange the pile. The rustling sound alerted Booth, who rushed to the site of the noise. Garrett jumped when he heard that familiar, menacing voice address him from the other side (of the plank barn wall), just a foot or two away: 'Young man, I advise you for your own good not to come here again.' It was Booth's second warning to him that night. There would not be a third, the assassin promised: 'If you do not leave at once I will shoot you.' Quickly, John Garrett dropped the pine kindling and retreated out of pistol range.

If they were gathering kindling, Booth realized, the manhunters did not plan on waiting until sunrise. They were going to burn the barn, and soon, probably. Booth decided to retake the initiative and stall the fire. He challenged his pursuers to honorable combat on open ground.

'Captain,' he called out to Baker, 'I know you to be a brave man, and I believe you to be honorable: I am a cripple; I have got but one leg. If you will withdraw your men in line one hundred yards from the door, I will come out and fight you.'

As a sign of good faith, Booth revealed that he had chosen, at least up to now, to spare Baker's life: 'Captain, I consider you to be a brave and honorable man: I have had half a dozen opportunities to shoot you, but I did not.'

Baker declined the glove: 'We did not come here to fight you, we simply came to make you a prisoner. We do not want any fight with you.' Neither did Secretary of War Edwin Stanton, who, back in Washington, awaited news from the manhunters. He wanted the assassin alive to interrogate him and expose fully the secrets of his grand conspiracy. Stanton, convinced that officials at the highest levels of the government of the Confederate States of America had participated in the assassination, wanted Booth to name his co-plotters. If Booth was dead, that would satisfy the nation's lust for vengeance, but not Stanton's curiosity. It was far better, the secretary of war believed, to take him alive, 'There would be plenty of time to hang him later, after the trial.'

Booth repeated his challenge but reduced the distance to give his antagonists more generous terms: 'If you'll take your men fifty yards from the door, I'll come out and fight you. Give me a chance for my life.'

Again Baker declined.

'Well, my brave boys, prepare a stretcher for me!' Booth jauntily replied.

Conger made up his mind and turned to Baker: 'We will fire the barn.'

'Yes,' his fellow detective agreed, 'the quicker the better.'

Conger bent over and lit the kindling. The pine twigs and needles, mixed with a little hay and highly combustible, burst into flames that licked the dry, weathered boards. Soon the barn's boards and timbers caught fire, and within minutes an entire corner of the barn blazed brightly. The fire illuminated the yard with a yellow-orange glow that flickered eerily across the faces of the men of the Sixteenth. Booth could see them clearly now, but held his fire.

As the fire gathered momentum, it also lit the inside of the barn so that now, for the first time, the soldiers could see their quarry in the gaps between the slats. Booth made a halfhearted attempt to suppress the flames by overturning a table on them, but that only fueled the rapidly advancing inferno. The assassin was trapped…

Booth moved to the center of the barn, where he stood awkwardly balancing the carbine in one hand, a pistol in the other, and a crutch under one arm. He glanced at the door and hopped forward, a crutch under his left arm and in his right hand the Spencer carbine, the butt plate balanced against his hip. 'One more stain on the old banner,' Booth cried out, conjuring up the Stars and Bars Confederate battle flag, perhaps 'imagining his own patriotic blood mingling with the vast ocean spilled by the South's quarter million dead.'

Unseen by Booth, Sergeant Boston Corbett watched the assassin's every move inside the barn; 'Immediately when the fire was lit…I could see him, but he could not see me.'… Now Booth was in easy range of Corbett's pistol. But the sergeant held his fire: 'I could have shot him…but as long as he was there, making no demonstration to hurt anyone, I did not shoot him, but kept my eye on him steadily.'

Booth moved again and leveled the carbine against his hip, as though he was preparing to bring it into firing position. Corbett poked the barrel of his revolver through the slit in the wall and aimed it at Booth. The sergeant described what happed next:

'Finding the fire gaining on him, he turned to the other side of the barn and got towards where the door was; and, as he got there, I saw him make a movement towards the floor. I supposed he was going to fight his way out. One of the men who was watching told me that (Booth) aimed his carbine at him. He was taking aim with the carbine, but at whom I could not say. My mind was upon him attentively to see that he did no harm; and, when I became impressed that it was time, I shot him. I took steady aim on my arm, and shot him through a large crack in the barn.'

Instantly Booth dropped the carbine and crumpled to his knees. Corbett's bullet had passed through (Booth's) neck and spinal column. Finally, after several attempts, Lincoln's assassin spoke: 'Tell mother, I die for my country.' Baker noted, 'He seemed to suffer extreme pain whenever he was moved, and would scowl, and would several times repeat: 'Kill me. Kill me.' 'We don't want to kill you,' Conger comforted him, 'we want you to get well.'

Conger walked away in search of the trigger-happy trooper. He returned soon but, it appeared to Baker, empty-handed.

'Where is the man?' (Baker asked.)

Conger laughed aloud and replied, 'I guess we had better let Providence and the Secretary of War take care of him.'

When Conger went off to find Booth's killer, Sergeant Corbett came forward, snapped to attention, saluted Conger, and proclaimed, 'Colonel, Providence directed me.' Corbett claimed, 'He had not shot Booth for vengeance, but because he believed the assassin was about to open fire on the soldiers. He did it to protect the lives of his fellow troopers,' he insisted. And, Corbett continued, 'he did not intend to kill Booth. He only wanted to inflict a disabling wound to render the assassin helpless, for capture.' Corbett exercised his own discretion as a noncommissioned officer and shot Booth: 'It was not through fear at all that I shot him, but because it was my impression that it was time the man was shot; for I thought he would do harm to our men in trying to fight his way out of that den if I did not.'

Booth died at sunrise."

In 1867, Howard University, originally housed in the First Congressional

Church of Washington, D.C., receives a Congressional charter to educate freedmen.

In 1868, the 14th Amendment to the Constitution is ratified, guaranteeing citizenship to all persons born in the U.S.

Dr. Samuel Mudd (a medical doctor who, as a lesser conspirator, had given Booth and Herold shelter and food after Lincoln's murder) was released from federal prison and allowed to return to his farm in 1869. Before he died, Mudd confessed the truth about the night of April 14, 1865, that he had known all along that the injured stranger at his door was John Wilkes Booth, Lincoln's assassin, and that he had misdirected the federal troops who were in pursuit. In 1906, Dr. Samuel Mudd's daughter published a collection of his letters, and in 1936, a Hollywood motion picture, *The Prisoner of Shark Island*, portrayed Mudd as an innocent country doctor obeying his Hippocratic Oath, deceived by Lincoln's assassin. That mythical image of Mudd's innocence was established in the collective mind of the country - his relatives and descendants continued to work for more than 100 years to perpetuate the myth.

In 1870, The 15th Amendment is ratified, guaranteeing the right to vote regardless of "race, color, or previous condition of servitude."

On December 20, 1870, Jefferson Franklin Long becomes the first Black American to be elected to Congress from the state of Georgia.

On February 20, 1895, Frederick Douglass and his wife Helen rode by carriage into Washington D.C. to attend a women's suffrage rally. When Douglass strode into the hall, the chairwoman interrupted the meeting, and all present rose as Susan B. Anthony and Anna Shaw escorted him to the podium.

After the animated women's suffrage meeting, Douglass and his wife returned to their home at Cedar Hill overlooking the city. After freshening up, the couple waited outside their house for a carriage to take them to the neighborhood Black church in the town of Anacostia - as they waited Douglass "began to mimic one of the day's earlier speakers by rising from his chair and then sinking to his knees in a heroic gesture. In an instant, Helen's delight became horror. Frederick crumpled to the floor (dead)."

Douglass (1818 - 1895) died instantly at age 77, probably from a ruptured cerebral aneurysm as he had snow white hair, a warning signal of a copper deficiency. His life spanned the terms of eight U.S. Presidents; he had become Chairman of the failed Freedman's Bank, a recruiter for the Union Army, Ambassador to Haiti, and, briefly, an advisor to Presidents Lincoln and Grant, however, he never achieved the status of an appointment to the Presidential Cabinet that had been his ultimate goal.

At Douglass' funeral, Robert Smalls - the former Congressman from South

Carolina stated, "The greatest of the race has fallen." Four days after his funeral, colored schools were closed and many thousands of school children visited Douglass' open coffin at the Metropolitan African Methodist Episcopal Church. Douglass' body was sent by train to Rochester where "his body laid in state in City Hall."

Booker Taliaferro Washington, the illegitimate son of a White man and a Negro slave was born in 1856, in Franklin County, Virginia. He graduated in 1875 from Hampton Institute, a Black vocational school, and for two years after his graduation, he was an instructor there.

In 1881 he founded Tuskegee Normal and Industrial Institute, which emphasized industrial training and became, under Washington's leadership, the foremost proponent of industrial education for Black Americans. In addition to being revered by the Black American for his lofty and tireless efforts on behalf of the Black population, Booker T. Washington was also accepted and respected by Whites from the North and the South because of his emphysis on the fact that "while the Negro should not be deprived by unfair means of the franchise, (he also believed that) political agitation alone would not save him":

> *"Think about it: we went into slavery pagans; we came out Christians. We went into slavery pieces of property; we came out American citizens. We went into slavery with chains clanking about our wrists; we came out with the American ballot in our hands.....Notwithstanding the cruelty and moral wrong of slavery, we are in a stronger and more hopeful condition, materially, intellectually, morally and religiously than is true of an equal number of Black people in any other portion of the globe.*
>
> *The wisest among my race understand that the agitation of questions of social equality is the extremist folly, and that progress in the enjoyment of all the privileges that will come to us must be the result of severe and constant struggle rather that of artificial forcing.*
>
> *The Negro should not be deprived by unfair means of the franchise, but political agitation alone will not save him. Back of the ballot, he must have property, industry, skill, economy, intelligence and character. No race without these elements can permanently succeed...We have a right to enter our complaints, but we shall make a fatal error if we yield to the temptation of believing that mere opposition to our wrongs will take the place of progressive, constructive action...Whether he will or will not, a White man respects a Negro who owns a two-story brick house."*

On September 18, 1895, Booker T. Washington delivers his "Atlanta Compromise" speech at the Atlanta Cotton States Exposition:

> *"Mr. President and Gentlemen of the Board of Directors and Citizens.*
> *One-third of the population of the South is of the Negro race. No enterprise seeking the*

material, civil, or moral welfare of this section can disregard this element of our population and reach the highest success. I but convey to you, Mr. President and Directors, the sentiment of the masses of my race when I say that in no way have the value, and manhood of the American Negro been more fittingly and generously recognized than by the managers of this magnificent Exposition at every stage of its progress. It is a recognition that will do more to cement the friendship of the two races than any occurrence since the dawn of our freedom.

Not only this, but the opportunity here afforded will awaken among us a new era of industrial progress. Ignorant and inexperienced, it is not strange that in the first years of our new life we began at the top instead of at the bottom; that a seat in Congress or the state legislature was more sought than real estate or industrial skill; that the political convention of stump speaking had more attractions than starting a dairy farm or truck garden.

A ship lost at sea for many days suddenly sighted a friendly vessel. From the mast of the unfortunate vessel was seen a signal, "Water, water; we die of thirst!" The answer from the friendly vessel at once came back, "Cast down your bucket where you are." A second time the signal, "Water, water; send us water!" ran up from the distressed vessel, and was answered, "Cast down your bucket where you are." "And a third and fourth signal for water was answered, "Cast down your bucket where you are." The captain of the distressed vessel, at last heeding the injunction, cast down his bucket, and it came up full of fresh, sparkling water from the mouth of the Amazon River. To those of my race who depend on bettering their condition in a foreign land or who underestimate the importance of cultivating friendly relations with the Southern White man, who is their next-door neighbor, I would say: "Cast down your bucket where you are" - cast it down in making friends in every manly way of the people of all races by whom we are surrounded.

Cast it down in agriculture, mechanics, in commerce, in domestic service, and in the professions. And in this connection it is well to bear in mind that whatever other sins the South may be called to bear, when it comes to business, pure and simple, it is in the South that the Negro is given a man's chance, in the commercial world, and in nothing is this Exposition more eloquent than in emphasizing this chance. Our greatest danger is that in the great leap from slavery to freedom we may overlook the fact that the masses of us are to live by the productions of our hands, and fail to keep in mind that we shall prosper in proportion as we learn to dignify and glorify common labour and put brains and skill into the common occupations of life; shall prosper in proportion as we learn to draw the line between the superficial and the substantial, the ornamental gewgaws of life and the useful. No race can prosper till it learns that there is as much dignity in tilling a field as in writing a poem. It is at the bottom of life we must begin, and not at the top. Nor should we permit our grievances to overshadow our opportunities.

To those of the White race who look to the incoming of those of foreign birth and strange tongue and habits for the prosperity of the South, were I permitted I would repeat what I say to my own race, "Cast down your bucket where you are." Cast it down among the eight million Negroes whose habits you know, whose fidelity and love you have tested in days when to have proved treacherous meant the ruin of you firesides. Cast down your bucket among these people who have, without strikes and labour wars, tilled your fields, cleared your forests, builded your railroads and cities, and brought forth treasures from the bowels of the earth, and helped make possible this magnificent representation of the progress of the South. Casting down your bucket among my people, helping and encouraging them as you are doing on these grounds, and to education of head, hand and heart, you will find that they will buy your surplus land, make blossom the waste places in your fields, and run your factories. While doing this, you can be sure in the future, as in the past, that you and your families will be surrounded by the most patient, faithful, law-abiding, and unresentful people the world has seen. As we have proved our loyalty to you in the past, in nursing your children, watching by the sickbed of your mothers and fathers, and often following them with tear-filled eyes to their graves, so in the future, in our humble way, we shall stand by you with a devotion that no foreigner can approach, ready to lay down our lives, if need be, in defense of yours, interlacing our industrial, commercial, civil, and religious life with yours in a way that shall make the interests of both races one. In all things that are purely social we can be as separate as the fingers (on one's hand), yet one as the hand in all things essential to mutual progress.

There is no defense or security for any of us except in the highest intelligence and development of all. If anywhere there are efforts tending to curtail the fullest growth of the Negro, let these efforts be turned into stimulating, encouraging, and making him the most useful and intelligent citizen. Effort or means so invested will pay a thousand percent interest. These efforts will be twice blessed - "blessing him that gives and him that takes."

There is no escape through the law of man or God from the inevitable: -

> The laws of changeless justice bind
> Opressor with oppressed;
> And close as sin and suffering joined
> We march to fate abreast.

Nearly sixteen millions of hands will aid you in pulling the load upward, or they will pull against you the load downward. We shall constitute one-third and more of the ignorance and crime of the South, or one-third its intelligence and progress; we shall contribute one-third to the business and the industrial prosperity of the South, or we shall prove a veritable body of death, stagnating, depressing, retarding every effort to advance the body politic.

Gentlemen of the Exposition, as we present to you our humble effort at an exhibition of our progress, you must not expect overmuch. Starting thirty years ago with ownership here and there in a few quilts and pumpkins and chickens (gathered from miscellaneous sources), remember the path that has led from these to the inventions and production of agricultural implements, buggies, steam engines, newspapers, books, statuary, carving, paintings, the management of drug-stores and banks, has not been trodden without contact with thorns *and thistles. While we take pride in what we exhibit as a result of our independent efforts, we do not for a moment forget that our part in this Exhibition would fall far short of your expectations but for the constant help that has come to our educational life, not only from the Southern states, but especially from Northern philanthropists, who have made their gifts a constant stream of blessing and encouragement.*

The wisest among my race understand that the agitation of questions of social equality is the extremist folly, and that progress in the enjoyment of all the privileges that will come to us must be the result of severe and constant struggle rather than of artificial forcing. No race that has anything to contribute to the markets of the world is long in any degree ostracized. It is important and right that all privileges of the law be ours, but it is vastly more important that we be prepared for the exercises of these privileges. The opportunity to earn a dollar in a factory just now is worth infinitely more than the opportunity to spend a dollar in an opera-house.

In conclusion, may I repeat that nothing in thirty years has given us more hope and encouragement, and drawn us so near to you of the White race, as this opportunity offered by the Exposition; and here bending, as it were, over the altar that represents the results of the struggles of your race and mine, both starting practically empty handed three decades ago. I pledge that in your effort to work out the great and intricate problem which God has laid at the doors of the South, you shall have at all times the patient, sympathetic help of my race; only let this be constantly in mind, that, while from representations in these buildings of the product of the field, of forrest, of mine, of factory, letters, and art, much good will come, yet far above and beyond material benefits will be that higher good, that, let us pray God, will come in a blotting out of sectional differences and racial animosities and suspicions, in a determination to administer absolute justice, in a willing obedience among all classes to the mandates of law. This, then, coupled with our material property, will bring into our beloved South a new heaven and a new earth."

On May 18, 1896, the *Plessy v. Ferguson* case decided by the U.S. Supreme Court upheld the principle of "separate but equal."

In 1908 the NAACP was founded.

On August 9, 1936 Jesse Owens wins four gold medals in the Berlin Olympics.

In June 1938, Joe Louis defeats Max Schmeling for the heavy weight championship of the world.

October 23, 1945, Brooklyn Dodgers sign Jackie Robinson and send him to the team's Montreal farm team.

November 1, 1945 marked the founding of *Ebony* magazine.

On March 21, 1946 Kenny Washington signs with the Los Angeles Rams and becomes the first Black player in professional football in 13 years. Three other Blacks, Woody Strode of the Rams and Ben Willis and Marion Motley of the Cleveland Browns signed in the same year.

On June 3, 1946, the U.S. Supreme Court in *Irene Morgan v. Commonwealth of Virginia*, bans segregation in interstate bus travel.

On December 5, 1946, President Harry S. Truman created the landmark Committee on Civil Rights. In October 1947, the committee issued a formal report, *To Secure These Rights*, that condemned racism in America.

April 10, 1947, Jackie Robinson joins the Brooklyn Dodgers. On April 15, 1947, Robinson played his first professional baseball game at Ebbetts Field and became the first Black player in the Major Leagues in modern times.

On July 26, 1948, in response to widespread Black protests and a threat of civil disobedience, President Truman issues two executive orders ending racial discrimination in federal employment and requiring equal treatment in the armed services.

On September 22, 1950, Ralph J. Bunch, the first Black to win a Nobel Prize, was awarded the Nobel Peace Prize for his successful resolution of the Israeli-Palestinian conflict.

On November 1, 1951, the publication of the first issue of *Jet* Magazine, marked the beginning of a weekly news coverage in Black America.

On May 17, 1954, in a unanimous decision, the *Brown v. Board of Education of Topeka* desegregation case, the U.S. Supreme Court overturns the "separate but equal" doctrine, "sounding the death knell" for legal segregation and Jim Crow laws in the U.S.

On May 10, 1955 Chuck Berry records "Maybelline," the musical piece that played a major role in the development of "rock 'n' roll." Berry and other Black stars, particularly Muddy Waters and Little Richard, were the major musical influences on the Beatles and other White groups.

On December 1, 1955, following in Frederick Douglass' footsteps in challenging the segregated train cars, Rosa Parks' refusal to give up her Montgomery, Alabama bus seat to a White man started the modern Civil Rights Movement and brought her the title, "Mother of the Civil Rights Movement." Rosa Parks was a NAACP activist who was well respected in Montgomery's Black community and a perfect symbol of the hardships caused by segregated buses. Martin Luther King Jr. stated, "She was one of the finest citizens of Montgomery - not one of the finest Negro citizens - but one of the finest citizens of Montgomery."

On December 5, 1955, the historic Montgomery Bus Boycott begins in Alabama. The Rev. Martin Luther King, Jr. was elected president of the boycott organization. Dr. King wrote in his book that, "Mrs. Parks' arrest was "the precipitating factor in the Montgomery Bus Boycott that lasted 381 days.

On August 29, 1957, the U.S. Congress passes the Civil Rights Act of 1957, the first federal civil rights legislation since 1875.

On September 25, 1957, President Eisenhower sends federal troops into Little Rock, Arkansas, to facilitate the integration of the Central High School. School children are escorted into the school by federal troops, an act that ended on May 10, 1955 Chuck Berry records "Maybelline," the musical piece that played a major role in the development of "rock 'n' roll." Berry and other Black stars, particularly Muddy Waters and Little Richard, were the major musical influences on the Beatles and other White groups effort to thwart the court ordered integration.

On December 17, 1959, Motown Records was founded, this recording institution helped change the understanding, marketing, and promotion of Black popular music.

On February 1, 1960, four North Carolina A&T students begin the Sit-in Movement at the lunch counter of a Greensboro, North Carolina 5 & 10 store.

In 1960, Wilma Rudolph became an Olympic legend by winning three Gold Medals at the 1960 Rome Olympics. She won the 100 meter, and the 200 meter races and she ran the anchor leg for the victorious 400 meter relay.

On May 4, 1961, 13 "Freedom Riders" begin the bus trip through the South to test compliance with laws banning segregation in interstate transportation. Black and White riders were bombed and severely beaten, but their movement exposed segregation in interstae transportation facilities.

On September 22, 1961, the Interstate Commerce Commission issues ruling prohibiting segregation on interstate buses and facilities.

The "Albany Movement" began as a spin-off of the Freedom Rides in the winter of 1961; a small collection of interracial groups, led by the Congress of Racial Equality (CORE), was founded by James Farmer as a nonviolent organization in Chicago in 1942.

Farmer, a graduate of Howard School of Divinity and race relations secretary for the pacifist Fellowship of Reconciliation, knew that many tactics necessary to fight the de facto segregation in the North were unacceptable to strict pacifists. Pacifists agreed with the use of the tactic of nonviolent passive resistance; however, many pacifists considered demonstrations aggressively provocative.

CORE chose to test the December 1960 Supreme Court decision in *Boynton v. Virginia*, which extended the prohibition of segregation in interstate travel to train and bus terminals. The ruling stated there should be no more "Colored" and "For Whites Only" waiting rooms; no more separate rest rooms, water fountains, lunch counters with separate facilities (with the facilities for Coloreds always inferior). It also stated that Blacks would no longer be confined to the front car of the trains, or seated at separate tables hidden behind a curtain in train dining cars - the typical Southern cultural standards of the times.

Unfortunately, the "For Whites Only" signs stayed up, especially in small Southern towns - local bureaucrats defied the U. S. Supreme Court ruling. Blacks who used the "For Whites Only" facilities in bus and train stations were arrested and brutally beaten.

This was the electrified environment that the Freedom Riders rode into in the spring of 1961 - they were committed to challenging the continued segregation on the buses, trains and in the terminals. Their goal was to force the executive branch of the federal government to enforce the *Boynton* decision.

The beatings and the arrests inflicted on the Freedom Riders during the spring of 1961 focused state, national and world attention on the Southern states in a manner that had not happened since the Montgomery Bus Boycott in 1955.

This public awareness forced the fledgling John F. Kennedy administration to take some action to protect the constitutional rights of the Freedom Riders, and to fully implement *Boynton* administratively with an Interstate Commerce Commission (ICC) order on September 22, 1961 directly prohibiting segregated facilities in interstate travel, effective November 1, 1961. This ICC order precipitated the demonstrations in Albany - a small, heretofore quiet southwestern Georgia town of 56,000 people (the population was 40% black). Albany was tightly governed by a traditional White "Good ole boy" oligarchy that was bent on resisting any threat to the local traditions and status quo.

Following the September 1961 ICC ruling, a small collection of Albany's Black pastors delivered a letter to the city government requesting meetings be held to discuss desegregation in Albany and requesting that there be progress toward compliance with the ICC's order. In reply, the *Albany Herald*, James Gray's ultraconservative newspaper, published a hostile editorial condemning the pastors for sending the letter. Following he editorial, the home of one of the pastors who had sent the letter was bombed.

The negative and violent response to a humble request from the local pastors that the city comply with federal law acted as a galvanizing force to the loose group of Black community leaders. Dr. William Anderson, a local osteopath, became the president of the Albany Movement; a coalition of community associations, ministers, NAACP members, and other individuals and organizations. A resolute activist, Dr. Anderson contacted SNCC workers in Atlanta who had been involved in a boycott of downtown Atlanta businesses that had refused to employ Black clerks the previous year, and asked them to come to Albany to help challenge the defiantly segregated bus stations.

Early in November 1961, in response to Dr. Anderson's request, SNCC sent six students - they boarded buses in Atlanta headed for Albany. As they arrived they attempted to use the Whites Only waiting room facilities and were promptly arrested. A handful of students from the local campus of Albany State, aware of the demonstrations, took the place of those arrested, and they themselves were quickly arrested.

Each wave of arrests resulted in another wave of students sitting in at the bus station in the main waiting area reserved for Whites - each wave was arrested. Dr. Anderson established a committee to publicize the demonstrations and obtain support for the incarcerated students.

The events in Albany soon reached a crisis; six weeks into the demonstration, some 2,000 students were in jail! The Albany jails were crammed beyond legal capacity with student demonstrators - although the demonstrations had been ignited by the single issue of Blacks being able to have access to the same facilities as Whites, by December the list of demands had grown significantly. Like Pharaoh, the city fathers of Albany were stiff-necked and refused to meet with Dr. Anderson and others in the Albany movement to resolve the problems.

The number of Black students in jail soon ran into the hundreds. Dr. Anderson decided to invite Martin Luther King, Jr. to speak at the Shiloh Baptist Church on the night of December 15 - Dr. King agreed to go to Albany, make a quick speech and return to Atlanta.

The next morning, Dr. King, Ralph Abernathy and Dr. Anderson led a crowd of 200 people to the front steps of the Albany City Hall to pray. The entire group was immediately arrested for trespassing and unceremoniously marched off to jail. Their arrests brought statewide, national, and international media scrutiny to Albany.

Many Freedom Marches, sit-ins, demonstrations, and boycotts followed the Albany demonstrations, however, it was the heavy-handed response by authorities in the 1963 Birmingham marches and boycotts that finally resulted in the federal government taking positive action.

Andy Young and his team met with the religious and business leaders of Birmingham to introduce themselves, let the community leaders (Black and White) know what was coming; Young felt the local business leaders "were not bad people, they were just people in a bad situation."

First they discussed the theory for the economic boycotts; Black citizens would be encouraged to stop spending their hard-earned money in stores where they could not get jobs or where they were required to submit to the humiliation of drinking at segregated water fountains or using "colored" toilets. Young also informed the business leaders that, "the demonstrations would continue and even escalate, until if need be, all Birmingham became a jail." It was made clear that the fear of jail or even death could no longer keep the Black community locked into a system that required them to accept a false inferiority, and in which White citizens enjoyed a superiority based solely on race; once again they spelled out our goals:

1) The desegregation of lunch counters, rest rooms, drinking fountains, and fitting rooms in all stores.

2) The hiring of Blacks on a nondiscriminatory basis as clerks and cashiers, not just as maids and janitors, throughout the business community.

3) The dropping of all charges against every citizen arrested in nonviolent demonstrations.

4) The formation of a biracial committee to develop a strategy for school desegregation and for a continuing dialogue on racial conflicts and tensions.

Easter Sunday arrived with Dr. King still in Jail; Andy Young led marches to the jail with 5,000 blacks to sing hymns to comfort those in jail. When they had reached a point two blocks from the jail, they noted that the Birmingham police had set up barricades with dogs to block them from reaching the jail. The barricades were backed up with fire trucks and firemen with hoses at the ready. Bull Connor, the chief of police shouted, "Y'all have to disperse this crowd. Turn this group around." However, there were 5,000 people behind them, so Andy asked everyone to get on their knees and pray.

Abruptly, Rev. Charles Billups, one of the most faithful and fearless leaders of the old ACMHR, jumped up and hollered, "The Lord is with this movement! Off your knees. Were going to the jail!" Everybody got up and headed for the barricades and the police who were waiting there. Bull Connor yelled, "Stop 'em, Stop 'em!" But not one of the police moved a muscle; even the dogs that had been growling, snapping and straining on their leads became calm. The protesters just marched right by them. Bull Connor yelled, "Turn on the hoses, turn on the hoses!" The firemen didn't move either. The firemen had tears in their eyes and they just let their hoses drop to the ground. Andrew Young recalled one old women, who, as she passed through the barricades shouted, "Great God Almighty done parted the Red Sea one mo' time!"

According to Andrew Young, "The Birmingham movement was the largest and most effective youth evangelism effort this country has ever seen." By Monday, April 29, the leaders were ready to kickoff large scale demonstrations utilizing high school students, and escalate them to their peak - the kids were ready to go to jail for the cause! They sent the athletic stars and the homecoming queens first, and the other students followed. They were preparing for a massive march on Thursday, May 2, which they labeled "D-Day" for Desegregation Day - the entire student bodies of Parker and Ulman and other high schools were committed to the demonstrations.

On "D-Day" 1,000 students marched into downtown Birmingham; about 900 were arrested. Two thousand five hundred more students lined up and were soon ready to march forward - soon their friends and younger siblings joined in. Bull Connor "went crazy" with the appearance of more than 2,000 kids demonstrating throughout the city and on Friday May 3, he made the ultimate decision - he ordered police and fire trucks into Kelly Ingram Park to quell the demonstrations.

Connor ordered the hoses unwound and the dogs brought to the front of the barricades. The kids kept marching and their singing of old freedom songs and chanting grew louder - suddenly Connor ordered the firemen to open and train their hoses on the marchers and the thousands of observers, he then ordered the police dog handlers to chase the frightened teens. The handlers unleashed their dogs - the police ran at the teen protesters, observers and newsmen, unceremoniously clubbing them with their night sticks. Live television coverage of the Birmingham police violence and brutality instantly went around the world.

At the same time, Alabama Governor George Wallace was creating his own problems by declaring he "would stand in the schoolhouse door and personally deny them entry before he would see the University of Alabama desegregated." The Federal Courts had decreed that Vivian Malone and James Hood were to be the first Black students to be enrolled at the University.

Following "D-Day", downtown Birmingham was in an economic meltdown and the night of Tuesday, May 7, the city fathers decided to negotiate a settlement. The United Auto Workers and the Maritime Workers Union posted bail to get all of the jailed adult and student demonstrators released and on May 10, President Kennedy scheduled a press conference to announce the Birmingham settlement. Ultimately it was the pressure of local economic sanctions that persuaded the Birmingham business establishment that the price of maintaining the segregation status quo was too high.

On October 1, 1962, escorted by 12,000 federal troops, James Meredith enters the University of Mississippi, effectively ending the state's defiance of federal laws.

On June 11, 1963, one month after the Birmingham agreement was signed, President Kennedy delivered a television address on civil rights, stating that he was going to introduce to Congress a comprehensive civil rights bill. The legislation forbade segregation and discrimination in public accommodations and transportation, education, and employment.

Just after midnight on June 12, 1963 Medgar Evers, the field secretary of the Mississippi branch of the NAACP, was murdered by a sniper - shot in the back in the driveway of his home.

The civil rights bill sent to Congress by President Kennedy was the most comprehensive package of civil rights proposals since Reconstruction. The Birmingham movement had given civil rights the moral high ground. The preparation of the actual legislation was up to the Justice Department and the NAACP's lobbyist, Clarence Mitchell. Mitchell, because of his efforts was given the honorary title of the "101st Senator." The legislation would face political and Constitutional barriers similar to those of the civil rights legislation of the 1870s (which had been struck down by an unsympathetic post-Civil War Supreme Court). Desegregation of transportation and other public services could be declared by Fiat under the federal power of the President to regulate interstate commerce. Employment discrimination in individual states was declared to be covered by the Fourteenth Amendment, which guarantees equal protection under the law.

There was, however, the matter of desegregating areas of life that had been relegated to "state's rights," especially schools and other local regulatory matters. Kennedy solved the problem by tying the standards of federally mandated segregation to eligibility and receipt of federal funding.

The March on Washington by 250,000 people, for Jobs and Freedom, took place on August 28, 1963. The march was originally conceived by the "Big Six" civil rights organizations, unions and some activist religious leaders:

Southern Christian Leadership Conference (SCLC)

Student Nonviolent Coordinating Committee (SNCC)

National Association for the Advancement of Colored People (NAACP)

National Council of Negro Women

Urban League

Congress of Racial Equality

On the morning of the 28th, people came by train and bus from the East and by bus from the South; they poured out onto Pennsylvania Avenue and they were singing freedom songs, "Ain't gonna let nobody turn me 'round, turn me 'round, ain't gonna let nobody turn me 'round; we're gonna keep on a-walkin', marching up to freedom land." Many celebrities gathered with the crowd at the steps of the Lincoln Memorial to listen to the speakers.

The last speaker was Martin Luther King, Jr. and he later wrote, "I started out reading the (prepared) speech, and read it down to a point. The audience's response was wonderful that day, and all of a sudden this thing came to me. The previous June, following a peaceful assemblage of thousands of people through the streets of downtown Detroit, Michigan, I delivered a speech in Cobo Hall, in which I used the phrase 'I have a dream.' I had used it many times before, and I just felt that I wanted to use it here. I don't know why. I hadn't thought about it before the speech. I used the phrase, and at that point I just turned aside from the manuscript altogether and didn't come back to it." He began with phrases from his "Bad Check" speech:

"I am happy to join with you today in what will go down in history as the greatest demonstration for freedom in the history of our nation.

Five score years ago, a great American, in whose symbolic shadow we stand today, signed the Emancipation Proclamation. This momentous decree came as a great beacon light of hope to millions of Negro slaves, who had been seared in the flames of withering injustice. It came as a joyous daybreak to end the long night of their captivity.

But one hundred years later, the Negro is still not free. One hundred years later, the life of the Negro is still sadly crippled by the manacles of segregation and the chains of discrimination. One hundred years later, the Negro lives on a lonely island of poverty in the midst of a vast ocean of material prosperity. One hundred years later the Negro is still languished in the corners of American society and finds himself an exile in his own land.

And so we've come here today to dramatize a shameful condition. In a sense we've come to our nation's capital to cash a check. When the architects of our republic wrote the magnificent words of the Constitution and the Declaration of Independence, they were signing a promissory note to which every American was to fall heir. This note was the promise that all men, yes Black men as well as White men, would be guaranteed the unalienable rights of life, liberty and the pursuit of happiness. It is obvious today that America has defaulted on this promissory note insofar as her citizens of color are concerned. Instead of honoring this sacred obligation, America has given the Negro people a bad check; a check which has come back marked 'insufficient funds.' We refuse to believe that there are insufficient funds in the great vaults of opportunity of this nation. And so we've come to cash this check, a check that will give us upon demand the riches of freedom and the security of justice.

We have also come to this hallowed spot to remind America of the fierce urgency of now. This is no time to engage in the luxury of cooling off or to take the tranquilizing drug of gradualism. Now is the time to make real the promises of democracy. Now is the time to rise from the dark and desolate valley of segregation to the sunlit path of racial justice. Now is the time to lift our nation from the quicksands of racial injustice to the solid rock of brotherhood. Now is the time to make justice a reality for all of God's children.

It would be fatal for the nation to overlook the urgency of the moment. This sweltering summer of the Negro's legitimate discontent will not pass until there is an invigorating autumn of freedom and equality. Nineteen sixty-three is not an end but a beginning. Those who hope that the Negro needed to blow off steam and will now be content will have a rude awakening if the nation returns to business as usual.

There will be neither rest nor tranquility in America until the Negro is granted his citizenship rights. The whirlwinds of revolt will continue to shake the foundations of our nation until the bright day of justice emerges.

But there is something that I must say to my people, who stand on the warm threshold which leads into the palace of justice: in the process of gaining our rightful place, we must not be guilty of wrongful deeds. Let us not seek to satisfy our thirst for freedom by drinking from the cup of bitterness and hatred. We must forever conduct our struggle on the high plane of dignity and discipline. We must not allow our creative protest to degenerate into physical violence. Again and again, we must rise to the majestic heights of meeting physical force with soul force.

The marvelous new militancy which has engulfed the Negro community must not lead us to a distrust of all White people, for many of our White brothers, as evidenced by their presence here today, have come to realize that their freedom is inextricably bound to our freedom. We cannot walk alone. And as we walk, we must make the pledge that we shall always march ahead. We cannot turn back.

There are those who are asking the devotees of civil rights, "When will you be satisfied?" We can never be satisfied as long as the Negro is the victim of the unspeakable horrors of police brutality. We can never be satisfied as long as our bodies, heavy with the fatigue of travel, cannot gain lodging in the motels of the highways and the hotels of the cities. We cannot be satisfied as long as the Negro's basic mobility is from a smaller ghetto to a larger one. We can never be satisfied as long as our children are stripped of their selfhood and robbed of their dignity by signs stating "For Whites Only." We cannot be satisfied as long as a Negro in Mississippi cannot vote and a Negro in New York believes he has nothing for which to vote. No, no, we are not satisfied and we will not be satisfied until justice rolls down like waters and righteousness like a mighty stream.

I am not unmindful that some of you have come here out of great trials and tribulations. Some of you have come fresh from narrow jail cells. Some of you have come from areas where your quest for freedom left you battered by the storms of persecution and staggered by the winds of police brutality. You have been the veterans of creative suffering. Continue to *work with the faith that unearned suffering is redemptive.*

Go back to Mississippi, go back to Alabama, go back to South Carolina, go back to Georgia, go back to Louisiana, go back to the slums and ghettos of our northern cities, knowing that somehow this situation can and will be changed.

Let us not wallow in the valley of despair. I say to you today, my friends: so even though we face the difficulties of today and tomorrow, I still have a dream. It is a dream deeply rooted in the American dream.

I have a dream that that one day on the red hills of Georgia the sons of former slaves and the sons of former slave owners will be able to sit down together at the table of brotherhood.

I have a dream that one day even the state of Mississippi, a state sweltering with the heat of injustice, sweltering with the heat of oppression, will be transformed into an oasis of freedom and justice.

I have a dream that my four little children will one day live in a nation where they will not be judged by the color of their skin but by the content of their character.

I have a dream today!

I have a dream that one day, down in Alabama, with its vicious racists, with its governor having his lips dripping with the words of interposition and nullification; one day right there in Alabama little Black boys and Black girls will be able to join hands with little White boys and White girls as sisters and brothers.

I have a dream today!

I have a dream that one day every valley shall be exalted, every hill and mountain shall be made low, the rough places will be made plain and the crooked places will be made straight and the glory of the Lord shall be revealed and all flesh will see it together.

This is our hope. This is the faith that I will go back to the South with. With this faith we will be able to hew out of the mountain of despair with a stone of hope.

With this faith we will be able to transform the jangling discords of our nation into a beautiful symphony of brotherhood. With this faith we will be able to work together, to pray together, to struggle together, to go to jail together, to stand up for freedom together, knowing that we will be free one day.

This will be the day, this will be the day when all of God's children will be able to sing with new meaning: 'My country 'tis of thee, sweet land of liberty, of thee I sing. Land where my fathers died, land of the Pilgrim's pride, from every mountain side, let freedom ring!' And if America is to be a great nation, this must become true.

And let freedom ring from the prodigious hilltops of New Hampshire .

Let freedom ring from the mighty mountains of New York.

Let freedom ring from the heightening Alleghenies of Pennsylvania.

Let freedom ring from the snow-capped Rockies of Colorado.

Let freedom ring from the curvaceous slopes of California.

But not only that.
Let freedom ring from Stone Mountain of Georgia.
Let freedom ring from Lookout Mountain of Tennessee.
Let freedom ring from every hill and molehill of Mississippi, from every mountainside, let freedom ring!
And when this happens, when we allow freedom to ring, when we let it ring from every village and every hamlet, from every state and every city, we will be able to speed up that day when all of God's children, Black men and White men, Jews and Gentiles, Protestants and Catholics, will be able to join hands and sing in the words of the old Negro spiritual, 'Free at last, free at last, Thank God almighty, we are free at last.' "

On September 15, 1963, four Black girls are killed in the bombing of the Sixteenth Street Baptist Church in Birmingham, Alabama.

President John F. Kennedy was assassinated by a sniper's bullet in Dallas, Texas on November 22, 1963.

On July 2, 1964, the Civil Rights Bill, complete with public accommodations and fair employment sections, is signed by President Lyndon B. Johnson.

On August 20, 1964, President Johnson signs the Economic Opportunity Act, launching Johnson's "War on Poverty."

On December 10, 1964 Martin Luther King Jr. was awarded the Nobel Peace Prize in Oslo, Norway.

On February 21, 1965, Malcolm X, the charismatic Black nationalist was assassinated at the Audubon Ballroom in Harlem. Three Black men were later arrested and convicted and sentenced to life imprisonment.

On March 21, 1965, thousands of marchers, led by Martin Luther King, Jr. and protected by federal troops, complete the first leg of the Selma-to-Montgomery march.

On August 6, 1965, President Johnson signs the Voting Rights Bill that authorized the suspension of literacy tests. Federal examiners were sent to the South under provisions of the bill.

On August 11, 1965, a "race riot" starts in the Watts section of Los Angeles and rages for six days. The Watts' riot was the first in a wave of major disturbances that forced a national reappraisal of racism in America.

On January 18, 1966, Robert Weaver is sworn in as Secretary of Housing and Urban Development and becomes the first Black member of a presidential cabinet.

On February 29, 1967, the Kerner Commission, issues its report on the racial riots in America - the report pointed to the emergence of two societies in America, "Black and White, separate and unequal."

On October 2, 1967, Thurgood Marshall becomes the first Black member of the U.S. Supreme Court.

On November 7, 1967, Carl Stokes of Cleveland and Richard Hatcher of Gary became the first Blacks elected mayors of major U.S. Cities.

On February 29, 1968, the National Advisory Commission on Civil Disorders (the Kerner Commission) stated in a formal report that White racism is the root cause of the race riots in American cities.

On April 4, 1968, Martin Luther King, Jr. was assassinated by a sniper while standing on the balcony of the Loraine Hotel in Memphis, Tennessee. The assassination ignited a national crisis with race riots in more than 100 cities and calls for racial renewal and repentance by both Black and White political leaders. President Johnson declared an official day of mourning for King.

At the time, Georgia boasted only a few Black legislators, and when they asked the then Governor Lester Maddox, a "fiery segregationist," if Dr. King's body could lie in honor in the state capitol.

Maddox not only swore he would never authorize a public tribute of King in the capitol Rotunda, he was outraged to see state flags, then characterized by the Confederate Cross, flying at half-staff in tribute to a Black man.

In 1983, President Ronald Regan, who had originally opposed the holiday as too costly, signed legislation officially marking Martin Luther King, Jr. Day as the third Monday in January.

Fifteen years later, after presenting 6,000,000 petitions to the U.S. Congress, Martin Luther King, Jr. Day was established in 1986.

On April 10, 1968, the U.S. Congress passes a Civil Rights Bill banning racial discrimination in the housing market and are making it a crime to interfere with civil rights workers.

On November 7, 1972, Andrew Young was the first Black American to be elected to the U.S. House of Representatives since Reconstruction.

The prologue of Andrew Young's book, *An Easy Burden*, summarizes the 1960s Civil Rights Movement - America's "second revolution" that brought the black American out of political and financial bondage:

'We have come so far, yet we still have a long way to go. 'Freedom is a constant struggle,' says the Negro spiritual. We've struggled so long, that we must be free. And we are free. That is the lesson of the American civil rights movement. We are as free as we dare to be.

There were many who made the American civil rights movement possible: men and women, preachers and lay people, students and workers, young and old. But in the 1960s, the Southern Christian Leadership Conference (SCLC), the organization that I was involved with during the civil rights movement, was largely made up of thirtyish, Southern-born, Negro preachers.

We were children of the New Deal of Franklin Delano Roosevelt. We spent our adolescence enjoying the rise of the United States as a defender of liberty and democracy in World War II. Our high school and university life was defined and colored by the social responsibility of the Marshall Plan, a sense of world community signaled by the founding of the United Nations and, yes, the successful liberation of India from British colonialism - without violence.

Even with the nuclear clouds above us, racial segregation surrounding us, and crippling seeds of inferiority sown within us by a thoroughly racist society, we were able to lay claim to a heritage of faith in God, confidence in the undiminished potential of our country, and hope for better tomorrows for ourselves and our children. We believed because we sensed the power and the grandeur of the ideals of this nation. We lived in the South, in the midst of its horror and shame, but our eyes were on the prize of freedom; we were willing to pay the price for freedom, we were willing to die for freedom, but we knew that the freedom to which we aspired could never be achieved by killing.

We began our struggle as a means of survival against the oppressive racism of our time. We were all confronted daily with disadvantages imposed on us simply by the color of our skin and the texture of our hair. Our religion taught us that we too were created in the image of God. Our school books taught us that we were "endowed by (our Creator) with certain unalienable rights." Yet our society determined to legally deprive us of self-respect, educational opportunity, political power, and economic access. Because we believed in this nation, we sought to remove the barriers that separated us from White society - not out of a need to be close to White people, but to gain the same access to society's benefits that they enjoyed. Whites and some Blacks assumed this would mean the assimilation of traditional White values and culture. But we knew there were no intrinsically "White values" and that in an open relationship the power and meaning of our Black experience would stand on its own merit and enrich the larger society.

We believed in spite of it all, that as children of God and agents of history we could redeem the soul of America. In the Old Testament, the redeemer was a kinsman who brought back land that one had lost. In the New Testament, the Redeemer is Jesus Christ, who paid for the sins of all believers with his life. The former slave and abolitionist Frederick Douglass described the effort to end slavery as a struggle to save "Black men's bodies and White men's souls." It was in this tradition that the preachers who founded the Southern Christian Leadership Conference decided its mission was "to redeem the soul of America." It was an ambitious mission for a small band of Negro preachers, a mission that could only be conceived in faith. That soul we saw less in America's actions than in its ideals: freedom, equality, justice. While we endured segregation, we knew that America had shed the blood of hundreds of thousands of its sons and daughters in a war that ended slavery. We knew that America had risen up out of the depths of a Great Depression to defeat fascism. We had cheered the exploits of Dorie Miller and the Tuskegee Airmen and other colored soldiers who refused to let racial segregation prevent them from offering their lives for freedom and for America, and we were inspired by their example. Dorie Miller was told he could only be a cook's helper, but he dared to believe he could shoot down enemy aircraft. The Tuskegee Airmen dared to believe Black men could fly.

We were thought to be naïve, but in truth we were visionary. We dared to believe that America could be healed of the gangrene of racism. We saw America as we could become, not just as we were. We believed that people could change, because we were constantly aware of how far we had come, personally. But most of all, we believed that a free society was constantly changing and that we could influence those changes to accommodate the needs and aspirations of our citizens, and that race, creed, gender, and national origin could be strengths rather than problems.

We began with the limited goal of ending racial segregation. But we came to understand segregation as just one aspect of the barrier confronting Black Americans in American Society. The March on Washington became a march for jobs and freedom, because in a nation based on free enterprise, access to jobs and money are an essential component of freedom.... As America made the world safe for democracy, we had to make America's democracy safe for the world.

Racism, war, and poverty were anchors dragging on our society, preventing us from reaching our full potential, as if anchors from a nineteenth-century sailing ship had been attached to the space shuttle. We accepted the challenges of detaching those anchors. We knew it was a burden, but we believed it was an easy burden in a country as great as ours. We believed that God didn't give anyone more burden than he or she had the strength to bear. Our faith made our burden light, because we never carried them alone. Our understanding and clarity of vision was a blessing, and I was taught that God requires us to use the gifts that we have been given. Racism, war, and poverty were heavy burdens, to challenge injustice was an easy burden.

We possessed a fundamental faith in democracy and free enterprise. We learned to address the nation through a free press; we made our claims on the economy by word and deed. We believed in our American heritage - a great people in a great nation that was ready to lead humankind in a new way of thinking and working. We believed in a future that we would help to create from our faith in spite of very real fears. Martin (Luther King, Jr.) expressed it for all of us when he constantly reminded us that "the moral arc of the universe is long, but it bends towards justice."

Each of us came to the civil rights movement by a different path and our backgrounds influenced our styles of leadership and approaches to the challenges we faced...."

On January 23-30, 1977, the ABC-TV dramatization of Alex Haley's *Roots* becomes the highest-rated drama in TV history and sparks a national "roots" craze.

On November 3, 1983, the Rev. Jesse L. Jackson, president of Operation

PUSH, announces that he will run for U.S. president. His first campaign generated unprecedented excitement; in his second campaign for president in 1988, he won four state primaries.

On September 20, 1984, The Cosby Show premieres on NBC-TV and changes the image of African-Americans and the viewing habits of White Americans.

On September 21, 1989, General Colin L. Powell is confirmed by the senate as chairman of the Joint Chiefs of Staff.

On November 7, 1989, L. Douglas Wilder of Virginia becomes the first Black elected governor.

On January 24, 1991, the uncontrolled AIDS epidemic is declared a major health threat to African-Americans by the U.S. Center for Disease Control. Officials said, "The disease, which forced a major re-evaluation of sexual relationships, was the leading cause of death among African-American women 15 to 44 years old in New York State and New Jersey." African-Amercan leaders cited the danger of addicts using infected needles and called for safe sex practices.

On March 3, 1991, the videotaped beating of motorist Rodney G. King by White Los Angeles police officers sparks an international uproar. Four White officers were indicted on March 14.

On June 27, 1991, Supreme Court Justice Thurgood Marshall announces his retirement and decries the increasingly conservative direction of the Court. On July 1, 1991, President Bush nominated Clarence Thomas, a conservative Black, then sitting on the U.S. District of Columbia Court of appeals, to fill the vacant seat.

On April 29, 1992, the acquittal of four White police officers in the Rodney King case ignites the biggest U.S. race riot since the urban explosions during the Civil War. Federal troops were called out to bring the riots under control. The Los Angeles Coroner's Office reported that 58 persons had died during the riots.

On May 18, 1993, Rita Dove became the first Black to be named Poet Laureate of the United States.

On May 9, 1994, as a result of an unprecedented voter turn-out in South Africa's first all-race elections on April 26 - 29, 1994, South Africa's new National Assembly unanimously elected Nelson Mandela President of South Africa.

On October, 16, 1995, the Million Man March, organized by Nation of Islam leader Minister Louis Farakhan and a coalition of religious and civil rights leaders, is held in Washington, D.C. The march was repeated in October 2005.

On December 17, 1996, Kofi Annan, longtime diplomat from Ghana, is named Secretary General of the United Nations.

On September 11, 1999, Serena Williams, age 17, became the first Black woman to win the U.S. Open tennis title since Althea Gibson's historic 1958 victory.

On July 11, 2000, the Rev. Vashti Murphy McKenzie is elected the first woman biship of the AME Church.

On Febuary 19, 2002, Vonetta Flowers, with teammate Jill Bakken, won a gold medal in the women's bobsled event at the Winter Olympics in Salt Lake City. She became the first Black athlete to win a gold medal at the Winter Olympics.

On March 26, 2002, the first class-action lawsuit for reparations was filed in U.S. District Court of New York City on behalf of descendants of Black American slaves.

On April 12, 2003, Army Specialist Shoshana Johnson, the first Black female Prisoner of War, was rescued by U.S. Marines. She was one of seven soldiers who were captured by Iraqi forces.

On October 26, 2005, Ken Williams, General Manager of the Chicago White Sox, held aloft the championship trophy after the team he put together won the World Series in a four-game sweep against the National League Champion Houston Astros. The White Sox hadn't won a World Series since 1917.

On Monday January 30, 2006 at 8:25 Pacific Time, Coretta Scott King, widow of murdered civil rights leader, Martin Luther King, Jr. died just days after arriving at an "alternative" health clinic in Mexico; she could have received the "very best of medical care" from the finest medical facilities in America - why did she flee to Mexico for treatment? She fled because she knew better than anyone that American hospitals are extremely dangerous institutions.

Coretta Scott King carried on her late husband's work to establish a color-blind society in America. Her body was laid in state in the Georgia State Capital (an honor denied Frederick Douglass and her murdered husband); and four U.S. Presidents (Carter; Bush, Sr; Clinton; George W. Bush) attended her funeral in Atlanta, Georgia.

In life and death, Coretta Scott King had attained the heights of political recognition and respect that had eluded Frederick Douglass and her husband Martin Luther King, Jr., and she leaves a legacy of positive proactivity for all to build on.

Chapter 3

"During the Civil War, one of my young masters was killed, and two were severly wounded. I recall the feeling of sorrow which existed among the slaves when they heard of the death of 'Mars' Billy. 'Mars' Billy had begged for mercy in the case of others when the overseer or master was thrashing them."

- Booker T. Washington
"Up From Slavery"

"Black Americans have shed their chains made of iron and the White only ballot, and yet, have again been enslaved by new slave masters - doctors in white coats with fraudulent chains of DNA and a conjured up black gene."

- Dr. Joel D. Wallach & Dr. Ma Lan

The History of Black Health Bondage: Emotional and Physical

With the dissolution of the Roman Empire it is clear that with the exception of the Iberian Peninsula, European interaction with Black Africa declined. As Jean Devisse, author of *The Image of --Blacks in Western Art*, said, "Particularly between the sixth and eleventh century the Occident fashioned an entire imagery based on prejudice and errors which 'cultivated' minds substituted, century after century, for objective thinking about Africa and Blacks. This situation sprang primarily from lack of knowledge which was sustained by the absence of physical contact between Africa and Europe."

From a medical-social perspective, the fourteenth to sixteenth centuries represented increasing contact between European societies and Africans through the evolution and development of the Atlantic, and to a lesser extent the Mediterranean, slave trade. The rise of the Ottoman Empire, the 13th to the early 20th centuries, particularly after the 1453 Moslem Turkish conquest of Constantinople, blocked the brisk Mediterranean slave trade in Slavs from the Balkan, Persian Gulf and Black Sea regions, rerouting the trade toward the African continent. Black slavery subsequently spread to Sicily, Italy, and the Iberian Peninsula. The growth and dominance of capitalism and the Age of Exploration, along with the Protestant Reformation, resulted in economic benefits and cultural traits that drove Western European societies into never seen before levels of corruption, wealth, greed, racism, and cruelty. Slavery, along with these major social developments, changed the medical ethical landscape and the delivery of health care to people of Black African descent.

The same Christians, who controlled the known world during the Age of Exploration, concluded the 800 year re-conquest of the Iberian Peninsula with Ferdinand and Isabella's capture of Granada in 1492. This took the form of the overthrow of a Moorish Moslem population by a White Christian one. The Spanish and Portuguese Christians shifted their attention and methods of dealing with non-White peoples outward and turned the Atlantic slave trade into big business. The Spanish and Portuguese hostile and aggressive brand of race relations and practices regarding non-White peoples, which had developed during the *Reconquista,* were brought to the Americas just as they brought with them the smallpox virus.

Black Africa gave 40 million to 100 million people to the slave trade - some 15 to 25 million were transported to the Americas. Descendents of this forced immigration are the African American citizens of the United States; Black, mulatto, and hybrid populations in the Caribbean; and Black, mulatto, and mixed African-European-Indian populations of central and South America.

Smallpox epidemics devastated Massachusetts in regular waves throughout the 90 years since its founding. A 1677 epidemic killed 700 people - 12 percent of the population. During the epidemic of 1702, during which, three of Cotton Mather's children were infected but survived. Cotton Mather, leader of the Puritan community, began to study smallpox. Several years later, Mather was shown the practice of vaccination by his Black slave, who had been vaccinated in Africa. Mather interviewed other Black slaves in Boston and learned that vaccination was a common practice in certain areas of Africa for hundreds of years.

In 1721, the HMS *Seahorse* pulled into Boston harbor from the West Indies carrying a new epidemic of smallpox. In a few short months 900 of Boston's citizens (out of 10,000) would be dead. Mather, who had trained as a physician before becoming a pastor, sent letters to the top ten practicing doctors in Boston to introduce them to the concept of the African vaccination against smallpox and pleading for them to use the procedure. Most of the doctors summarily rejected the practice. One doctor, Dr. William Douglas, dismissed the practice of inoculation for smallpox as, "the practice of Greek old women."

A significant amount of energy and time has been made of Black differences in America compared to Whites and other cultures for almost 400 years - this concept has been most evident in the arena disease and health care. These differences have been used through a biomedical path as the basis for justification for the hierarchies and casting of society (in particular the medical profession); and they have been used as "yardsticks" to arrive at priorities and percentages of resource distribution for health care. The extremes of these policies include unethical experimentation, surgical exploitation, and sterilization; the culture of racism and discrimination in the health system; and overt discrimination in the health professions are all influenced by this "difference" factor. Myrdal has even suggested that, "America's traditional policy of health care *nilhism* regarding African-Americans may represent an underlying public policy of eliminating the Black race in the United States." Most of these concepts, beliefs, and practices became institutionalized in our health care system before the Civil War.

There has always been a wide variety of human kind from the phenotypic (superficial external appearance) standpoint. The human race, such as, breeds-of-dogs, have an identical pool of genes, biology and physiology and suffer from the same diseases, yet may look different on the surface.

Medical historian Todd Savitt has consistently recorded in his research and publications, "Jews are less prone to contract tuberculosis, but more subject to Niemann-Pick Disease and Gaucher's Disease." He points out that Swedes exhibit high rates of sarcoidosis, porphyria, and pernicious anemia; whereas the White South Africans of Dutch decent commonly are stricken with porphyria cutanea tarda. Eighteenth and early nineteenth-century physicians recorded these facts, and in particular as they related to Blacks - it was in their financial and political interest.

Physicians, who provided health care for large colonies of Black slaves, recorded that they exhibited immunity to a variety of fevers. The resistance seemed to favor the newly arrived African Blacks following the "breaking-in" period. Typically it was difficult or impossible to differentiate these fevers according to origin - this was beyond the scientific capabilities of the eighteenth and nineteenth-century physicians - anthropological and medical historians retrospectively can only provide "educated etiological guesses today." The life threatening fevers that Africans appeared to have resistance to included yellow fever, sleeping sickness, and malaria. Clinically producing recurrent fevers, these diseases were often misdiagnosed and confused with each other.

Yellow fever is a viral disease of humans and monkeys that is transmitted by the blood sucking *Aedes* mosquito. The disease is known by more than a 100 names, however, it is commonly referred to as "yellow jack"; the "Bay of Benin Fever," each name reflecting its geographical point of origin; the "Black Vomit," referring to a common clinical sign produced by the vomiting of digested blood; and "bilios remittent," referring to the pathophysiological cyclical recurrence of jaundice and fever. It is called yellow fever because of the jaundice (a yellow cast given to the skin and the whites of the eyes that is produced by high circulating levels of bile pigments) that was associated with the disease.

Following considerable historical and epidemiological wrangling, the general consensus currently is that yellow fever originated as an endemic disease in monkeys and was carried across the Atlantic and brought to the New World following Columbus's arrival. Both the disease and the *Aedes* mosquito (which originated in Africa) were established in the Americas during the years of the Atlantic slave trade.

Symptoms of yellow fever exhibit an acute and sudden onset of fever followed by a severe headache. Horrific pain is followed by vomiting large quantities of black "coffee grounds" blood caused by the digestion of blood released into the stomach by a viral gastritis. As many as 50 percent of the fatalities, that occur from yellow fever, are from the victims "vomiting themselves to death." Survivors of yellow fever possess immunity for life. Infected children typically have a mild form of the disease and acquire permanent immunity - Black slaves from the endemic areas in West Africa were notably resistant to the epidemics of yellow fever - an immunity that was correctly observed and recorded by the 18th and 19th century physicians.

Sleeping sickness, now known to be caused by microscopic, spindle-shaped parasites (*Trypanosoma gambiense* and *T. rhodesience*), that are characterized by an undulating membrane. This disease was known as the "narcotic dropsy" and the "sleeping distemper" by slavers on the West African coast.

The parasite is transmitted through the bite of the tsetse fly (*Glossina*), which injects the parasite into the victim through its tubular mouth parts as it feeds on blood. The legendary disease shows up as an intermittent fever, headache, and pain in the limbs. The injected parasites spread to lymph glands in the back of the neck (a sign that slavers used as a screen to identify infected victims), followed by the victim developing the "sleeping sickness." After the parasite spreads to the brain, the victim sleeps as if in a coma; they cannot care for themselves; they become covered with sores, and die of pneumonia, dysentery, or starvation. Infected Blacks were thought to be mentally slow and lethargic or extremely homesick when the disease was observed during the days of the Atlantic slave trade. It is possible that the behaviors and lack of mental acuity associated with this illness may have generated the misconceptions of White superiority and African inferiority by Europeans.

Africans that originated from the endemic regions infested with tsetse flies and sleeping sickness in West Africa and the Congo developed some degree of immunity to the disease. Again, the 18th century doctors correctly observed that African Blacks did have some degree of protection against the disease that American born Blacks did not.

Between 1730 and 1812, malaria was known as "intermittent" or "remittent" fever. Its other names included "fever and chills," "marsh fever," and "autumnal fever." Malaria was eventually proven to be caused by a *Plasmodium spp.*, a one-celled parasite that colonizes red blood cells. After being injected into the human bloodstream by an infested *Anopheles* mosquito, the immature parasite invades liver cells, multiplies, and reenters the bloodstream by bursting through the walls of the host cells. They multiply and then reinvade red blood cells, rupturing and destroying them - this stage produces chills and fever.

As the body defends itself through the efforts of phagocytic white blood cells, which phagocytize (engulfs) the parasite, capillaries in the lymph nodes, spleen, and other vital organs become choked with red blood cell debris, engorged parasite laden phagocytes, and large numbers of free floating parasites that progresses to organ failure and death. The three major forms of the disease are due to *Plasmodium falciparum* (infection lasts 6 - 8 months), *P. vivax* (infection multiplies for 5 years), and *P. malariae* (infection can last up to 30 years).

The clinical onset of malaria is characterized by the appearance of severe chills unrelieved by many layers of blankets, followed by waves of extremely high fever, frequent nausea, vomiting, and severe headaches. Profuse sweating for up to 5 hours occurs during the break in the fever, which is then followed by severe weakness and prostration. The break in the fever can last from one (*P. falciparum*) to four (*P. vivax*) days while the parasites go through another cycle of multiplication in the host's bloodstream. This cycle can recur multiple times during a several week period, and then recur months or years later depending on the victim's state of health and the individual species of the causative parasite. Following each wave of parasite reproduction, the host is further weakened and susceptible to secondary infections.

Planters were only concerned about fevers so far as they could kill their slaves, disable his laborers during the harvest season, and could relapse, causing extended work absenteeism and even death of a chattel slave. Some acquired immunity to malaria was possible when slaves were exposed to repeated infections of the parasite over a several year period.

Recent medical research has revealed that red blood cells lacking a factor called the "Duffy antigen" are resistant to *P. vivax*. Up to 90 percent of West Africans lack the Duffy antigens on their red blood cells, as do approximately 70 percent of Black Americans. This hematologic antigen is asymptomatic and is extremely rare in other racial groups.

Two other abnormal hemoglobin conditions, sickle cell disease (serious form of anemia) and sickle cell trait (the asymptomatic carrier form of the anemia that is generally thought to be transmitted genetically to a subsequent generation), result in a decreased severity of clinical illness from the falciparum form of malaria. Deficiency of the enzyme glucose-6-phosphate dehydrogenase (G-6-PD deficiency) also results in some malarial resistance. Since up to 22 percent of Africans transported to the New World brought sickle cell traits and up to 20 percent brought G-6-PD deficiency traits; it is estimated that 30-40 percent of the slaves were protected from the various forms of malaria as a result of these traits.

The clinical manifestations of the sickle cell disease syndrome include organ failure, loss of bone mass, stroke, anemia, suppressed immune system, increased susceptibility to infectious diseases, joint pain, stunted or delayed growth and sexual maturation, leg ulcers, loss of appetite and the sense of smell - all of these symptoms can also be elicited by deficiencies of specific nutrients such as vitamins, amino acids, major minerals, micro-trace minerals and enzymes.

While working on a large, multi-million dollar, NIH training grant (The Center for the Biology of Natural Systems) at Washington University, St. Louis, Mo., (Wallach) was able to identify sickle cell anemia in white-tailed deer and further discovered that it could be reversed by the supplementation of the trace mineral selenium.

Since 1991, we (Dr. Wallach and Dr. Ma Lan) have worked with the Sickle Cell Foundation of Georgia through their genetic councilor, Phil Oliver. We learned that by providing all of the essential nutrients on a daily basis and adding extra selenium to the individuals supplement program that their sickle cell disease goes into "remission," they generally have an improvement in their quality of life, and they do not suffer painful or life threatening "attacks."

Sickle cell patients on our supplement program claim more energy, better sleep, fewer pain attacks, fewer hospital visits, significant increases in hemoglobin and hematocrit levels, feel more rested after sleep, increased appetite, significant increase in physical strength and less susceptibility to infections.

It is obvious from our experience that the sickle cell problem is not the simple genetic disease that it was thought to be - rather the clinical expression of the sickle cell trait may be a manifestation of a deficiency disease.

Immediately following the end of the Civil War, President Lincoln was assassinated.

Under the supervision of the Congress and President Andrew Johnson, reassertion of private entrepreneurial dominance and White Southern resistance followed. It was an expansive and fluid period for institutions and individuals located in the North. For Southerners it was chaotic.

Reconstruction itself created conflict and adversity. Following the suggestions of the late President Lincoln, the Congress agonized and finally passed the Thirteenth (enacted 1865, ratified 1865) and Fourteenth (enacted 1866, ratified 1868) Amendments to the Constitution, which abolished slavery and began the process of ensuring citizenship and civil rights for all citizens. The Fifteenth Amendment to the Constitution followed (1870), guaranteeing ex-slaves' right to vote. Rights granted to Black Americans by these amendments were quickly neutralized by non-enforcement by the federal government and rogue rulings by recalcitrant local and federal courts.

In collusion with President Andrew Johnson, the South resisted the important social and political changes proposed by the Northern-dominated Congress. Historians Lincoln, Hughes, and Meltzer described the congressional response:

Aroused by the refusal of most Southern states to ratify the Fourteenth Amendment protecting Negro citizenship, by the revival of the Black Codes of slavery days and by growing violence against the Negro, the Stevens Committee won Congressional approval for its Reconstruction Act of 1867.

The Stevens Committee represented the so-called Radical Republicans. They imposed martial law, divided the South into five military districts, and proclaimed universal manhood suffrage. They also required the drafting of new state constitutions and required ratification of the Fourteenth Amendment by all states for readmission to the Union. The committee proposed weak efforts, which never came to pass, to sell or lease abandoned federal lands acquired as spoils of war to the freedmen.

Violent White protest flared up in the South, along with turmoil, racial violence, and the proliferation of mythology which still surrounds the 21st century's discussions of the Reconstruction Era. In response to massive social and institutional collapse and dislocation in the South, disproportionately affecting Blacks and poor whites, Congress passed the Freedmen's Bureau Legislation on March 3, 1865.

The first serious federal aid program emphasized education, the provision of rations for the destitute, and enforcement of the freedmen's newly won legal and citizenship rights. Medical programs grew out of the necessities of the battlefield and, later urban crises.

As far as Black American health options were concerned, the Reconstruction and post-Reconstruction eras were a disaster. As new waves of epidemics, poor health, sickness, and death swept through the postwar South, along with an increase in tuberculosis morbidity and mortality. J. O. Breeden summed up the Black health status: "A higher incidence of tuberculosis was one indication of the deteriorating health of the former slaves. Left to their own devices for survival after the collapse of Reconstruction, freedmen developed excessively high rates of sickness and death."

President Lincoln viewed abandoned Negroes as "a laborless, landless and homeless class (trapped) in a hazy realm between bondage and freedom." Having little or no belongings, the few ex-slaves with craft skills were almost universally blocked from using them by working-class Whites. Less than 10 percent of the freedmen could read or write. Blocked from access to education or training, few Blacks were able to apply for or gain access to the trades or professions.

Government Reconstruction programs were enormous and multifaceted efforts in the area of health care. Although the government had begun providing health care services to limited groups of merchant seamen in the previous century, the Freedmen's Bureau activities were unique in U.S. history. These health programs represented the first large government effort to provide health care for massive numbers of the civilian population.

America entered the Gilded Age (1870 - 1890). The year 1870 began a weakening of Northern resolve, commitment or interest in the problems of Black Americans, a discontinuance of most of the Freedmen's Bureau services, a resumption of the dominance by American business of governmental, political, and economic institutions that had been attained during the Antebellum Period. It was as if the Civil War had served as only a brief hiatus of "business as usual."

The Hayes-Tilden Compromise of 1877 was a political agreement between conservative Southern Democrats and Republicans to resolve a disputed 1876 presidential election in the Electoral College and Congress. Elected president despite losing the popular vote, Hayes agreed to formally end Reconstruction and to withdraw Union troops from the South. This resulted in the Black American population again depending on the mercies of their former owners, and for the most part ended Black suffrage, encouraged enactment of new Jim Crow Laws, and spawned a reign of terror on the Black community. Effectively, the "solid South" was created.

After the Hayes-Tilden Compromise of 1877, America moved toward a conservative regrouping of assets and the withdrawal of Union troops from the South. The "Black problem" was effectively returned to Southerners and was transformed into "states rights," or a series of Black political issues to be dealt with locally. This included providing health care to an ignorant population whose medical services had historically been the responsibility of themselves and their former owners. Most Southern charitable and public institutions for the indigent such as hospitals, dispensaries, and mental institutions refused to provide services to Blacks.

The Progressive Era (1890 - 1920) was a 30 year time of aggressive social and political intervention by wealthy White Americans who believed that through the use of scientific and social knowledge they could eliminate America's social and financial concerns. For Black Americans the Progressive Era became one of the most racially restrictive chapters in U.S. history. As America entered the 1890s, Benjamin Bawley, a scholar of this period, wrote in, *A Social History of the American Negro*, that, "The Negro was already down, he was now to be trampled upon." In 1886, in New York, Henry W. Grady, the well respected Atlanta Constitution newspaper editor, and part owner, preached a doctrine of "The New South." He convinced the nation that the South "was on the move politically and economically and that the Black problem was a local matter that the North had concerned itself with for too long." The North was "greatly relieved and receptive" to his message.

Booker T. Washington, in a series of speeches between 1894 and 1904, earned recognition as the national leader of the American Blacks, replacing Frederick Douglass, who had died in February 1895. As Rayford Logan noted, "The Atlanta Compromise" speech delivered on November 18, 1895, was Washington's high water mark: "The national fame that Washington achieved overnight by his Atlanta speech constitutes an excellent yardstick for measuring the victory of 'The New South,' since he accepted (a) subordinate place for Negroes in American life."

Disenfranchisement, starting with Mississippi in 1890 and South Carolina in 1895 as examples, resulted in the stripping away the Negro vote over the entire South. Federal, state, and local court decisions stripped away Black access to public accommodations, voting, property, and civil rights.

With regard to health care, the plans suggested by General Howard, first president of Howard University between 1869 and 1874, and Dr. Hubbard, Meharry's founder, were successful. The production of Black health professionals began to speed up. Meharry Medical College and Howard University

School of Medicine functioned as the sole sources of trained Black medical and health care professionals between 1910 and 1970.

Black patients continued their traditional roles (the practice began during slavery with the rise of clinical training, anatomic dissection, and clinical research in medicine) as being over utilized for medical demonstration, dissection, and risky surgical and experimental purposes.

In the South, where two-thirds of the Black population struggled through World War II, Black Americans were folded into the "semi-feudal tenant-sharecropper quagmire that had replaced slavery." With the exception of a small band of Negro professional and middle-class businessmen, the great majority of Southern city-dwellers were unskilled workers or domestic servants. Their endless poverty compounded their health crisis, where public hospitals and clinics were either nonexistent or grossly deprived. Similar to the West in the nineteenth century, the North in the twentieth century became a safety valve and route of escape from hopeless oppression: "Almost a half-million Negroes, responding to the siren call of economic security and freedom, left the eleven states of the Old Confederacy from 1910 to 1920. Nearly 800,000 more moved away during the twenties and were followed by another 400,000 during the thirties."

One Northern manifestation of basic Black health care needs included the overwhelming overload of Black patients of the public facilities in Northern cities, characterized by the Harlem Hospital Center in New York City:

> *The demands made on Harlem's out-patient clinic were staggering. From 1920 to 1932, dispensary visits increased by more than 300 percent, from roughly 80,000 to 250,000....(S)o overcrowded were its facilities that the syphilis clinic was forced to exclude new patients and limit old ones to no more than 300 per session. Similarly, the bed capacity of Harlem Hospital was inadequate to meet even the barest needs of the neighborhood.*

Poor health outcomes crushing Blacks and the poor were "scientifically" rationalized as being genetically and hereditarily predetermined. Segregation, involuntary sterilization, nihilistic public health and educational policies, and incarceration were considered "solutions" for the nation's poor, disabled, mentally challenged, or racially "inferior" populations and the problems they created.

The Great Depression, however, and the rise of Hitler and Nazi Germany, which promoted similar ideologies and policies, helped to slow and neutralize the increase of these hateful practices in America. By the end of World War II many of these activities had gone underground or had been almost completely discredited.

The health care environment perpetuated the U.S. tradition of misusing

Black, poor, socially disadvantaged (prisoners), and disabled (mentally challenged children) patients for medical experimentation, eugenics, or demonstration need. These practices were justified and defended on the grounds of "scientific research," the health professions need for "teaching purposes," or limiting defective genes (and limiting the welfare rolls as a result).

As late as the mid-1920s, highly respected African American social scientists such as E. Franklin Frazier argued that White physicians regarded their patients as "simply experimental material." This distance between medical ethics and U.S. health system practices happened on several levels, including but not limited to utilizing uninformed or poorly informed patient populations for research that result in injury or, at the very least, compromise their health outcomes; performing excessive or unnecessary surgery on patients, often under coercion or without their consent, especially for eugenic purposes; over-utilizing patients and tailoring their care and treatment on the basis of the professional training or research requirements of the personnel or institutional (surgical demonstration or "teaching and training material") instead of real medical needs driven by the requirements of the individual patient case; and denying, inadequately treating, or abusing patients in need of simple basic care or services because they fail to have rare diseases, "uninteresting" or "routine" cases or do not meet the standards for research protocols.

Between 1930 and 1945, the picture of this misuse and abuse changed as the research excuse for these practices became more accepted. The latter was largely a result of the Flexner/Johns Hopkins model for medical education and biomedical research that had been enacted at a network of major American medical facilities. The infamous Tuskegee syphilis experiment, initiated in the 1930s, is an example:

Initially implemented as part of a U.S. Public Health Service/Rosenwald Fund rural syphilis public health and treatment program in the late 1920s, the non-treatment phase of approximately 400 syphilitic Black men with 200 uninfected controls began in 1932 in Macon County, Alabama (Tuskegee, the county seat, is home of the famous Tuskegee Institute). The purpose was to study the effects of syphilis on untreated African-American men. Fueled by patient deception, professional paternalism, blocking patients from receiving penicillin after World War II, and coming to view the patients as laboratory animals, the experiment continued for 40 years. It resulted in 100 deaths from untreated syphilis, scores of blind and demented participants from the ravages of syphilis, numerous presentations at medical meetings, and more than 13 scientific papers. It was scientifically flawed from the start, and most of the subjects received some treatment in order to render them noninfectious early in the study.

The Tuskegee experiment, an unethical, exploitive experiment in which treatment for syphilis was withheld from almost 500 rural illiterate, poverty-stricken Black men, was conducted for more than 40 years, beginning in the early 1930s. For more than 30 years it was clear that the experiment was subjecting the men to excess morbidity and mortality as the Tuskegee medical researchers deceptively told the men they were being treated.

The ethical considerations, and the practice of overusing Black American patients for inhumane and unethical purposes, continued. Dr. John A. Kenny, one of the most influential and highly respected physicians in the United States, exposed perspective to the enormity of the problem during that era. In his 1941 plea "that a monument be raised and dedicated to the nameless Negroes who have contributed so much to surgery by the "guinea pig," route, he said:

In our discussion of the Negro's contribution to surgery, there is one phase not to be overlooked. That is what I may vulgarly, but at the same time seriously, term the "guinea pig" phase....one of that practically endless list of "guinea pigs."..... (U)ntold thousands of....Negroes have been used to promote the cause of science. Many a heroic operation performed for the first time on a nameless Negro, is today classical. Even Negro physicians, surgeons and nurses, at times wince at the scenes...of Negroes used for experimental and teaching surgery.

Despite the desperate health conditions in which Black Americans found themselves as they stepped into the 1890s, there had been some progress in general health care for them.

Benjamin Brawley said that, by the beginning of the Progressive Era, "the pendulum had swung fully backward, and in the years from 1890 to 1895 were in some ways the darkest that the race has experienced since emancipation. Lynch law and the Democrats were in force, and by February 1893, Black lynching occurred almost daily."

By 1900, there were more than 1,000 Black physicians practicing in America. There were eight Black medical schools, at least nine nursing schools, and two dental and pharmacy schools graduating Black American health professionals each year. After being rejected for membership several times during the Gilded Age by the American Medical Association (AMA), a Black medical profession organized nationally, creating the National Medical Association (NMA) in 1895, which also developed state and local chapters.

Under the auspices of the Hill-Burton Act (1946 - 1974) the federal government spent $3.7 billion, which was matched by $9.1 billion from the private sector for a total of $1.3 trillion dollars to erect and upgrade the private hospital infrastructure in the Southern United States after World War II to meet the needs of returning World War II veterans. It promoted government-funded, legally sanctioned, segregated health facilities until legal battles resulted in anti-discrimination provisions in 1964.

As recently as 1989, many hospitals in New York State had failed to fulfill their Hill-Burton Act obligations to provide health services to indigent Blacks, even though they were located in predominantly impoverished Black communities.

The period between 1812 and 1861 was the Age of Jackson. It was a time of grand and enormous expansion in America. The policies of President Andrew Jackson (1767 - 1845), a Tennessee-born soldier, politician, and planter, were critical and important to the African American.

Jackson was almost single-handedly responsible for resolving the national political and Constitutional debate concerning conflicts between the belief that "all men are created equal" and permanent Black chattel slavery and the rights of Native Americans. Jackson determined that both groups were to be "subjugated to permanent slavery and dispossession" under the "aegis of official national government policy." He created the political economy and social infrastructure for the non-White minorities for 200 years.

Between 1803 and 1860 the young developing nation quadrupled in land mass and its economy grew even faster. Market and technological advances and revolutions pulsed through the receptive economy like the "perfect storm." These growing pains generated a division between the industrial North and the slave based agricultural economy of the South that spawned the Civil War. These events had a dramatic effect on the health care systems for the Whites and Blacks. Even though the general health of Americans improved, the Blacks and Native Americans continued to suffer a decline in general health and access to health care institutions.

While there was an explosive national expansion and general increase in personal wealth between 1812 and 1861, Black longevity, mortality, and fertility showed only minimal improvement for the initial 18 years of this period and then they collapsed after 1830. The lie of the "contented well cared for slave" is unraveled by the slave health deficit that continued and worsened during the Jacksonian and Antebellum periods. The Antebellum Period exhibited the typical "improved health status goes hand in hand with generalized prosperity," however the general benefit to the White population did not spill over to the Black population.

The winning of the War of 1812 stoked an intense pride in the new nation and elevated "Old Hickory" (Andrew Jackson) to a legendary and mythical national frontier hero in Indian fighting and jingoism. This time in history, combined with Jackson's devastating victory against the British at the Battle of New Orleans (1815) set in motion the North American expansion; occupation of vast expanses of land acquired in the Louisiana Purchase (1803); and the expansion in the 1840s eventually resulted in the occupation of all the United States' current territories (except Alaska and Hawaii) by 1850. This tidal wave-like expansion established the concept of community and government social and health system programs and development.

Politically, the 1828 election of Andrew Jackson to the presidency of the United States, was a result of the almost complete popular rejection of Alexander Hamilton's concepts of Federalism, that promoted a strong centralized national government in favor of almost total reliance on the individual and the rejection of the "elite-rule." Jackson's policies also were characterized by the ruthless national policies of Native American displacement and extermination for the "sake of national expansion, and the entrenchment of the slave system for the commercial and ideological reasons." The spoken cover of "moral certitude and implied egalitarianism" was in fact just the opposite of America's increasing political and marketing aggressiveness, exploitation, socioeconomic inequities, and military-driven domestic and foreign policies. The American character was based on "individualism and survival of the fittest," a theme that was also perpetuated in the healthcare system. These events and policies of exclusion drove the Blacks in America into developing their own family and community health systems that were below the radar and beyond the reach of the White healthcare systems.

Even more basic than the adverse individual effects on the peoples of the two suppressed and "inferior" minorities (Blacks and Native Americans), Indian extermination and Black chattel slavery drove the United States' westward expansion and the metamorphosis from an agricultural to an industrial economy.

The creation of a "new" Democratic Party in 1826, was a symptom of the rekindling of the concept of "rule by the common man," (if he was White) and frontiersman style westward expansion.

Presidents Jackson, Tyler and Polk encouraged free-booting privateers such as the well known Army Captain John C. Freemont, General Stephen Kearny, and Navy Commodore Robert F. Stockton - their raiding and slaving activities drove national westward expansion. Annexation of Texas (1845), the Mexican War (1846), the take over of the Bear Flag Republic (California 1848) and the creation of a diplomatic impasse over the Oregon Territory (this led to an annexation of Oregon) completed the formation of the Continental United States. These policies threw gasoline on the fires of the North-South political and economic differences and ultimately led to the bloody Civil War.

These westward expansions by Americans continued to perpetuate and encourage home health care and the importance of and the dependency on traditional healers for another three generations. Health system arrangements for Mexican and Native Americans were added to those already established for the Black and poor White Americans.

Many of American medicine's movements towards professionalism occurred in the 20 years prior to the Civil War. Blacks, Native Americans and women were systematically excluded from the formal training necessary to obtain a university generated medical degree and the benefits of membership to the profession. Restrictions against Blacks and women were a reflection of the cultural restrictions of the multiracial relationships of a Jacksonian America. As Tocqueville stated in *Democracy in America* and as Takaki expanded on:

During the Age of Jackson, Blacks were not regarded as "sons of nature" or the subjects of "melancholy reflections"; nor were they "obstacles" which had to be removed beyond the Mississippi River or destroyed. Rather Blacks lived in the settled areas of the United States, within White civilization, in physical proximity to Whites. As workers, Blacks possessed the labor slaveholders appropriated in order to cultivate the "vacant lands" they had taken from the Indians and to produce surplus for the market. Thus Blacks had a unique future in America: Unlike Indians, they were not to be expelled but to be even more securely chained to White society and its political economy......"Free" in the North and enslaved in the South, Blacks had different regional relationships to the process of production.

The American medical system was a reflection of the American political and social systems, and typically excluded people based on race (Blacks, Native Americans, Mexicans), gender (females), and religion (Jews). The only medical schools that admitted these minorities were the Thomsonians, Eclectics, and Homeopathic. Black practitioners inspired by the slave "do it yourself system" were often times welcomed by slave owners who saved money by paying the Black healers less than he would have paid a White doctor, plus the slave would lose fewer working days.

The first Black to have a formal medical education in the United States was James McCune Smith (1811 - 1865). Born of a free mother in 1811 in New York City, Smith's father, an ex-slave, was a successful merchant. Smith received his primary education at the New African Free School on Mulberry Street, which had been established by the New York Manumission Society in 1787. As early as age 11, Smith obtained notoriety by delivering the welcoming address when General Lafayette visited the school in 1824. Lafayette's visit was a manifestation of his advocacy of educating Negro youth for productive citizenship. Nevertheless, after being denied admission to institutions of higher learning in his own country, Smith entered the University of Glasgow in 1832. While there he earned the B.A. degree in 1835, the M.A. degree in 1836, and the M.D. degree in 1837. Smith immediately returned to New York, opened and developed a very successful medical practice, and opened the doors of two very well respected pharmacies.

Smith was extremely successful financially and professionally and set standards for Black physicians that Bousfield characterizes: "He set a pattern generally followed by colored doctors ever since: he became a leader of his people, and was an ardent abolitionist."

Smith authored and published numerous scientific papers, became an expert in medicine, statistics and politics and clearly was regarded as a national leader of Black Americans by 1843.

David John Peck became the first Black American to earn an M.D. degree from an American medical school. Born in Pittsburgh, Pennsylvania, he became a protégé of Martin Robinson Delany, who practiced medicine and was a dominant Black leader and abolitionist in Pittsburgh. Peck had been a member of several youth groups that had been formed by Delany, including the Juvenile Anti-Slavery Society, chartered in Pittsburgh on July 7, 1838. Peck later entered Rush Medical College in Chicago, Illinois and graduated in 1847.

Peck encountered difficulties in trying to establish a medical practice in Philadelphia and New York. It was reported: "In February 1848 when another of Delany's young men, David Peck, left for Philadelphia to practice medicine and was kicked out of Thomas' Auction Store at a sale of medical books, Foster had the comment: 'We presume this gross insult was perpetrated on a young man of education, simply to curry favor with the Southern students who were in attendance.'" Another example of Peck's exclusion in New York during the winter of 1851 - 1852, where, "Like many another young black, then and now, he was asking, 'Education - for what?'"

Dr. John Sweat Rock (1825 - 1866) entered a medical apprenticeship with Doctors Sharp and Gibbon in Salem, New Jersey, between 1844 and 1848, While teaching school, Rock was denied admission to medical school, though he more than met the requirements of that era. By 1850 he had completed a second apprenticeship with Dr. Harbert, he also mastered dentistry and set up a dental practice in Philadelphia. He was eventually allowed to attend the required two years of medical lectures at American Medical College in Philadelphia, earning an M.D. degree in 1852. By age 27 Rock was a fully trained teacher, dentist, and physician.

Rock moved to Boston in 1853, where he practiced medicine and dentistry for seven years. He was the second Black to be admitted to the Massachusetts Medical Society (1850s); he became heavily involved with the Abolitionist Movement and treated slaves moving through the "Underground Railroad."

Rock became a nationally acclaimed orator, speaking on the *Unity of Human Races* before the Massachusetts legislature in 1856, on *"The Light and Shadows of Ancient and Modern Tribes of Africa"* in Philadelphia in 1857; and at Faneuil Hall in Boston for Crispus Attacks Day on March 5, 1858. In that frequently quoted speech, Rock coined the phrase and developed the theme that *"Black is Beautiful."*

Incapacitated by tuberculosis, Rock discontinued his medical and dental practices by 1860 and began to study law. Rock passed his Bar exam to practice law on September 14, 1861. He became very active in the Negro Convention of Colored Men held at the Wesleyan Methodist Church in Boston, October 4 - 7, 1864, Rock and George L. Ruffin were the two publishers of the proceedings. Rock pushed Black participation in the Civil War by recruiting a major portion of the men for the 54th and 55th Massachusetts Infantry Regiments.

Rock's admission to practice before the U.S. Supreme Court led to his becoming the first Black lawyer to be received on the floor of the U.S. House of Representatives. Rock died a year later from the complications of tuberculosis.

According to Bole, "2.4 million slaves (during the Jacksonian and the Antebellum Periods) of the nation's 3.9 million slaves lived in the Deep South, it is clear that most slaves lived on plantations in close proximity to numerous other slaves…(T)his proved to be a cultural fact of great significance."

The growing concentration of slaves ultimately required that more slave hospitals be built, more slave hospitals were built in the cities, and a slave health system grew and developed separately, more elaborate and more organized. Not only were more regular (both medical school and apprentice-trained) physicians contracted, more slave health personnel participated in health care delivery in the form of granny midwives, granny nurses, root doctors and slave healers. Larger slave colonies were able to preserve and encourage the more traditional African spiritual healers, conjure men, root doctors, and voodoo doctors.

Classically, the plantation owner or his wife was responsible for treating the sick slaves, on some plantations the overseer took over this responsibility. A medicine chest and health books such as *Gunn's Domestic Medicine, Poor Man's Friend; The Planter's and Mariner's Medical Companion; The Plantation and Family Physician; A Work for Families Generally and for Southern Slave Owners Especially; Embracing the Peculiarities and Diseases, the Medical and Hygienic Management of Negroes, Together* with the Causes, Symptoms, and Treatment of the Principal Diseases to Whites and Blacks. Local physicians were called to help with only severe or unusual cases.

Many plantation slave hospitals were "adequate"; however, many would be described as "Hell holes." The following is a description of a plantation infirmary on the Butler Island Plantation on the Georgia coast near Savannah. It was the property of Pierce Butler and the description was abstracted from a letter written by his new bride, one Fanny Kemble, a well known actress of the Antebellum Period, to her friend Elizabeth Sedgwick in 1834:

The infirmary is a large two-story wooden building containing four large rooms. The first I entered was half dark, some of the windows are glazed but encrusted with dirt and the shuttered openings were closed to keep out the cold. In the enormous chimney a few feeble embers glimmered and here many of the sick women were cowering on wooden settles, the poor wretches too ill to rise, lay strewed about on the earthen floor without bed, pillow or mattress. Here, in their hour of sickness and suffering, lay those whose health and strength are spent in unrequited labor for us, those whose husbands, fathers, brothers and sons were, at that hour, sweating over the earth whose produce was to buy for us all the luxuries which health care revel in, all the comforts which can alleviate sickness....Here lay women expecting the agonies of childbirth, others who had just brought their off spring into the world, others groaning over the pain and disappointment of miscarriages-here lay some burning with fever, or chilled with cold and aching with rheumatism upon the cold and hard ground, in droughts and dampness, dirt, noise and stench - here they lay like brute beasts, all absorbed in physical suffering...I told old Rose, the midwife, to open some of the shutters and myself went to the fireplace to build up the fire, but as I lifted a log, there was a universal cry of horror, and old Rose tried to snatch it from me, exclaiming: "Let alone, Missis-let be! What for you lift wood? You have nigger enough, Missis, to do it!" I made Rose tiddy up the miserable apartment. It was all I could do. The other rooms, one of them for sick men, were in the same deplorable condition of filth, disorder and misery; the floor was the only bed and scanty begrimed rags of blankets the only covering. And this is the hospital of an estate where the owners are supposed to be humane, the overseer efficient and kind, and the negroes well cared for! I left this refuge for Mr. Butler's sick dependents with my clothes covered with dust and full of vermin....I went again today to the infirmary and was happy to perceive there had been some faint attempt at cleaning, in compliance with my desires. I remonstrated with one of the mothers, a woman named Harriet, who was ill herself, upon the horribly dirty condition of the baby and she assured me it was impossible for the mothers to keep their children clean, that they went out to work at daybreak and did not get their tasks done til evening and then they were too worn out to do anything but throw themselves down and sleep...In another room a woman was lying on the floor in a fit of epilepsy, barking most violently; she excited no particular attention, the women said was subject to fits; she lay barking like an enraged animal. I stood in profound ignorance, sickened by the sight of suffering which I knew not how to alleviate. How I wished that...I had been taught something of sickness and health, that I might have known how to assist these poor creatures and direct their ignorant nurses. The swarms of fleas are incredible; I have never come away from the infirmary without longing to throw myself into the water and my clothes into the fire.

Eight Black physicians were recruited by the Union Army and they served during the Civil War. They were Alexander T. Augusta, Charles B. Purvis, Alpheus Tucker, John Rapier, William Ellis, Anderson R. Abbott, William Powell, and John Vancerille DeGrasse. W. Montague Cobb's revelation: "The recruitment of these officers appears to have resulted from a tour of the nation's medical schools, particularly those in New England, by Dr. J.V.C. Smith, a prominent physician of the time who sought to obtain competent young Negro medical graduates to serve as surgeons with the Negro units."

Reconstruction, at the governmental relief level, began in March 1865 with the passage of a compromise bill "which lumped supervision of refugees, freedmen, and abandoned lands in one agency of the War Department." Called the Freedmen's Bureau, Major General Oliver Howard, whose reputation for piety had won him the nick-name 'the Christian soldier', was picked to head the bureau.

Union Army Black physicians were all restricted to service with either Black units or to Freedmen's Bureau facilities serving Black populations. While in the army they were all subjected to frequent acts of overt or covert racial discrimination. Typically the Black physicians performed very well. Alexander T. Augusta, the Virginia-born Canadian medical school graduate referred to previously, was decorated and rose to the rank of Lieutenant Colonel, a rank that was not reached by any other Black American over the next 70 years.

As the Civil War ground on and finally ended, critics could look at the progress of health programs for Black Americans in a positive way. Just about all observers agreed that the Freedmen's Bureau health activities had a positive effect on Black health. Howard Ashley White declared, "The medical services of the Freedmen's Bureau were among its most constructive activities. Frederick Douglass, a former slave who published a newspaper in Washington, gave the Freedmen's Bureau credit for lowering the national Negro death rate from 30 percent to 4 percent."

The Freedmen's Bureau approach to Black American health was a revolutionary phenomenon. Before the Civil War, the provision of health services to a dependent Black population had been an almost exclusively private enterprise. Poor health care services, substandard Black health status and results were of interest only to the slaveholder. The slave owner could decide to provide or withhold effective health care for his chattel slaves. When Union Army generals approached the federal government with the idea of providing health and support services to the newly freed and contraband slaves, a new concept had been proposed. Legislatively and logistically the U.S. Congress participated for the first time. Black American's health became a legitimate concern of the U.S. government. Even though the Bureau and its administrators knew there was no other program to replace the health programs, by 1872 government-sponsored health care for ex-slaves was finished. James H. Jones reported the opinions of physicians on the effects of the Civil War and the emancipation of Blacks:

When the Civil War erupted, physicians in both the North and the South warned that freedom would mean extinction for Blacks. While other groups discussed the future of the free Blacks, physicians debated whether the race as such had a future. They saw the emancipation of the slaves as a watershed in Black health, the chief result of which was likely to be a decline in health that was so drastic as to endanger the survival of the race.

The precipitous and cataclysmic deterioration in slave health immediately after the war can be attributed to several factors including the sudden severing of all relationships of slave owners with their former chattel slaves. An ex-slave gave this account in Ben Botkin's *Lay My Burden Down: A Folk History of Slavery*:

When freedom came, my mama said Old Master called all of 'em to his house, and said, "You all free, we ain't got nothing to do with you no more. Go on away. We don't whup you no more, go on your way." My mama said they go on off, then they come back and stand around, just looking at him and Old Mistress. They give'em something to eat and he say, "Go on away, you don't belong to us no more. You been freed." They go away and they kept coming back. They didn't have no place to go and nothing to eat. From what she said, they had a terrible time. She said it was bad times. Some took sick and had no 'tention and died. Seemed like it was four or five years before they got to places they could live. They all got scattered....Old Master every time they go back say, "You all go on away. You been set free. You have to look out for yourselves now."

Circumstances were aggravated by the fact that Negro slaves in the United States were freed with no education, financial means, and very limited skills for a competitive labor market.

The Vanderbilt University Medical School successfully stalled the predominantly Black Meharry Medical College's full participation in training programs at Nashville General Hospital from 1893 until the early 1990s. Vanderbilt continues to block Meharry's participation in the staffing or training programs involving the federally funded Nashville VA Hospital and the publicly financed Children's Hospital. In 1998 Vanderbilt moved back in to assume control over the new city hospital Meharry virtually donated to Nashville.

In the North, where Black's gained more access to public hospitals in the post World War II era, growth of the public facilities and services was accentuated and exaggerated by increasing residential and class segregation, "White flight" from the inner cities, and the blossoming of White suburbs. The malignancy of expanding health empires focusing around academic health centers, capitalized on these problems as city center ghettoes were rendered more vulnerable to institutional manipulation due to their increasing deficits in education, community leadership, and political influence peddling. These problems fanned the flames of inequitable race-and class-based tiering of the health system.

The academic health centers satisfied their institutional, financial (jobs), research, educational, and prestige needs and yearnings while ignoring basic community health priorities. Many of these "pork barrel" programs, again driven primarily by academic health center priorities, took on the look of 19th century Western European-based colonial blueprints for providing social services. In the process, large, increasingly Black, public aid populations became "training material" for the medical school and research infrastructure, which continued its tradition of being dysfunctional ombudsmen for the poor, frequently non-White, populations. As Barbara and John Ehrenreich observed regarding the disturbing cultural and social distancing between Black patients and White doctors-in-training in large city hospitals:

As interns, young doctors get their training by practicing on the hospital ward and clinic patients - generally non-White. Later they (the doctors), make their money by practicing for a paying clientele - generally White. White patients are "customers"; Black patients are "teaching material." White patients pay for their care with their money; black patients pay with their dignity and comfort (and lives).

The federal government became a broad influential force in the United States health care system following World War II through its financial influence on the institutional health care, health education, and research infrastructures. Before the mid-1960s it proved to be poorly coordinated and susceptible to outside control by interest groups, including corporations, lobbyists, and educational institutions. A prime example is Mary Lasker's and Mary Mahoney's private, lay lobby for scientific research - the American Society for the Control of Cancer (ASCC, later the American Cancer Society [ACS]). The ACS became so powerful that it not only determined the policies of the National Cancer Institute (NCI), but it also manipulated U.S. Presidents, Congress, and Surgeon Generals in the pursuit of its agendas. Agenda-setting by such elite organizations and the institutions they represented had little to do with the enormous number of unfulfilled health service needs of the American population. As Paul Starr observed:

Gleaming palaces of modern science, replete with the most advanced specialty services, now stood next to neighborhoods that had been medically abandoned, that had no doctors for everyday needs, and where the most elementary public health and preventive care was frequently unavailable. In the 1960s many began to observe that abundance and scarcity in medicine were (found) side by side.

Another reason for the government's failure to create socially focused goals and objectives relative to the health system's race and class inequities and inequalities was that its enormous participation was divided and parsed through a grid of competing agencies and institutions. Federal health programs included, but were not limited to, 64 United States Public Health Service (USPHS) agencies; three Food and Drug Administration (FDA) agencies; a Veterans' Administration (VA) consisting of a string of 166 hospitals, a $1.5 billion budget, 5,000 full-time and 2,000 part-time physicians treating 86,000 patients daily; a Department of Defense (DOD) health service; Office of Economic Opportunity (OEO) health programs and clinics; Department of Agriculture meat inspection programs; Atomic Energy Commission (AEC) health programs; and health programs administered through the Bureau of Indian Affairs.

Compounding this fragmentation of the federal founding into competing programs - there were no aggressive lobbies or focus groups that lobbied on behalf of the people. Even the designating of cabinet status with the formation of the Department of Health, Education and Welfare (DHEW or HEW) in 1953 did not correct the power imbalance. Groups, including underrepresented minorities, senior citizens, children, welfare recipients, and social workers had no powerful lobbying or political groups representing them on Capitol Hill before 1965. Powerful, wealthy interest groups including the AMA, the hospital industry, the insurance industry, and the tobacco industry were competitors against these neglected groups and their health interests. The dramatic and devastating problems perpetuated by these imbalances remain yet today.

In spite of AMA and medical establishment resistance, by the 1960s, Black Americans and the poor enjoyed improved access to a selective and impersonalized version of medical care through government-sponsored health programs such as the Kerr-Mills program (1960), providing government health funding for the elderly poor, passage of Medicare and Medicaid (1965), and improved postwar government-sponsored programs at academic health centers and their affiliated public and teaching hospitals. Despite the good intentions of some public health and health reform advocates, medical-social assessment of this care revealed that it had not lost the historical characteristics of health care for inner-city or poor people in America: "The whole history of medical care of the poor in America suggests that there has not ever been any well-thought-out plan, but rather health programs have taken the path of least resistance." And the myth of "good care for the poor" was perpetuated: "In the process we have disguised this kind of medical care by saying that charity patients receive outstanding medical care….This, like most folk sayings, is only half true because the poor do not receive adequate care - as can be demonstrated statistically or by actual observation of the kind of health care offered."

From a public health view, socioeconomic status and health tend to parallel each other. Understanding the unfavorable epidemiologic state of disadvantaged groups in the United States including Blacks is difficult when it is stripped of its demographic and vital statistics variables. Moreover, as Nicolette Hart reiterates incorrectly in the last two editions of the *Oxford Textbook of Public Health*, race is a determinant of health and disease: "Through a genetic attribute, fixed at conception and generally irreversible, a racial inheritance is also a sociopolitical-economic and cultural variable and a fundamental source of social and health stratification.

Despite signs of material and statistical progress, the National Research Council reported: "In the 1960s Blacks deeply resented their continuing second-class status. Despite their gains…Blacks in general did not share the affluent life styles of the White majority." This frustration - "another postwar dream deferred" - spilled over into the health system and was reflected in the persistence of disparate Black American health status and outcome. As the National Research Council noted: "During much of the period covered….there was open segregation of medical facilities in the United States. In the 25-year period before 1965, persistent barriers to access to preventive, primary, and hospital care influenced the quality of life and the patterns of illness observed among blacks." Improvements in Black access to public and personal health care, to quality hospitalization, to quality preventive health services, and to culturally competent and sensitive health providers were the gains of a health care Civil Rights Movement that had its roots in the 1945 to 1965 period.

One of the dark secrets of the American biomedical and health care systems between 1960 and 1980 was the "epidemic" of forced sterilizations and unethical surgery. Why the Tuskegee Syphilis study raised such an outcry and the forced sterilizations "rated hardly a whimper" is a story of medical racism. Most of the victims of this sterilization, unethical surgical epidemic "were the traditional targets of the scientific racist, Galton-orientated, hereditarian, social Darwinist, biological-determinist influenced U.S. scientific and health system - Black Americans, Hispanic/Latino Americans, lower-middle-class and working-class families unable to afford the costs of proper medical care, the mentally challenged, the disabled, the incarcerated, the indigent, institutionalized children, and the unemployed."

By 1980 the United States' sterilization laws had been in place for more than 70 years (the first such law had been enacted in Indiana in 1907). Driven by Sir Francis Galton's International Eugenics movement, 30 states and Puerto Rico ultimately passed similar forced sterilization laws; most of these sterilization laws were based on the Model Eugenical Sterilization Law drafted before 1922 by Harry H. Laughlin, superintendent of the Eugenics Record Office (ERO) and coeditor of the *Eugenical News* - he also authored a book entitled, *Eugenical Sterilization in the United States.*

The Model Law required each state to appoint a state eugenicist responsible for enforcing compulsory sterilization laws. These laws were directed at the "feebleminded," insane, and criminalistic (including the delinquent and wayward); epileptic; inebriate (including drug addicts); diseased (including patients with tuberculosis, the syphilitic, the leprous, and others with chronic infectious and legally segregable diseases), blind, deaf, deformed and physically disabled, and dependent orphans, "ne'er-do-wells," the homeless, tramps and paupers - the state eugenicist's jurisdiction included all the above people he judged to be members of "socially inadequate classes."

Of the 63,678 people sterilized under the eugenic laws between 1907 and 1964, 33,374 (52.4 percent) "were sterilized against their will for being adjudged feebleminded or mentally retarded, which in most of these states was defined as having an IQ test score of 70 or lower."

Beginning with the Great Depression and World War II, "involuntary sterilization in the South had increasingly been performed on institutionalized Blacks." As Dorothy Roberts reported: "The demise of Jim Crow (laws) had ironically opened the doors of state institutions to Blacks, who (then) took the place of poor Whites as the main target of the eugenicist's scalpel."

In 1955 South Carolina's State Hospital reported that all 23 persons sterilized over the previous year were Black women. Of the nearly 8,000 "mentally deficient persons" sterilized by the North Carolina Eugenics Commission between the 1930s and 1940s, 5,000 were Black. The State Hospital for Negroes in Goldsboro, where all of the doctors and most of the staff were White, routinely operated on Black patients confined there for being criminally insane, feebleminded, or epileptic.

Before World War II, Black men there were castrated or given vasectomies for being convicted of attempted rape, for being considered "unruly" by hospital authorities, or to make them "easier to handle." None were asked for their consent.

According to Chase: "These victims of Galton's obsessive fantasies represented...the smallest part of the actual number of Americans who have in the (20th) century been subjected to forced eugenic sterilization operations by state and federal agencies." Ironically, by the 1960s, when the first generation of mandatory sterilization laws were repealed, a wave of new laws assaulting reproductive rights and a massive and unprecedented wave of forced sterilizations - many of them paid for by the government and facilitated by new health financing mechanisms, often hidden under the cloak of "expanded health services for the poor, and carried out by health delivery system institutions already in place swept the country." These programs differentially affected and were executed on Black American women.

In 1974 it was argued before Federal District Judge Gerhard Gesell, in a case brought on behalf of poor victims of involuntary sterilizations performed in hospitals and clinics participating in federally funded family-planning programs, that: "over the last few years, an estimated 100,000 to 150,000 low-income persons have been sterilized annually under federally funded programs." "A study discovered that nearly half of the women sterilized were Black." In the 1970s Robert's observations revealed, "Most sterilizations of Black women were not performed under the auspices of eugenic laws. The violence was committed by doctors paid by the government to provide health care for these women."

These operations were occurring at the same time that sterilization became the fastest growing form of birth control in the United States, reaching a peak of 1,102,000 in 1972 and dropping off to 936,000 in 1974.

Government officials estimated that an additional 250,000 sterilizations annually, hidden in hospital records as hysterectomies, could be added to the previous total. Blacks were disproportionately represented in these populations, and a new dimension compounded the system's potential for abuse: "Teaching hospitals performed unnecessary hysterectomies on poor Black women as practice for their medical residents. This type of abuse was so pervasive in the South that these operations came to be known as "Mississippi appendectomies."

Since the failed health reform efforts of 1994, continued expansion of an

American health care system driven by market forces, entrepreneurism, overspecialization, and inefficient utilization of medical technology has undercut illusions of predicted cost savings, forced HMO failures, and initiated more rationing of health care. More evidence of the deteriorating health system environment is underscored by the observations of former Surgeon General Dr. David Satcher, "that of the $1.5 trillion (then) spent on health care, less than one percent is expended on prevention."

December 8, 2004, *The Los Angeles Times* featured a front page story that revealed the current state of the "modern" Black American hospital system. The story described the terrible conditions at the King/Drew Hospital and "how whole departments fail a hospital's patients. A culture of mismanagement pervades nursing, orthopedic surgery, the residency program and the pharmacy. Individual employees' shortcomings often made matters worse."

"Patients languished unattended by nurses."

"There was so much 'stuff' at that place (King/Drew)... You couldn't focus on patient care."

According to *The Los Angeles Times*, "Mistakes and lax supervision have debilitated King/Drew's pharmacy and doctor training programs, which affect nearly every patient. The Department of Orthopedic Surgery was crippled by employee misbehavior, absenteeism, profiteering, even the commission of felonies."

At King/Drew Hospital, "it was every doctor, every nurse and every pharmacist for themselves - the patients are neglected to the status of a vehicle that the hospital staff rode to obtain money, drugs, sex and power - it was and still is a modern Sodom and Gomorrah."

In 2005, it was reported by multiple organizations including Ralph Nader, U.S. News and World Report, the CDC, the Harvard School of Public Health, the John Hopkins School of Public Health, the USA Today, that 300,000 Americans are killed each year by licensed medical doctors in hospitals alone by medical negligence; 1.3 million physical injuries are inflicted on American patients by medical doctors in hospitals each year; 2,000,000 infections are inflicted on Americans by medical doctors in hospitals each year, and despite "heroic intravenous antibiotics" and round the clock nursing care 90,000 to 100,000 die; each year there are 2.2 million untoward or bad drug reactions perpetrated on American hospital patients by careless doctors, of which 140,000 to 200,000 die - a whopping total of 5.8 million "casualties" inflicted on their customers annually - killed, injured and infected at the hands of licensed medical

doctors in their work place and they have never received an **OSHA ticket. Of course the Black patient is carrying the brunt of these deaths, injuries and infections.**

According to the World Health Organization and the Center for Disease Control in Atlanta Georgia in April 1990, America ranked 17th in the world in health and longevity; in June 2000 America ranked 24th in health and longevity; and in August 2005 America ranked 46th in health and longevity - hardly a sign that we, Black and White, are receiving the appropriate "bang for the health buck."

While everyone knows what the problem is, few will pick the correct answer out of a multiple choice survey on how to solve the problem. The quote from Albert Einstein says it all, "Insanity is when one does the same thing over and over and expects a different outcome." The medical doctor's idea of prevention is more brick and mortar infrastructure, more and more dangerous drugs, and more physical exams and treatments for Blacks based on their presumption that Blacks are plagued with "genetically transmitted" diseases such as hypertension, cardiovascular diseases, diabetes, cancer, obesity, arthritis, osteoporosis, etc. - diseases that *Time, Newsweek and U.S. News and World Report* magazines declare have now reached epidemic numbers of new cases each year.

In fact the numbers of new cases for all of these chronic degenerative diseases can be reduced significantly or eliminated in a short period of time with simple dietary changes and disease-specific nutritional supplement programs. Most of the individuals already afflicted with these degenerative diseases (the exception being cancer) can eliminate their diseases with disease-specific supplement programs.

It is a natural phenomenon for humans to cling to a familiar but failed system regarding any subject. So what causes American Blacks (and American Whites for that matter) to follow a failed, corrupt and dangerous medical system like lemmings, over the cliff en mass to our financial destruction, demise and death.

As unlikely as it seems, the original 1933 version of the movie King Kong sheds light on the plight of the 20th and 21st century Black patient and further points to the path to free themselves from the bondage of modern medicine.

The King Kong story line (written by Merian C. Cooper and Edgar Wallace) takes place on a tramp steamer and a remote "Skull Island" where a motley team plans to make a low budget movie during the Great Depression.

Indigenous natives kidnap and offer the blond and blue eyed Ann Darrow (played by Fay Wray), a hungry Vaudeville want-to-be, as a sacrifice to appease the rage of the last of a giant gorilla race - King Kong. Kong, curious about this blond human, allows Ann Darrow to live and hustles her off to his jungle domain.

Darrow is terrified and fears for her life, even as Kong duals with a variety of Jurassic Age reptiles that want to devour her. The sailors from the steamer form a rescue party to save Darrow, and she later has to watch helplessly as Kong kills them all except for the male lead.

Kong is eventually tranquilized, captured and taken back to New York and displayed as a stage curiosity to a very upscale audience in a grand concert hall. Kong brakes his chains, jumps into the audience, and kidnaps Ann Darrow a second time. To evade the pesky humans trying to recapture him and save Darrow, Kong climbs the the heights of the Empire State Building.

During the climb to the top of the building, Kong places Darrow on a ledge so he can get a better grip to hoist himself up; and Darrow in her terror and efforts to escape, slips and falls towards her certain death, however, Kong saves her by grabbing her as she fell.

Army Air Corps biplanes arrive, circle Kong and begin to fire at him with their machine guns to rescue Darrow, and to everyone's surprise Darrow attempts to wave off the planes to save Kong!

Kong is finally fatally shot and he falls to his death on the street, more than 100 floors below. The producer of the Skull Island movie and leader of the adventurers exclaimed, "It wasn't the planes that got him, it was beauty (that) killed the beast."

The most important feature of the movie King Kong was a human behavior recognized in ancient times and defined and named in modern times - The Stockholm syndrome.

At 10:15 a.m. on August 23, 1973, three women and one man were taken hostage in Sveriges Kreditbank, one of the largest banks in Stockholm, Sweden. The perpetrators sprayed the bank with machine gun fire and announced that "The party has just begun."

The hostages were held for five and a half days by two escaped convicts who initially terrorized them and then later showed them some small kindnesses. The leader of the gang, 32 year old Jan-Erik Olsson, held the hostages for 131 hours in an 11 x 47 foot vault.

To the world's surprise, all of the hostages strongly resisted the government's efforts to rescue them and were quite eager to defend their captors. Indeed, several months later, long after the hostages had been saved by the police, they still had warm feelings for the men who had threatened their lives. Two of the original women hostages eventually became engaged to their captors.

In similar instances the captives raised money for their captor's legal defense and testified in their behalf at their trial.

The Stockholm bank robbery forced journalists and social scientists to research the event and to determine whether the emotional bonding between captors and captives was a "freak" incident or a common phenomenon in oppressive situations. Psychiatrist Nils Bejerot coined the term "Stockholm syndrome."

The investigators discovered that the behavior, known as the Stockholm syndrome, is a common result if the following conditions are met:

* Perceived threat to survival and the belief that one's captor is willing and able to act on that threat. Captives begin to identify with their captors; at least at first, this is a defensive mechanism based on the idea that the captor will not hurt them if they are cooperative and even positive and supportive. The captive often seeks to win favor with the captor in an almost child-like manner.

* The captive often realizes that action taken by his would-be rescuers is very likely to hurt or kill him instead of obtaining his release. Attempts at rescue may turn a presently tolerable situation into a lethal one. If the bullets of the authorities don't get him, quite possibly those of the provoked captor will.

* Long term captivity builds even stronger attachment to the captor as he becomes known as an individual human with his own problems and aspirations (particularly in political or ideological situations); longer captivity also allows the captive to become familiar with the captors point of view and the history of his grievances against authority. He may come to believe that the captor's position is just.

* The captive seeks to distance himself emotionally from his plight by denying that it is actually taking place. He fancies that it is all a bad dream; or loses himself in long periods of sleep, or in delusions of magically being rescued. He may try to forget the situation by engaging in useless but time consuming busy work. Depending on his degree of identification with the captor, he may deny that the captor is at fault, holding that the would-be rescuers and their insistence on punishing the captor are the ones really to blame for his situation.

* The captive's perception of small kindnesses from the captor within an environment of terror.

* Isolation from perspectives other than those of the captors.

* Perceived inability to escape.

The Stockholm syndrome is a survival mechanism. "The syndrome begins with a sudden and shocking capture, terror and infantilism (where) you cannot eat, talk, move or use the toilet without permission," says FBI psychiatrist Frank Ochberg. He continued, "But then somebody gives you permission to talk, eat and move and live. It is not a reflex for life, but rather a sense of gratitude."

The individuals or groups of people who get it perceive they are fighting for their lives. Psychologist Dee Graham has stated that the Stockholm syndrome also occurs on a societal level.

In the most famous case of the Stockholm syndrome, Patty Hearst, the granddaughter of the publishing baron William Randolph Hearst, was kidnapped by radicals within the leftist Symbianese Liberation Army in 1974. She then robbed a San Francisco bank together with her captors, having been brainwashed into denouncing her capitalist roots.

Hearst, herself claimed, "I knew that the real choice was the one which Cin had mentioned earlier; to join them or to be executed. They would never release me. They could not. I knew too much about them. He was testing me and I must pass the test or die."

She was sentenced to seven years in prison for her part in the robbery, but had her sentence commuted by then U. S. President Jimmy Carter.

William Sargant, a British expert in mind control who interviewed Hearst before her trial, concluded that a person whose nervous system is under constant pressure or threat can display "paradoxical cerebral activity," that is, "bad can become good and good can become bad."

Groups of people and individuals who have demonstrated the Stockholm syndrome include:

1) 14 year old Elizabeth Smart, who was kidnapped on June 5, 2002 was so terrorized by her captor Brian "Emmanuel" David Mitchell, that she failed to ask for help, call out or draw attention to herself even in very public situations with clear opportunity for escape.

2) 78 percent of the Palestinian people voted for the self proclaimed terrorist group Hamas during their 2006 national parliamentary elections to the surprise of the world and even to the surprise of Hamas.

3) Domestic violence 911 calls: abused wife will often attack police trying to arrest her abusive husband.

4) Concentration camp prisoners; prisoners of war; hijacking and carjacking victims; cult members; prostitutes by pimps; altar boys by priests; battered wives by husbands; physically and emotionally abused children by parents; incest victims by older relatives; nurses by doctors; slaves by slave masters; patients by doctors, etc.

In the mid 19th century, many Blacks adamantly refused to leave their masters, even when they were granted freedom. Though in a sense, slaves were confined to the area which their master controlled and had the lingering fear of violence, they could still claim that certain areas of their lives were their own.

Slaves were not generally as directly threatened as hostages. Even so, the legacy of domination and abuse manifested itself in the "one sided relationship where American Black slaves remained devoted to their master despite the cruelties they had endured.

"Indeed, the regulation of behavior and the resultant adjustment that was made had a direct influence on the consequent formation of a slave's personality."

In his autobiography, *Up From Slavery*, Booker T. Washington offered a classic example of the Stockholm Syndrome in slaves:

"One may get the idea from what I have said, that there was bitter feeling toward the White people on the part of my race, because of the fact that most of the White population was away fighting in a war which would result in keeping the Negro in slavery if the South was successful. In the case of the slaves on our place this was not true, and it was not true of any large portion of the slave population in the South where the Negro was treated with anything like decency. During the Civil War one of my young masters was killed, and two were severely wounded. I recall the feeling of sorrow which existed among the slaves when they heard of the death of 'Mars Billy.' It was no sham sorrow but real. Some of the slaves had nursed 'Mars Billy'; others had played with him when he was a child. 'Mars Billy' had begged for mercy in the case of others when the overseer or master was thrashing them. The sorrow in the slave quarter was only second to that in the 'big house.'

When the two young masters were brought home wounded, the sympathy of the slaves was shown in several ways. They were just as anxious to assist in the nursing as the family relatives of the wounded. Some of the slaves would even beg for the privilege of sitting up at night to nurse their wounded masters."

Consequently the domination pattern of those with money and power, typically European over the African is still prevalent today, as parts of society still holds that they (Black Americans) are inferior, as would be in a master and slave relationship.

It is now an easy leap to understand how a patient and in particular a Black patient can be consciously put into the captive emotional state known as the Stockholm syndrome by the doctor (both White and Black doctors equally).

Patients are put into a stark, small isolated examining room. The patient is oftentimes left alone for long periods of time, causing them to feel ignored, and then when the doctor or nurse reappears the patient feels relieved and becomes happy. After a long isolation (10 to 30 minutes or more) the appearance of the doctor may seem like a welcome form of human contact.

Every feature of the examining room reinforces the fact that the doctor is in control and the patient is dependent for everything - the paper gown to cover the patients naked and vulnerable body, a glass of water, a tissue, a visit to the restroom, the room temperature (usually very cold) are all under the doctor's control.

Seating in the doctor's office or examining room is strategically arranged to ensure the patient's cooperation; the doctor sitting in close proximity with the patient. To intensify the patient's anxiety the doctor consciously moves "nose to nose" into the patient's personal space - the doctor will back away and give relief only when the patient agrees to taking expensive, severe and dangerous treatments (i.e.- prescription drugs, surgery, invasive tests, chemotherapy, etc.).

The doctor gives candy or free drug samples as the patient leaves the office as a reward for accepting the doctor's diagnosis and treatment plan - the patient's health insurance dollars are often bought with drug samples given to the doctor free of charge by the pharmaceutical companies.

From the doctor's view the patient begins to develop the Stockholm Syndrome in which the patient is now under total control of the doctor and his cohorts (i.e. - specialists, laboratories, hospitals, nurses, therapists and the pharmaceutical companies). The Stockholm syndrome can be initiated following as little as ten minutes of isolation, especially when the patient believes or has been told he or she has a painful, disabling, life threatening or fatal disease.

Doctors take acting classes to learn how to communicate compassion to terrified patients with the right word or a soft touch or pat on the arm, thus initiating the Stockholm syndrome in the sensitized patient. While increasing the patient's dependence, the doctor works as an actor to build trust by pretending that they care for the patient or the patient's plight, and that he wants to hear the patient's story and that he understands. The doctor works to become the patient's only source of physical, mental and emotional salvation, when the patient perceives (rightly or wrongly) that his or her condition is severe or life threatening.

Black athletes oftentimes become superstars, however, fame and fortune frequently comes with a price - a high rate of disabilities and sudden death.

In the 1992 Olympics in Barcelona, observers were shocked to note that West African Blacks and African American Blacks won every Gold Medal in all men's track events up to the 400 meter hurdles. And East African and North African Blacks won all of the men's track events from the 800 meter through the marathon. This feat was repeated in the 1993 World Track and Field Championships in Germany; Black men were victorious in every sprint and long distance race.

The results were predicted by Amby Burfoot, executive editor of *Runner's World*, in an article entitled *White Men Can't Run*. Since 1932 Black men have been establishing a hegemony on the highest honors in Olympic and world championship track events. In 1983, Blacks won half of the 33 available track medals; in 1987 they won 19; in 1991, they won 29 - in those three years Asians won only one medal.

According to Burfoot, "On the all-time list for the 100 meters, 44 of the top 50 performers are sprinters of West African origin. The highest ranking White (runner) stands in 16th place."

Unfortunately, Black athletes drop dead suddenly or die at an early age more often than Whites (i.e- Jesse Owens, Wilma Rudolph, Wilt Chamberlin, Reggie Lewis, Walter Peyton, Cory Stringer, Renalda Pierce, etc.).

The Medical Committee for Human Rights was a group of Northern volunteer doctors and nurses who had gone to Selma, Alabama to support and treat injured civil rights marchers.

When one looks at selected mortality rates, by race (the data was collected from the National Center for Health Statistics, 1990s) the African American has a "particularly disadvantaged mortality experience." The age-standardized risk of death in the American Black male is 1.6 times greater than that of White males and in Black females 1.8 that of White females. In comparison, Black females have 1.5 times the age standardized mortality risk of White females. The life expectancy for White females who lived on the average 5.5 years longer than Black females; and White males live 7.4 years longer than Black males.

In 1988 the mortality rate for Black infants in America for both males and females was 2.1 times that of White infants; and the post natal death rate was 2.0 times greater in American Blacks than in Whites.

The annual income of the average Black employee in America is only 60 percent of that of Whites. The Black unemployment rate is nearly double that of Americans as a whole. One third of American Blacks fall into the economic classification of the poor compared with about 10 percent of Whites. One half of all Black children live in poverty. The proportion of Black male high school graduates who go on to college is lower in 2005 than it was in 1975. There are more young Black males in prison than there are in college. Murder is the leading cause of death for Black males between the ages of 15 and 34.

Black Americans make up 12 percent of the American population, yet they account for more than 35 percent of all AIDS cases in America. This fact alone causes a great paranoia and belief that the American health care system is an instrument of oppressive racism - which in fact it is.

Almost 50 percent of all Black American families are headed by single women. More than 65 percent of all American Black children are illegitimate.

Chapter 4

"It is utterly exhausting being Black in America - physically, mentally and emotionally. There is no respite or escape from your badge of color."

- **Marian Wright Edelman**

"Evolutionary trends in the health system's subculture, having roots and precursors stretching back to Mesopotamian, Egyptian, and Greco-Roman times, have led to profound race and class problems plaguing the contemporary U.S. health system."

- **An American Health Dilemma**

"Insanity is when we keep doing the same thing and expecting a different result."

- **Albert Einstein**

History of Black Medicine

The health practices of the slaves and freedmen were different from those of the Europeans as a result of their exclusion from "civilized and learned" health care systems, private and public. Slaves were denied access to private and public hospitals based on their race. On the face of this, ignorantly and emotionally, one could pity the chattel Black slaves who were excluded from the health system of the times, forced to take care of themselves with home remedies, and suffering the humiliation of eating (the superior) the cooking by-products such as the vitamin and mineral rich vegetable broth, while their White masters ate the boiled and nutrient leached vegetables; one could also pity them for having to eat the skin, tendons and bones of slaughtered animals while the master ate the filet; one could also pity them for being forced to use home remedies as hospital admission to filthy germ-filled wards was denied; one might even pity the Black physician who was denied licensure because he was unable to complete one year of the hospital training required to become licensed.

However, in the first half of the 20th century Black Americans lived longer than White Americans. This disparity and inverse expected result was attributed, by the scientific community, to the process of "natural selection" that occurred as the weaker slaves died enroute from Africa to the New World. It is of great interest that the same genes that were given credit for the longer life and better health of the early 20th century Blacks are, in the last half of the 20th century and in the beginning of the 21st century, being blamed for the inferior health that Black Americans have had from the last half of the 20th century to 2006.

In fact by 1950, wood as a fuel, the source of nutritional minerals (plant minerals left over as the carbon of the wood was burned) had been replaced by electricity, natural gas, propane, kerosene, liquid paraffin and heating oils, and as a result, wood ashes (plant minerals) were no longer available in modern urban centers as a source of nutritional minerals.

This precipitous decline in the health status of the Black American can be illustrated by the longevity history of the family of Dr. Jennifer Daniels:

"My paternal grandparents were born of slaves. My paternal grandfather lived into his mid-90s. My paternal grandmother lived into her early 90s. All 10 of their children were born at home. Five of their 10 children died of "natural causes." My uncles died at 33, 56 and 62. My aunts died at ages 56 and 67. While some are still living, none has reached the age of 80. This is an average life expectancy of 92 years for my grand parents and and average life span of 55 years for their children - genes cannot explain these discrepancies - obviously the second generation are missing the mineral nutrients that their ancestors received in abundance from the by-product of daily living - wood ashes (plant minerals) which were placed in the garden as fertilizer, mixed in their food as culinary ashes and used to cut the more valuable table salt - 10 parts wood ashes to 1 part salt."

Amongst the good things, including political freedom, access to the vote, educational freedom, and some degree of financial freedom, the Civil Rights Movement gave Black Americans access to White doctors and the deadly environment of the modern urban hospital and the deadly

mineral deficient diet of the middle class Whites.

A fundamental flaw lies in certain false beliefs of the Black community - "We must have access to everything the Whites have because all that they have is better." They mistakenly believed that the diet that Whites ate and the health care that Whites received were superior to the Black health care and diets and by getting the food and access to the medicines that Whites had historically kept for themselves would give great value and benefit to the Black community.

On May 3, 2006, a study was published, in the *Journal of the American Medical Association*, that compared a large group of 55 to 64 year old White Americans to a similar group of middle aged White British citizens: the study revealed that White Americans had twice the rate of diabetes, 50 percent more hypertension and twice the cancer rate of the British. The study was done by Dr. Michael Marmot, an epidemiologist at the University College of London. The study looked at the White populations only because the authors felt that the low average age of Americans was due to the low average age of the Black population of America. The authors noted, "Startling new research shows that White, middle-aged-to-older Americans - even those who are rich - are less healthy than their peers in England, a finding that *flummoxed* some experts."

No one in positions of authority in the Black leadership could have predicted the wave of suffering and illness that would be unleashed on Black Americans in their quest for health equality, and without critical evaluation, brought into the failed and corrupt White health care system and the failed and ignorant White dietary infrastructure - the Four Food Group concept and the Seven Food Group Pyramid.

Since prehistoric times, medicine and health care have been an important human practice. Since the beginning, those who dispensed medicines and administered healing have always been held in the highest of esteem and given priestly, god-like power and influence in primitive and still today in modern societies.

Western medical science and health care as we understand them are traced back to the ancient river valleys of two river systems. Both of these valleys were found on the pre-African land mass of the supercontinent known as Pangaea 130 million years ago. The civilizations that grew up on and around these river systems can trace their beginnings mythically before 6000 B.C. and through the written record to 4000 B.C.

The culture credited with the earliest of written medical practices, was found in the southwest Asian region known as Mesopotamia, which translates to "between the rivers." The two rivers, the Tigris and the Euphrates, originate in the mountains of Asia Minor and flow through Iraq and Kuwait into the

Persian Gulf.

A second people credited with the production of medical writings were the Egyptians, whose culture developed on the banks of the legendary Nile River in northeastern Africa.

The prehistoric beginnings of American medicine and health care from these two regions were born of medicine's early religious and mystical base. The Egyptian and Mesopotamian formats were only two of the blueprints of what is referred to as "archaic medicine." Additional models of early medicine that is thought of as archaic include the ancient Chinese, Indian, Central American, South American and more recently a few sub-Saharan African systems - all other systems are thought of as being "primitive medicine."

Archaic medicine recorded its practices and results to ensure reproducible health care and for the benefit of future health care givers. Early medicine men and physicians were oftentimes priests that also carried messages from their gods to royalty and the common people - this concept was injected into the Christian Era.

By contrast, the Greeks were more successful in separating religion and medicine; although Greek medicine dominated (500 B.C. - A.D. 500) the temple complexes that functioned as religious spas, sanitariums and hospitals. The collapse of the Roman Empire and the invasion of barbarism through Europe drove medicine back to the protection of the Church.

The first indications of a formal medical system are found in the records of Mesopotamia dating back to 3000 B.C.. Some of these early medical records, treatment methods and medical-legal rules are found in the Code of Hammurabi which is dated at 1700 B.C.. By comparison Mesopotamian medical writings are more mystical and less rational (in modern terms) than Egyptian medical writings. There are writings that clearly indicate a class hierarchy in both the Mesopotamian and Egyptians regarding the availability of health services. Systems directing health care "tiering" are the models now used by the American health care systems. These "status based" health policies were most evident in Mesopotamia, where slaves received significantly lower standards of treatment, given by poorly trained physicians and at reduced fee scales.

Mesopotamian medical theory was based on the belief that disease was a punishment from the gods because of some sin or trespass committed. Physicians were therefore responsible for getting divine guidance and had extra priestly functions.

Generally, Mesopotamian physicians were trained in "schools" located near temples, however, in Nippur and multiple locations in Sumer there were specialized institutions separated from the temples that were in effect medical schools.

Mesopotamian medicine placed major emphasis in the area of demonological and divine causes of disease. Some benefits were derived from these theories in that a great deal of effort was directed toward personal hygiene - quarantine, isolation of the sick and merging the social disability with the "sick role" - these practices were passed on to modern times through Hebrew and Greek medical practices.

Commonly used plant medicines included hyoscyamus, opium, belladonna, hellebore and mandrake. The Mesopotamian physicians were tightly controlled and kept in line by harsh punitive measures for malpractice which were clearly laid out in the Code of Hammurabi; however, Mesopotamian physicians had no rules for maintaining ethical behavior or practice or for treating patients equally or equitably.

About 6000 B.C. Egypt, "a complex, highly technical, multiracial civilization, blossomed in northeastern Africa along the 4,000-mile length of the Nile River." By 3000 B.C. the Egyptians had mastered the use of paper, ink, pens, and the writing skills necessary to record for posterity their medical experience and thoughts. According to Thorwald, "The effect of Egyptian (not Greek) medical theory and traditions has been all encompassing":

Many decades were to pass before this unrealistic view was corrected and it was recognized that a body of medical experience and knowledge had existed long before the Greeks; that the Greeks had, in fact - with the "vitality of bastards" as a modern medical historian expressed it - absorbed everything they could from older sources.

Egyptian medicine provided a tradition of medical specialties, diagnostic procedures, drugs, and the written descriptions of diseases, medical data, anatomy; and a code of medical-social responsibility to provide health care to all members of society in an ethical and even-handed way. They also left a tradition of conscious elitism and professional secrecy - practices that negatively impact health care in America and in all industrialized nations today.

The Egyptian medical traditions were steeped in religion; therefore, the earliest Egyptian physicians were also priests. Egyptian physicians were held in high regard by lords as well as commoners and were trained at schools attached to religious temples dedicated to their gods.

Imhotep was the chief physician of Pharaoh Zoser around 2980 B.C. and is considered to be one of the founding fathers of Egyptian medicine. According to Sir William Osler, Imhotep "was the first figure of a physician to stand out clearly from the mist of antiquity." Imhotep was also an architect, priest and scribe. Sometime later Imhotep was deified and his teachings, theories and philosophies were to dominate Egyptian medicine for 2,500 years.

Egyptian medicine was segmented into specialties, with some physicians becoming doctors of the eyes, others became specialists in the care of the abdomen and yet others skilled in the care of the anus. Homer, as early as 1000 B.C., exclaimed that "Egyptians were the finest of physicians," and Herodotus, in 500 B.C. again confirmed this observation. Egyptian physicians treated both medical and surgical conditions, including infectious diseases, tuberculosis, disease from water and food-borne contamination, parasitic infestations; night blindness, cataracts and trachoma; atherosclerosis; women's diseases; pneumonia; appendicitis; arthritis and gout; kidney and bladder stones; cirrhosis of the liver; hernias; and tumors of the ovaries and bones.

Diagnosis arrived at by Egyptian physicians were made from histories collected from patients and from detailed physical examinations and the study of sputum, feces, and other body fluids. Diseases were treated with many different "drugs" and modalities including purges and enemas and a wide variety of medicinal plants, herbs, minerals, metals, and other "drugs" with narcotic and antibiotic effects.

The Egyptians conserved their collective knowledge by keeping a library of religious and medical treatise. Egyptians wrote medical textbooks in the form scrolls or papyri as early as 4000 B.C. These papyri make up the most complete collection of ancient medical texts; amongst the most well known include the Edwin Smith (1600 B.C.) and the Ebers papyri (1550 B.C.). The Smith papyri is predominantly a surgical text while the Ebers papyri is a vast collection of medical problems and therapies. The Kahun gynecological papyri, authored about 1900 B.C., deals with contraception, determination of the sex of the child during pregnancy, infertility, premature labor, amenorrhea, dysmenorrhea, venereal diseases, and inflammation of external and internal genitalia.

The Egyptians provided medical care and services to all of the population regardless of class, race, or social status through a formal system of state-salaried physicians; these included sanitation inspections, formal assignments to temples, the care of slaves and peasants and military assignments.

As early as the 1920s scholars such as J. A. Rogers and W. Montague Cobb insisted that Imhotep was Black; these efforts were ignored, discredited or marginalized by many orthodox scholars. Evidence now supports the belief that many Egyptians in the highest positions were Black; ancient Black populations were not related genetically or politically to the Arabs that predominate in Egypt today. Black sub-Saharan populations were very closely related to ancient Egypt and were intimately involved with the sophisticated infrastructure of Egypt.

Greek philosophers, however, are rightfully given credit for introducing the concepts of empiricism, objectivity and logic. Guided by philosopher-scientists including Thales (640 - 546 B.C.), Anaximander (560 B.C.), Anaximenes (546 B.C.) and Pythagoras (530 B.C.), the Greek approach to medicine and life in general deemphasized the mystical, magical and superstitious - replacing these primitive views with a "concrete and natural law" belief.

Greeks held the prevailing thought in medicine for 1,000 years between 500 B.C. to A.D. 500. Until current times, the thinking was that Western medicine and health care were Greek institutions that were started during the Golden Age about 500 B.C. Such a view is understandable when one appreciates the extensive Greek "medical borrowings" from the Mesopotamian and Egyptian medical treasure chests. This medical cultural "kidnapping" was successfully completed by 400 B.C. when Alexander the Great installed Ptolemy as Egypt's Pharaoh and Alexandria as the center of all Western knowledge and medical training.

By the time of the Roman Empire, the myth of Greek preeminence as the single originators of Western civilization, science and medicine was overwhelming. The Romans, being politically astute, "adopted and despised" the Greek's scholarly leadership. Some of the most revered and gifted Greek philosophers, physicians and teachers were held as Roman slaves. It would "require 19th century European scholars to finally obliterate the African's Egyptian contribution to civilization and medicine" and award the place of honor to the Greeks.

Before the complete dominance of the Mediterranean basin by the Greeks, slaves were considered biologically and intellectually equal to all other humans and race was not, at least in writings, a consideration.

The economic dependence of Greek civilization on the "institution of slavery" added a negative influence to Western culture. The Greek philosophers, Plato and Aristotle, who are traditionally considered to be the philosophical fathers of modern science and medicine, "began to arbitrarily place slaves of all races into a status of lower rank within the human race; they speculated that slaves were inherently inferior and less intelligent - they also added specific color prejudice towards Blacks and Asians."

After beginning as "itinerant, haphazardly-trained, synthetic adherents" of Mycenian, Cretan, Egyptian, and Asian medical traditions, Greek physicians began to change and to establish a distinct identity by 600 B.C. Pre-Socratic philosophers like Pythagoras, in a quest for harmony, explored medicine in great detail. "Spawned by a litter of Greek medical schools at Croton," where Pythagoras dwelt: in Sicily; in Cyrene; in Asia Minor and the Archipelago at

Rhodes; and in Cnidus and Cos, Hippocrates (460 - 370 B.C.) emerged as the 'ideal' physician."

Hippocrates, a contemporary of Plato, was a legendary practitioner of medicine who traveled throughout Egypt and the Levant "performing medical miracles." Hippocrates was perhaps the most famous medical practitioner and teacher of medicine of his time; he was born in Cos and he was a physician member of the Asclepiad cult. His immortality is based on his writings, which are found in the Hippocratic Corpus, a large encyclopedic collection of medical monographs, textbooks, manuals, speeches, extracts and notes. His corpus, which originates from a variety of sources and authors, show that Greek medicine had become "a highly developed healing art which had succeeded in ridding itself of the magical and religious elements that still clung to ancient oriental medicine, and that it was guided by observations and experiment."

After the establishment of the Greek school of medicine at Alexandria, which collected and disseminated Hippocrates' corpus, his fame outstripped other legendary Greek physicians such as Praxagoras and Chrysippus. This unprecedented media blitz established Hippocrates as the virtual deity of Western medicine.

The Hippocratic "empirical, objective approach to medicine developed into the medical scientific method. By the time of the dominance of the cults and 'schools' of medicine (associations of philosophers, medical teachers, practitioners and students) at Cnidos and Cos in the fifth century B.C., Hippocratic physicians approached both diseases and sick patients as 'natural' phenomena.

They applied the principles of hypotheses, meticulous observation, and empiricism to their patients and their disease processes. This approach existed bedside, and often complemented, the religious spa-like approach to illness perpetuated by the more ancient Asclepiad temple complexes."

The Greek contribution to modern Western medicine and health care "was extremely positive at the professional, didactic and therapeutic levels. However, its medical-social contributions to health care are not generally viewed in a positive manner. Many authorities have noted that the Greeks institutionalized arrogance, social distancing, professional self-interest, class exclusivity, and cult-like behavior as acceptable norms within the medical profession; established a professionally focused, highly individualistic, societally irrelevant, paternalistic, materialistic, amoral medical ethic; laid the groundwork for the biomedical sciences to become invoked in the hierarchical ranking of humanity; established a scientific climate of intolerance toward deviation from Western Classical physical norms; began the process of 'couching racist ideology in pseudoscientific guise'; and encouraged a professional approach toward health (care) delivery and health services reflecting Greek society's slavery and its medical profession's self-serving and weak social covenant. A close look at the Hippocratic Oath and corpus by medical ethicists reveal these characteristics. The public perception and trust in the medical profession's lofty ideals, dogged commitment to patients, and rigorous ethical codes are often misguided, or at the very least, misunderstood."

Medical ethicists have pointed out that the "Hippocratic Oath is a highly individualistic contract between independent agents, demonstrating little bonding, commitment, or concern with social well-being." Much like a religious order, physicians swear to maintain 'trade secrets,' vow to cover up for each other's mistakes or deficiencies, and pledge to preferentially channel the educational process to each other's children. The medical profession has done an excellent public relations job in the utilization of this relatively selfish, elitist, and autocratic oath.

Much of this ideology is reflected in how the Greeks delivered and distributed health services. Members of the Greek medical profession traveled widely in pursuit of fees from patients. Trained professionals had little concern for the poor, slaves, or lower classes. Both Plato and Aristotle described the hierarchy of Greek physicians and the different ways they practiced on different classes of people. As M. I. Finley stated about Plato's description of Greek medicine:

> *There were actually two sorts of doctors…the free and their slave assistants, and "in most cases" it was the latter who treated slaves. That the slave's fees were substantially less is a further implication from the way Plato develops the difference between the two "kinds" of medical practice.*

The less fortunate got less sophisticated, less scientific care. Most fully trained physicians worked on a strictly fee-for-service basis and courted upper-class patients.

Evidence that the idealization of ancient Greek civilization has not always been put to good use in the United States was its application as a defense of the antebellum South's slave based plantation system in the nineteenth century.

Moreover, Greek attitudes toward hierarchies, typologies, and categories spilled over into their medical science. Greek physicians Herophilus (300 B.C.) and Erasistratus (260 B.C.) of Alexandria were possibly the first Western physicians reputed to use prisoners for vivisection at a time when that practice was banned universally. As Celsus (14-37), the Roman scholar-historian, wrote of their experimentation on the defenseless:

Herophilos and Erasistratos....laid open men whilst alive - criminals received out of prison from the kings - and whilst they were still breathing, observed parts which beforehand nature had concealed, their position, colour, shape, size, arrangement, hardness, softness, smoothness, relation, process and depressions of each, and whether any part is inserted or is received into another.

The utilization of the poor, defenseless (slaves), and disenfranchised for medical experimentation and demonstration purposes had begun in Western medicine. Slaves and criminals were especially convenient grist for the mill of the medical community. Later, the teachings and doctrines of the Christian church, with its prohibition on dissection and murder, would inhibit the medical profession in this practice. In Europe, physicians were commonly attacked and mobbed for practicing human dissection, experimentation, and suspected grave-robbing until the nineteenth century in Europe. Later, African American slaves, who were routinely exploited for such purposes, would benefit from far less societal or religious protection.

"Hippocrates passed away; Alexandria sprang up, Greek medicine discovered the laboratory. And all this time the Romans had no physicians at all." Pliny said, "*non rem antique damnabant, sed artem*; it was not medicine itself that the forefathers condemned, but medicine as a profession...chiefly because they refused to pay fees to profiteers in order to save their own lives."

Majno stated, "For six hundred years the frugal Romans carried on with folk remedies. Surely there was no reason to pay for those." Pliny echoed, "The Roman people for more than six hundred years were not without medical art but were without physicians." Throughout Roman history, medicine remained a profession dominated by foreigners - the Greeks, Egyptians and the Jews most of whom were thought to be slaves. It was only in 293 B.C. when a devastating plague appeared that the Romans sent an urgent envoy to Epidauros, the famed Greek healing center, did their medical isolation come to an end.

From 250 B.C. to A.D. 600, a transition and consolidation took place between the ancient Greek medical art and the European Renaissance. Arabic medical dominance during the early Middle Ages served as another.

Galen (A.D. 129 - A.D. 199) was the dominant individual in Roman medicine. "He was an amalgamator, and synthesizer of the major currents of Greek philosophy, medicine, surgery, and therapeutics." Unfortunately Galen was legendary for his anti-Black prejudices and his contributions to scientific racism. His encyclopedic written record would be preserved as he traveled through Oriental, Christian and Arab cultures, elevating him to the level of a "medical deity."

Galen's humoral theories, anatomical books and physiological interpretations remained unchallenged until the work of the Italian physician-anatomist Vesalius in 1543 and English physician-physiologist Harvey in 1628 disproved some of Galen's original work - Galen's work had remained unchallenged for

45 generations.

Galen effectively threw gasoline on the fires of racism and class by continuing to speak and write in negative and anti-Black ways:

> *He mentions ten specific attributes of the Black man, which are all found in him and in no other; frizzy hair, thin eyebrows, broad nostrils, thick lips, pointed teeth, smelly skin, black eyes, furrowed hands and feet, a long penis and great merriment. Galen says "that merriment dominates the Black man because of his defective brain, whence also the weakness of his intelligence."*

As for Africa, health has always been a limiting problem. Ransford stated, "The great mass of Africa, that part lying within the tropics, has carried a more grievous burden of disease than any other area of the world, and it very largely determined the history of this vast region." Black Africa extends from 15 degrees north south to the Cape of Good Hope - it dominates an excess of three-fourths of the "dark continent."

Black Africa is significantly different compared with the Mediterranean littoral and the high Ethiopian plateau climatically, politically, and culturally and has been so since before recorded history. A considerable percentage of the continental interior is guarded from the eyes of civilization by infested swamps and dense tropical forests and opaque shields of vegetation on a hot, stifling, steamy coastal plain. The bosom of the tropics have historically provided an ideal hatchery for insects, the parasites of malaria, sleeping sickness, the virus of yellow fever, bilharzias (blood flukes), hook worms, filariasis, and river blindness. Contributing to "the mystery of Black Africa was the reality that these diseases were untouchable, either in prevention or by cure, by European or Arabic medicines - and the Black African appeared to have learned to survive these diseases whilst other races had not."

Despite European beliefs, African life spans were in general short and infant mortality was exceptionally high. Infectious disease and parasites were significant barriers to population growth and expansion; and stimulants of high fertility rate, polygamy and extended families. Africans developed both active and passive vaccine immunity to coexist with their diseases. Geological isolation between clans, villages, tribes and other cultures reduced the risk of epidemics from outside disease to susceptible people. The appearance of the Atlantic slave industry in the 1500s pierced the isolation and brought Arabic and European diseases to Black Africa.

While the Atlantic slave trade produced catastrophic effects on the entire African continent, these events are usually ignored. Realistic estimates of slave mortality are considerably higher than those originally based on ship's logs and port registers. The death toll caused by the disruptive events throughout Black Africa (mortality estimated to be 50%); and following the slaves arrival in the New World (estimates up to 30% during the first year after arrival) are not usually included. Davidson and Mazrui noted, "Africa lost millions of vital skilled workers, artisans, farmers, hunters, reproductive-age women, and children - people in their prime years."

Large numbers of slaves were captured and bought to supply the triangular trade between Europe, Africa and the New World colonies; and because of the growing demand, the slave trade, like any other industry became more efficient and more systematized. The slave wars, round-ups, and long treks from the interior of the "Dark Continent" to the coastal ports produced high mortality. The growth industry of slavery demanded deeper and more disruptive incursions into the unknown territories of the Black African centers; greater numbers and longer marches traveled by slave coffles; greater concentrations of slaves in holding pens, slave castles, and on ships drove the death rates in the captives and purchased chattel to 50% and beyond before they even departed their home territories for the New World.

Europeans brought with them new diseases including tuberculosis, syphilis, smallpox, and measles. The method of capturing and purchasing slaves engendered slave wars; herding the captive slaves into dense packs and driving them in slave coffles from the interior to the coast "redistributed and then homogenized" isolated local African diseases throughout large populations of susceptible and helpless tribal Africans. These events produced epidemics and drove the spread of previously limited and geographically isolated diseases into the captive Blacks. Through their chains of slave castles and trading posts up and down the West African coasts, the Portuguese and Spanish, followed by the English, Dutch and French mixed and blended the formally isolated clans, tribal and empires populations in slave barracoons, storage ships, and castles - "this endless crush of sweat and filth contributed significantly to an endless wave of death."

The Atlantic slave trade was a new epidemiologic nightmare for an African continent already historically loaded with more than its share of mysterious diseases. These epidemics are credited with the 18th and 19th century depopulations of vast land areas on the Dark Continent. According to Basil Davidson, a prominent African scholar, "Sociologically and epidemiologically, the coming of the Europeans in the fifteenth and sixteenth centuries was the worst thing to happen to Black Africa."

In the early days of the Atlantic slave trade, European physicians could do very little to reduce disease mortality and morbidity, however medical support became quite advanced and extremely well organized later in the 16th and early 17th centuries when Spain and Portugal were the main perpetrators of slavery. If one compares the early English slave ports with the Spanish-operated port early in the era of the Atlantic slave trade, the English ports were primitive and chaotic relative to Cartegena and other Spanish ports where slaves and slave ships were subject to rigorous health inspections; and Spanish embarkation ports and slave markets "instead of being quartered in the towns of Spanish America, new slaves were kept on outlying farms and restored to health before they were sold."

By the end of the 17th century as the Dutch, British and French became the dominant slavers, most of the Spanish health practices had been abandoned. The British considered medical support of the slave trade essential, however, financial considerations rather than moral or health care needs of the slaves were the pre-eminent concerns of the White doctor - Black patient system.

The slave ship's own surgeons (usually the second highest paid person on the ship behind the captain) adopted the concept of the Black African's inferiority. The most catastrophic phase of the slave trade was the Middle Passage aboard ships from their African origins to their arrival in the New World. Sanitation was non-existent aboard the ships; the human cargo was stacked like "spoons" on shelf-like decks - they had to lay down and sleep in their own urine and feces.

Diseases common to the Middle Passage included dysentery, diarrhea, ophthalmia, malaria, scurvy, parasites, yaws, typhoid fever, small pox, yellow fever and measles. The slaves also suffered from chaffing sores from their shackles, ulcers, wounds and injuries that were caused by fights and the "laying on of the lash."

Slaves often tried to commit suicide by throwing themselves over the side of the slave ship or by going on hunger strikes.

The absence of simple training regarding personal hygiene and a lack of soap for hand scrubbing, utensil and dish washing led to the spread of and high rates of gastro enteric disease. Existence in the slave compounds known as "slave quarters" was crowded, filthy and miserable; their water supplies were contaminated with urine and feces; intestinal parasites were rapidly spread throughout the quarter.

The pervasive crowding and lack of sanitation led to a horrific stench and endemic hoards of flies that in turn carried bacterial, viral and parasitic infections from cesspools to humans, including tuberculosis, cholera (*Vibrio*), typhoid fever and food poisoning (*Salmonella*), bacterial dysentery (*Shigella*), viral hepatitis, amoebic dysentery (*Entameba histolytica*).

Diphtheria, scarlet fever, strep throat, rheumatic fever, influenza and pneumonia came in killer waves that would wipe out the entire population of children in the quarter.

Slaves were reported to have a notable incidence of brucellosis or "undulant fever" or "Malta fever," a disease of livestock that produced an intermittent fever in humans (often mistaken for malaria) that usually spiked in reported cases during the beef and swine killing season in the fall.

Leptospirosis (mud fever), a bacterial disease, was frequently contracted by slaves getting animal urine contaminated water (streams, ponds, rivers, swamps, etc.) into their mouth, eyes or nasal passages.

Anthrax was another disease common to domestic animals and slaves. Slaves usually contracted the disease by inhalation of the spores while skinning infected animals; anthrax caused skin infections, meningitis and pneumonia.

Venereal disease including gonorrhea and syphilis were common amongst the slaves because it was cheaper to breed and raise slaves than it was to buy them, so many plantations created another income stream by requiring that all Black women must be pregnant - in effect slave "breeding farms" were created.

Heat stroke was common in the hot summer months because salt was expensive and not usually "wasted" on slaves.

Nutritional diseases were so common as to be considered "normal" in the Black race. The slave ration was rich in calories (4,000 to 6,000 Kcal per day) which were necessary to support the hard labor they were forced to perform. The staple diet contained 1/2 pound of pork and 1 1/2 pound of corn meal each day. The slave was expected to supplement his daily diet on his own by gardening, foraging, fishing and trapping. Slaves could also do extra chores to obtain molasses, sweet potatoes, cabbage, collard greens, turnips and turnip greens; however, these seasonal supplements did not supply sufficient levels of niacin (vitamin B3) and the amino acid tryptophan to prevent pellagra which was common in the slave quarter. The cause of pellagra, a disease that affects the skin, gastrointestinal tract and central nervous system was eventually elucidated by Public Health Service epidemiologist Joseph Goldberger, who began researching pellagra in 1914.

Differentially affecting Blacks, by the 1920s, pellagra initially was thought to be caused by an infectious agent (this resulted in the construction of a chain of federal "retardation centers" throughout the South), was finally found to be caused by the nutritionally deficient diet composed of corn meal, sorghum, and salt pork that most Black Americans were forced to survive on in the South. The addition of fresh meat, poultry, grain, fresh vegetables, milk and eggs prevented the disease. Later, the simple use of B-Complex supplements (originally in the form of brewer's yeast) practically eliminated the disease - by the 1940s, pellagra deaths in the Black community finally dropped below 20 per 100,000.

Riboflavin (vitamin B2) deficiency often caused "sore mouth" in slaves. The slave diet was notoriously short in vitamin A and the mineral calcium.

Vitamin A deficiency resulted in "sore eye," night blindness and corneal ulceration and blindness in slave children (vitamin A deficiency is thought to be the cause of Ray Charles' blindness). "Cachexia Africana" or wet beri-beri (thiamine or vitamin B1 deficiency) caused weight loss, muscle wasting, diarrhea, anemia, congestive heart failure and death.

Miscarriages and infertility were common as were congenital birth defects (caused by nutritional deficiencies during early pregnancy) of every description including polydactyly (extra fingers or toes), hernias, Down's syndrome, cleft lip and palate, spina bifida, etc.

Sudden deaths in Black infants were attributed to "smothering" or "overlaying," current thinking is that these sudden deaths were actually cases of "SIDS" or Sudden Infant Death Syndrome. Today SIDS is known to be caused by a selenium deficiency in the suckling infant being fed canned formulas instead of breast milk.

Geophagia, commonly known as clay eating or pica was reported in nearly all newly arriving slaves (particularly common in pregnant women), indicated multiple mineral deficiencies. Slaves who put wood ashes (the plant minerals that are left when the carbon in the wood fuel for cooking and heating is burned away) in their gardens as a fertilizer, mixed them in their food as "culinary ashes" or "pot ash," and cut their salt, 10 parts wood ash to 1 part salt, did not exhibit pica and cribbing and did not develop mineral deficiency diseases.

The uncommonly sturdy bones of Black women and the reduced rate of osteoporosis in slaves compared to White women was origionally attributed to "primitive" genetic influences. It is now understood that the high mineral, especially calcium and boron, content of collard greens and other garden vegetables and weeds (fertilized with plant minerals from wood ash sources) was the actual reason for their strong bones.

Slaves were typically reduced to drinking the cooking water from the boiled vegetables while the slave master and his household ate the vegetables themselves, and to boiling the chicken bones, goat bones, pork bones and fish bones with vinegar into a mineral-rich soup while the master ate the mineral deficient high meat diet. Today we know that boiled vegetables release much of their vitamin and mineral content into the cooking water and that there is more mineral nutrition in bone soup than in the roast beef.

The master and his family were unwittingly being malnourished in terms of micronutrients while the slave was getting the superior vitamin and mineral nutrition from what was considered "garbage." The disparity in mineral and vitamin intake was reflected in the physical and constitutional superiority of the slave. This disparity in strength and stamina between the Black man and the White man was attributed to the "animal-like" genes of the Black man.

Because clothes and bedding were rarely changed or washed, skin infections and parasite infestations were common, including impetigo, rats ate appendages of slave children during the night, killed new babies, and were themselves infested with fleas that transmitted disease including bubonic plague, murine typhus (*Rickettsia mooseri*), scrub typhus (*R. prowazeki*) and tape worm.

Various types of nematode (roundworms), cestode (tapeworm) and trematode (fluke) were common including ascariasis (roundworms) that also caused malnutrition and anemia.

Out of necessity chattel slaves developed their own health system that lasted more than 246 years. They embraced slave midwives, root doctors, healers and magicians that had their origins from either Africa, Arabia, India or as a result of their association with Native American slaves. Blacks were the primary providers of these slave health services; however, planters, the overseers, and their wives also administered to the sick and injured Blacks.

Medical/scientific racism was referenced as the scientific justification for the enslavement of 95 percent of more than 2,000,000 Black people in North America and viciously subjugating the remainder. Northern and Southern physicians using European biological, anthropological and ethnological "sciences" in the 18th and 19th centuries produced large volumes of "data" that "documented the Negro's (inferiority and) differences."

These negative racial attitudes within the life sciences had to affect the health status expectations regarding Blacks, the efforts exerted to ensure equal health service delivery to Blacks, and the professional and policy responses to the poor health status of patients of Black African descent - the result has been devastating for Black people in the past and continues into the 21st century.

The first Black healer to be "recognized" in North America was an elderly Southern slave who was freed after he revealed the ingredients in an herbal formula that was successful in treating syphilis in slaves. Lieutenant Governor Gooch of Virginia reported:

> *"(He) met with a negro, a very old man, who has performed many wonderful cures of diseases. For the sake of his freedom, he has revealed the medicine, a concoction of roots and bark...There is no room to doubt of its being a certain remedy here, and of singular use (in the treatment of syphilis) among the negroes, it is well worth the price (60 British pounds)*

of the negro's freedom, since it is now known how to cure slaves without mercury."

The first Black healer, Simon, to be written up in a public media appeared in the Philadelphia *Pennsylvania Gazette* in 1740 after escaping slavery. He was noted for his skills in "bleeding and drawing teeth, pretending to be a great doctor among his people."

Kenneth Ludmerer, author of *Learning to Heal*, says, "Blacks .. ...faced much greater obstacles that mirrored the problems they encountered elsewhere in...American life. Before the Civil War, physicians in the North openly denied Blacks entrance to the profession. In the South, Blacks were sometimes permitted to practice folk and herbal remedies on fellow Blacks and slaves but were not allowed to receive formal medical instruction or treat Whites.

Caesar, a Negro slave, authored the first medical paper (a snakebite remedy published in the *Massachusetts Magazine* in 1792) by an African American. It has been estimated by numerous Black historians that there were thousands or tens of thousands of Black traditional folk medicine healers, conjure men, root doctors, spiritual healers, magicians, granny nurses and slave midwives that provided "health services" in the Black slave quarters and in effect contributed to the very survival of the Negro people in the New World.

Lucas Santomee (a Dutch trained Black physician) arrived in New Netherlands early in the 1600s; no other university trained Black physician appeared in the United States until 177 years later when James McCune Smith (1813 - 1865) showed up in New York City in 1837 - he had earned his B.S., M.S. and M.D. degrees from the University of Glasgow.

According to Byrd and Clayton:

"**As far as a voice from university-trained African American healers in English North America in the intervening years is concerned, the silence is deafining. The facts are emblematic of the relationship between the mainstream health providers and the Black population and Black healers. A national pattern of health care involving Black dependency on trained White health providers, rather than self sufficiency, was established and remains today. Although the exact social mechanisms, medical educational deficiencies, and political economic landscapes have changed, the end results have been the same. The representation of Black physicians has remained at the 2-3 percent levels for the past century, and proportional and equitable representation for African Americans in the prevailing health policy environment has been a structural impossibility.**"

In the North, Black healers and Black physicians were a rare commodity. An example of an apprentice-trained Black physician in the North was James Derham of Philadelphia (less than 10 percent of the New World's physicians held the M.D. or any university degree for that matter); between 25 and 50 percent were apprentice trained. So Derham was in the main stream of colonial America. Derham was bought as a child by the well-known Philadelphia physician John Kearsley, Jr. who trained the young boy in various aspects of health care.

After Kearsley's death "relating to treasonable activities" in 1777, Derham was sold by the estate to another physician, who again sold him to another physician and they each taught him something about mixing medicines and treating patients. Dr. Robert Dove, of New Orleans, Derham's final owner, allowed him to purchase his freedom. Derham was so well trained that he impressed Dr. Benjamin Rush, a prominent physician who was a signer of the Declaration of Independence and the new nations first Surgeon General.

Rush said of Derham's knowledge, "I have conversed with him upon most of the acute and epidemic diseases of the country where he lives, and was pleased to find him perfectly acquainted with the modern simple mode of practice in those diseases. I expected to have suggested some new medicines to him, but he suggested many more to me."

Between 1730 and 1812, major advances occurred in the White medical world, however, many of the new "discoveries" were long held cures bought or extorted from unworldly and innocent healers. The most legendary "drug" to be identified in the 18th century was digitalis, which was part of a mixture of 23 herbs long used by an "English witch" for treating congestive heart failure and dropsy. After many years of studying the herbal mix, William Withering (1741- 1799) identified the specific active ingredient as foxglove (*Digitalis purpura*) in 1785.

Treatments, for mental illnesses, were documented by Frenchman Phillipe Pinel (1745-1826), Englishman William Tuke (1732-1822), and American Benjamin Rush (1745-1813).

Of public health importance was the 1798 acceptance of the procedure for vaccination for smallpox (a procedure presented in 1721 to the Royal College by Cotton Mather - he learned the procedure from his Black slave; a procedure that had been used in Black Africa for more than 500 years) put forth by Edward Jenner (1749-1823). Credit for bringing Jenner's cowpox vaccination for smallpox experiments into wide clinical use went to Dr. Benjamin Waterhouse (1754-1846).

British Royal Naval Surgeon James Lind (1716-1794) proved the effectiveness of citrus fruit and green vegetables for preventing and curing scurvy (vitamin C deficiency).

The Black inferiority myth was perpetuated in the academic community by Dr. Charles Caldwell (1722-1853), a student of Dr. Benjamin Rush, a graduate of the University of Pennsylvania, and a professor of natural history from the same university. A nationally respected lecturer and medical academician, later in his career, Caldwell became the most respected phrenologist in America.

Caldwell participated in a series of debates against Reverend Samuel Stanhope Smith, the early 19th century promoter of a single creation of White and Black men (monogenesis) and the environmental causes of racial differences. Smith considered himself "the first introducer of true medical science into the Mississippi Valley, because of his founding of two Southern medical schools in Kentucky, one at Transylvania University in Lexington and the other at the University of Louisville.

Plantation owner's wives are commonly depicted as frail, weak and sickly, requiring Black wet nurses to breast feed and raise their White babies.

When the plantation owner was ill and deemed to have an incurable disease by the White doctor, he would oftentimes sneak down to the slave quarters in the dark of the night to get a cure. The slave cures were a combination of Native American, African folk, Arabic, European and island voodoo remedies. Slave medicines and cures had to be easy to get, easy to produce and real cheap because they didn't have any money.

Chapter 5

"Some seek not gold, but there lives not a man who does not need salt."

- Cassiodorus
Roman Statesman

"Hypertension in Blacks not genetic."

- Dr. Richard S. Cooper
BMC Medicine
January 5, 2005

High Blood Pressure in Blacks

The December 6, 2004 issue of *Time* magazine declared on the cover - "America's HIGH BLOOD PRESSURE crisis is spinning out of control." Despite a whole collection of calcium channel blockers, Beta blockers, diuretics, weight loss programs, and growing fitness center memberships, the numbers of people with uncontrolled hypertension, and the numbers of new cases of hypertension in children - in particular in the Black community - continues to rise.

As of December 2004, one in three American adults has high blood pressure; more men than women suffer from high blood pressure and African Americans have a 43 percent greater chance of developing high blood pressure than Whites.

The February 5, 2006 issue of *The Indianapolis Star*, featured a front page article entitled, *Heavy Kids Getting Grown-up Diseases*, that stated, "The signs of the hypertension epidemic (in American children) was first detected in the 1990s, (however, the medical profession was) slow to react." Scary diagnosis, such as, high blood pressure, clogged arteries, and diabetes, were now being reported in eight to 15 year old kids - primarily Black kids.

Even a simple superficial look at the current medical methods of managing hypertension tells us that "it ain't workin." It is certainly long overdue, that we reach for a different "recipe" to deal with hypertension. The White and the Black government and private medical systems have all failed because they have limited their approach to managing the symptoms of hypertension with drugs rather than eliminating hypertension by fixing the nutritional deficiency cause.

The Problem:

Typical of the descriptive medical view of hypertension and techno-babble, is Gillum's lofty statement:

"Hypertension acting in concert with other risk factors determines many patterns of cardiovascular mortality and morbidity, (and) captures hypertensive disease's unique contribution to U.S. mortality and morbidity, which often relates to, and works in concert with, heart and cerebrovascular diseases."

The prevalence of hypertensive disease (HD) and hypertensive heart disease (HHD) as secondary causes of death in 20:1 ratios for the former, and 1:1 ratios with other causes, respectively, speak to the prevalence and importance of these relationships.

Although there are considerable geographic variations in the racial prevalence and incidence of HD and HHD - which for Blacks seem to be between 1.4 to 2 times the White rates - a sampling of age-adjusted HD and HHD mortality in the middle of the period indicated that Black death rates related to these causes may be as high as four and five times White death rates for both genders. At the very least, "Comparing Black women and men to the total population, one sees a nearly twofold difference in death rates," according to Charles Francis, director of the Department of Medicine at Harlem Hospital Center, speaking at a 1992 NHLBI conference, "Minority Health Issues for an Emerging Majority." Although age-adjusted death rates per 100,000 declined for HD and HHD in each sex and race group between 1979 and 1988 - for Black males, HD - 13.3 percent, HHD -14.3 percent; for Black females, HD -10.6 percent, HHD -17.4 percent; the percentage declines in Whites were more dramatic: White males, HD -21.8 percent, HHD -23.7 percent; White females HD -23.0, HHD -25.5 percent. Moreover, survey and sampling data during the era indicated higher percentages of Whites with blood pressures controlled by treatment than Blacks.

Symptoms and effects of hypertension:

Hypertension is blood pressure that stays at or above 140/90. The first number is the systolic pressure which represents the force of the blood against the blood vessel (arteries) walls as the heart contracts. The second number is the diastolic pressure which represents the force against the blood vessel (arteries) walls as the heart relaxes.

Normal blood pressure is below 140/90 or slightly lower. Some physicians believe blood pressure above 120/80 is "prehypertension."

Symptoms of high blood pressure can be vague or non-existent, however, they can include but are not limited to headache, fatigue, nausea, sweating, vision changes, shortness of breath, chest pain (angina) and cold extremities.

Complications can include stroke, heart attack, kidney failure, siezures, detached retina and increased risks of ruptured aneurysms. In pregnant women hypertension is associated with the toxemia of pregnancy, pre-eclampsia, premature births or miscarriages.

Salt:

Contrary to popular belief and medical dogma, salt consumption has little or nothing to do with the genesis or perpetuation of hypertension. At the July 1997 meeting of the American Heart Association in Portland, Oregon, a paper was presented that stated, "Doctors lack proof that too much salt is unhealthful." The authors went on to say, "After years of telling healthy people that too much salt isn't good for them, researchers still don't have solid evidence to back up that claim."

A great deal of controversy was raised by the 1997 "Sodium Task Force" study which showed that too little dietary salt actually increases your odds of having a heart attack by 600 percent. The study, which followed 3,000 middle-aged Americans, found that the people with the lowest salt intake had the highest risk of heart attacks.

The National Heart, Lung, and Blood Institute, recommends that Americans limit their dietary sodium, the mineral that composes 40 percent of table salt, to 2,400 mg per day - about one teaspoon of salt.

The 1997 Sodium Task Force study indicated that, individuals who limited their sodium intake to 1,000 mg a day as the NIH recommends, had six-times more heart attacks than those who consume 2,400 mg per day!

There are many complaints of edema or swelling of the ankles, fingers and face following the consumption of table salt. If heart disease, liver disease and kidney disease are not present, then the cause of the edema is almost always a low level of blood protein. Invariably, these individuals complaining of edema have given up eating eggs at the direction of their physician "to help lower cholesterol." In fact eating four to six poached or soft scrambled eggs (in butter not margarine) per day will effectively raise blood protein and eliminate the edema.

Genetics:

Contrary to popular belief and medical dogma, hypertension is not genetic, but rather hypertension is a simple mineral deficiency disease. On February 1999, the journal, *Scientific American,* ran a cover article that looked at hypertention in African Americans. The article featured a blood pressure study including Third World Nigerian tribes still living in the remote bush country and African Americans of Nigerian decent in the U.S.

An examination of the tribal Nigerians revealed that they had an average of seven percent of the individuals tested affected with hypertension, while there was a 33 percent rate of hypertension in the U.S. urban individuals of Nigerian decent - from this simple study one could determine immediately that high blood pressure in Blacks was not genetic. The authors themselves stated, "The findings suggest that hypertension may largely be a disease of modern life; and, that genes....do not account for the high rates of hypertension in African-Americans."

If hypertension was genetic in Blacks, the results of the Nigerian study would have shown similar rates of hypertension in Nigerians in the bush and in the U.S., either seven percent and seven percent or 33 percent and 33 percent - the disparity of seven percent in the bush and 33 percent in the city shows clearly that genetics are not a factor!

What then causes the difference in the hypertension rates between the tribal and the urban Nigerians? The tribal Nigerians still add wood ashes (plant minerals that are left over when the carbon in the wood is burned away) from their heating and cooking fires to their gardens as fertilizer, they still add ashes, a.k.a. plant minerals, to their food as "culinary ashes" and they still cut salt with wood ashes 10:1 - while their city cousins use electricity and propane as fuel, thereby lacking a source of plant minerals and typically do not proactively supplement with plant mineral supplements.

January 5, 2005, the journal *BMC Medicine*, published an article that stated - "High Blood Pressure in Blacks Not Genetic."

The authors, led by Dr. Richard S. Cooper, of Loyola University, went on to state, "Although genetic factors are often blamed (for the high rate of hypertension in Blacks), new research suggests that this racial gap (in the rate of hypertension between Whites and Blacks) is largely due to environmental - and ...preventable factors."

They continued:

"If racial origin played a major role in high blood pressure, then rates of the condition for each race would be expected to be about the same regardless of where people lived. Instead, the researchers found wide variation rates, ranging from 14 percent for Blacks in some geographic regions to 44 percent in other places. For Whites, the rates ranged from 27 percent to 55 percent depending on where people lived."

Calcium:

Dogs, cats, parakeets, turkeys, pigs, cows, monkeys, and all other animals can get high blood pressure. Practically speaking, however, pets, laboratory animals and farm animals don't get high blood pressure, not because they can't, but rather, because the calcium and other essential nutrients necessary to prevent and reverse hypertension are added to their commercially designed feed.

Supplemental calcium and certain essential dietary cofactors can prevent and reverse simple uncomplicated hypertention.*

Amounts of Metallic Calcium in a 1,000 mg Tablet or Capsule

Calcium Source	mg available
Calcium gluconate	90
Calcium carbonate	400
Calcium acetate	230

Calcium citrate	210
Calcium lactate	140
Cow's milk (1,000 mg fluid)	10
Wood ash (mg/G)	271 - 307
Calcium as a colloidal chelate (1 fluid oz)	1,200

*Hypertension caused by kidney disease requires an additional, yet simple, effort added to the mineral mix to bring blood pressure into the normal healthy range.

The Hypertension Program

1. 90 essential nutrients

2. 2,500 mg of available calcium (as a colloidal chelate).

3. Selenium

4. Antioxidants

      Green tea

      Grape seed extract

      Tomato extract

      Exotic fruit juices

Chapter 6

"Cultural historians have traced the many dishes associated with the American South that come almost unchanged from Africa: gumbo (the Bantu word for okra), chilis, pilau, and just about anything deep fried."

- Andrew Curry,
U.S. News & World Report
August 2005

"It's not the amount of fat you eat; it's the kind of fat you eat."

- Dr. Frank Hu
Harvard School of Public Health
November 20, 1997

Cardiovascular Disease in Blacks

The Old South, found southeast of a line running from the Chesapeake Bay to central Texas is known as the "heart attack, stroke and cancer belt" of America. In December of 1997, the Harvard School of Public Health, released the results of a study that looked at longevity in America county by county. The Harvard study revealed a very clear line of demarcation showing that Americans in the upper mid-west and the plains states lived almost 20 years longer than those in the "heart attack, stroke and cancer belt" of the 11 states in the Old South.

The difference is in the cooking. In the upper mid-west and the plains states, people cook primarily by roasting and stewing; by contrast, in

the heart attack, stroke and cancer belt of the Old South, people cook primarily by frying. Fried food consumption equals heart disease, stroke and cancer.

Heart disease:

Elevated cholesterol and/or triglycerides do not contribute to the cause or genesis of coronary artery disease, arteriosclerosis, or atherosclerosis, cardiomyopathy or myocardial infarctions in any way - yet, considerable effort ($117 billion is spent annually) is spent for cholesterol testing alone.

"Heart attack" death is caused by a collection of nutritional deficiency diseases and is not caused in any way by genetics, but rather it is a collection of nutritional deficiencies. The most common type of heart attack death is caused by a coronary thrombosis (the plugging of a coronary artery by a blood clot) or a myocardial infarction (the blocking of blood supply to a zone in the heart by atherosclerotic plaques). Thrombosis and blood clots are caused by the abnormal stickiness of platelets and red blood cells which is caused by a catastrophic **deficiency of omega-3 essential fatty acids**.

Wallach petitioned the FDA to obtain a health claim for product labels regarding the health benefits of Omega-3 esential fatty acids; and eventually obtained the claim: "This product contains Omega-3 essential fatty acids which have been shown to significantly reduce the risk of stroke and thrombotic heart attack."

The second most common cause of "heart attack" is a hypertrophic cardiomyopathy heart attack - death of significant areas of the heart muscle as a result of a **selenium deficiency**. Selenium is a trace mineral that is required by the heart muscle cells to protect them from free radical damage.

Free radicals are produced by the frying of foods using margarines, cooking oils or burnt animal fats which results in the production of trans-fatty acids or heterocyclic amines.

Meats cooked well done and burnt animal fats produce another type of heart-dangerous free radical called heterocyclic amines.

A classic example of a cardiomyopathy heart attack was the tragic 1993 death of Reggie Lewis, the 28 year old captain of the Boston Celtics. He collapsed during a playoff game against the Charlotte Hornets because of a cardiomyopathy heart attack, he initially survived. The Celtics hired a group of twelve cardiologists dubbed "The Dream Team" of cardiology to save Reggie and get him back on the floor. They considered heart transplant, installing a pacemaker and drugs to control his heart rythym, but before they decided on a treatment,

Reggie died of a second cardiomyopathy heart attack. No one gave Reggie one dollar's worth of selenium and as a result he died.

January 1995, one and one half years after Lewis' death, Dr. W. Thomas Nessa, an avid runner of the Boston Marathon, and considered to be a "premiere" sports medicine cardiologist and the head of the "Dream Team" of Cardiologist who treated Reggie Lewis, died of a cardiomyopathy heart attack himself at age 48.

Heart disease, combined in all its forms is the leading cause of death in America - causing 31.7 percent of total U.S. deaths in 1996. Heart disease contributed the largest majority to the White male and female advantage in life expectancies compared to Blacks. Even though there have been highly publicized improvements in heart disease mortality, the disparities between the heart disease outcomes of White and Black Americans have increased significantly between 1990 and 2000.

According to Michael Horan, director of the Division of Heart and Vascular Diseases at the National Heart, Lung, and Blood Institute (NHLBI), reported on cardiovascular disease (CVD) mortality in Blacks in 1992, "Blacks die of heart failure 2.5 times more frequently, than Whites and seven times more frequently than Asians."

Paralleling the rise in racial disparities in the overall death rates from 1.5 in 1960 to 1.6 in 1995, the 1960 Black/White heart disease death rate ratio was 1.2, rising to 1.5 in 1995. As Richard F. Gillum had recorded by the early 1990s, death rates for heart disease were higher for Blacks, especially for males of younger ages, beginning in the 1 to 4 year old age group, and, "at younger ages, rates were higher in Black women than White women." The Black/White mortality ratio for all causes of death rose from 1.5 in 1980 to 1.7 in 1995 for Black males. Black male heart disease death rates, which were 49.3 percent higher than White male death rates in 1980, rose to 66.5 percent higher than White rates by 1995. For Black females, the Black/White heart disease death rate ratio rose steadily from 1.4 in 1980 to 1.6 in 1995. Black female heart disease death rates, which were 49.4 percent higher than White female heart disease death rates in 1980, rose to 64.7 percent higher in 1995.

During these years, the medical myths about coronary heart disease (CHD) in Blacks were revealed for the first time in *The Report of the Secretary's Task Force on Black and Minority Health*. The Secretary's Task Force consensus findings drew the following conclusions:

1. Instead of CHD being uncommon in Blacks, CHD is the leading cause of death in U.S. Blacks.

2. Instead of acute myocardial infarction (AMI) being rare in Blacks, AMI hospitalization rates are high in Blacks with higher case fatality rates than Whites.

3. Despite the myth of angina being rare in Blacks, they have high prevalence rates of angina in the United States.

4. Despite the myth of a White preponderance of CHD compared to Blacks, U.S. CHD mortality and prevalence rates are similar in Black and White males, with Black females having higher CHD mortality and prevalence rates than White females.

Heart disease is the number one killer of women; a woman has a 50 percent chance of dying from her first cardiac event compared with a 30 percent chance for males; of those who survive their first heart attack, 38 percent will die within a year compared with 25 percent of men; 46 percent of women are disabled by heart failure after a heart attack compared with 22 percent of men.

5. Despite the myth that Blacks are immune to CHD, they proved to be relatively susceptible in the United States.

Stroke:

The current information on stroke of all types, with wide racial rate differences, is mixed. The prevalence, incidence, and hospitalization rates for stroke, the third leading cause of death, were higher in Blacks than in Whites in current surveys. Additionally, as Horan of the NHLBI stated, "Blacks die of stroke (at a rate) three times more frequently than Whites." The overall mortality rates for cerebrovascular diseases (strokes) dropped 35 percent between 1980 and 1995. However, the long-term decline in stroke mortality rates, which had accelerated in 1973, began slowing after 1980 in contrast with the spectacular 44 percent decline in stroke mortality between 1965 and 1980. The Black/White mortality ratio increased over 15 years from 1.8 (Black death rates 80.3 percent higher than Whites) in 1980 to 1.9 in 1985 and 1990 (respective Black death rates 85.3 percent and 89.8 percent higher than White rates), declining slightly to 1.8 (Black death rates 82.2 percent higher than White rates) by 1995. Further, as Gillum stated: "Race ratios were much higher for ill-defined stroke (IDS)....This suggests that access to diagnostic services such as CT scanning was poorer for Blacks and did not improve over the decade." The male/female sex ratios for sample subgroups in Blacks (male/female about 1.3 for intracranial hemorrhage [IH], 1.2 for thromboembolic stroke [TES] and IDS) and Whites (male/female, IH 1.3, TES 1.4, and IDS 1.4) were similar.

Age-adjusted hospital discharge rates for first-listed cerebrovascular disease in the NHDS were 30 percent higher in Blacks, and the "limited published data suggest poorer survivorship after acute stroke in Blacks than Whites," according to the Handbook of Black American Health.

The early warning signals that one is at high risk for a stroke or heart attack (coronary thrombosis) caused by a blood clot or thrombosis include cracked cuticles, hang nails, cracks on the sides of the index fingers, ends of the thumbs and heels that indicate a **deficiency of the Omega-3 essential fatty acids**. The systemic effect of an Omega-3 deficiency results in abnormal stickiness of the platelets and red blood cells which will result in a thrombosis or blood clot.

Wallach petitioned and procured a product claim for Omega-3 essential fatty acids from the FDA, that, in effect the claim allows us to say that, "This product contains Omega-3 essential fatty acids, which have been shown to reduce the risk of stroke and heart attack."

Cardiomyopathy: Cardiomyopathy or hypertrophic cardiomyopathy, are common forms of heart disease that are caused by a deficiency of the trace mineral selenium. Supplementation with the trace mineral selenium can significantly reduce the risk of, prevent and reverse early cardiomyopathy.

Coronary artery disease: Coronary artery disease, arteriosclerosis and atherosclerosis are not caused by elevated cholesterol or elevated triglycerides as the medical system claims.

Elevated blood cholesterol and triglycerides are indicators of a deficiency of niacin (vitamin B3), Omega-3 essential fatty acids, chromium, vanadium, early hypothyroidism and early diabetes.

Plugged arteries are not caused by elevated cholesterol, elevated triglycerides, elevated homocystine (produced by a folic acid deficiency) or bacteria that infest the gums and mouth.

Artery disease in fact is caused by high intakes of free radicals (fried foods, alcohol, caffeine, meat cooked well down, burnt animal fat, consumption of margarine, cooking oils) and trans-fatty acids. High levels of circulating antioxidants protect against free radical damage to the intima or lining of the arteries.

Free radicals from any source can damage circulating cholesterol so that HDL (high density lipo-protein or good cholesterol) is converted to the dangerous LDL (low density lipo-protein or bad cholesterol).

Ruptured aneurysms:

Ruptured aneurysms are caused by a **deficiency of the mineral copper** and several associated co-factors. Copper deficiency produces a breakdown of the elastic fibers in the blood vessels of the body.

A breakdown of the elastic fibers in the veins as a result of a copper deficiency results in the formation of "spider veins," varicose veins and hemorrhoids. A breakdown of the elastic fibers in the arteries produces a balloon or bubble in the weaker points on an artery resulting in an aneurysm.

The rupture of a small aneurysm in the brain produces a subdural hemorrhage or bleeding type of stroke and in the eye results in a detached retina. The rupture of a large aneurysm in the brain, coronary artery, aorta or pulmonary artery results in extreme disability or instant death.

Easily observed external early signs of copper deficiency include white, gray or siver hair and a breakdown of the elastic fibers in the skin. The loss of hair color is the result of a deficieny of copper which is required for the conversion of the amino acid tyrosine to melanin. The loss of elasticity of the skin, veins and arteries is the result of a deficiency of copper which results in a failure of the enzyme lycyl oxidase, which is required for the conversion of elastin into the elastic fibers necessary for blood vessel wall health.

A tragic example of a ruptured aneurysm occurred, June 2004, in a young Black woman, was the death of 19 year old Ronalda Pierce. Pierce was a freshman at Florida State University and at 6 foot 5 inches tall, agile, smart and good looking was the darling of the FSU women's basketball team.

Her financial future as a high draft choice WNBA player was assured - unfortunately no one paid attention to her essential mineral needs and she died of a ruptured aortic aneurysm - a simple copper deficiency at age 19.

Cardiovascular Health program

1. No fried or burnt foods, no margarines or cooking oils

2. No carbonated drinks

3. Limit caffeine intake

4. Limit alcohol intake

5. Supplement with all 90 essential nutrients

6. Selenium 600 mcg per day

7. Omega-3 (3 percent of total calorie intake) 10 - 15 Gm/day.

8. Antioxidants

>   Green tea

>   Grape seed extract

>   Tomato extract

>   Exotic fruit juices

Chapter 7

"I die by the help of too many physicians; it was the crowd of physicians that killed me."

- Alexander the Great, on his death bed.

Diabetes in Blacks

The number of Americans with diabetes in 1980 was 5.8 million, in 2002 the numbers rose to 18.2 million with an estimated 17 million American diabetics undiagnosed or in the prediabetes stage.

Between 1988 and 1994, 45.7 percent of Americans over the age of 18 years with diabetes were obese and between 1999 and 2002, 54.8 percent of Americans with diabetes were obese.

On June 20, 1999, *The Huntsville Times*, reported that Black and Hispanic children are more prone to developing adult onset type II diabetes than White kids, that can lead to heart attacks, strokes, blindness and amputations. According to Dr. Robin S. Goland, co-director of the Naomi Berrie Diabetes Center, New York, "Type II diabetes was practically unheard of in young people until the last few years and its recent appearance is alarming."

A UCSD, San Diego, California study assessed 58 children and teenagers of different ethnicities who had been diagnosed with type II diabetes. All except one were overweight, more than 50 percent were Hispanic and 19 percent were Black.

In the Naomi Berrie study, investigators looked at 19 obese children; nearly half were Hispanic and 37 percent were Black.

In the year 2000, according to the June 1, 2001 issue of the *U.S. News and World Report*, there was an epidemic of new diabetics in the U.S. - a whopping 1,000,000 new cases. In 2005, there were 1,600,000 new cases of diabetes in the U.S. - more than a 50 percent increase in new cases of diabetes in only five years - and as expected the Black community and other minorities suffered the most.

The USDA reported that 100 years ago Americans consumed one pound of sugar per person per year; by 2004, Americans consumed one half pound of sugar per person per day. The sources of sugar came from dry cereals, toaster pop up pastries and waffles, pancakes, breads, doughnuts, juices and soft drinks.

On June 11, 2004, Matthias B. Schulze, presented the results of an eight year Harvard Nurses Health Study on 91,000 nurses to the American Diabetes Association's 64th scientific sessions. Women in the study who drank at least one sugar-sweetened soda a day were 85 percent more likely to develop type II diabetes than those who didn't.

The Malone-Heckler report brought attention on the alarming excess morbidity and mortality that minorities suffered from diabetes. Diabetes is the fifth most common cause of death due to disease in Black Americans and the sixth leading cause of death due to disease in the overall population, which reflected the fact that diabetes prevalence, morbidity, and mortality are at least twice as high among Black Americans as those of the U.S. White population.

Facts show that, "(F)rom 1963 to 1985, the rates of known diabetes in the United States doubled for Whites, but tripled for Black Americans" and that "African American males had a lower rate than White males from 1963 to 1973; but after 1975, there was a crossover such that the rate (of diabetes) for Black males became higher than the rate for White males."

Since the Secretary's Task Force report, Black diabetes mellitus death rates have been increasing from 20.1, to 24.8, to 25.3, to 26.8, to 27.4, to 28.5 deaths per 100,000 population in 1985, 1990, 1992, 1993, 1994, and 1995, respectively. And Black/White mortality differentials have increased from 2.3 (133.7 percent higher in Blacks than Whites), to 2.4 (143.6 percent higher than White rates) times the White rates in 1985, 1990, and 1995 respectively. The final NCHS data for 1996 revealed so significant improvements.

The complications of diabetes, such as cardiovascular disease and stroke, diabetic kidney disease and end-stage kidney disease (Black ESRD rate is 2.9 times the White rate), the highest rates of blindness due to diabetes between the ages of 20 and 74, and lower extremity amputations (Black LEA rates 1.5 to 2.0 times White rates) remain considerably higher in Blacks.

Limited research on minority group factors influencing diabetes and its complications has been done, despite the unknown relationships between personal characteristics such as genetic, age, sex, and history of glucose intolerance and lifestyle factors such as exercise and obesity that influence the rate of appearance of, and racial/ethnic variations and differentials in (Latino/Hispanic American and Native American populations), diabetes mellitus. The differential toll that diabetes suffers on the Back American community has been overtly obvious for several decades.

Adult onset type II diabetes (insulin resistant diabetes) is not a genetic disease in Blacks or Whites, rather diabetes is a simple mineral deficiency disease. Proven in animal studies using laboratory animals, pet animals and farm animals and reported in 1957, it was confirmed that type II diabetes was preventable and curable by the use of mineral supplements and dietary manipulations - the mineral deficiency etiology of type II diabetes was demonstrated in humans by researchers from the University of B.C., Vancouver, Canada in 1977, 20 years later.

Insufficient dietary intakes, or reduced absorption efficiency of chromium, vanadium and other mineral cofactors increased blood levels of sugar and insulin, increased glycosuria, elevated serum cholesterol and triglycerides, increased incidence of arterial plaque, increased risk of peripheral neuropathy, produced dementia and decreased fertility and lowered sperm count.

Increased blood levels of insulin produces hypoglycemia, hyperinsulinemia, narcolepsy, anxiety, panic attacks, pre-diabetes and adult onset type II diabetes (insulin resistant diabetes).

Adult onset type II diabetics produce more and have higher levels of insulin than non-diabetics - adult onset type II diabetes is not an insulin problem; rather it is a simple mineral deficiency problem.

The relationship between chromium, vanadium, insulin and heart disease shows why the most common cause of death in diabetics is cardiovascular disease. This relationship is described by Walter Mertz, M.D., who reported that chromium was an essential nutrient in 1955 - he was soon appointed to the Chairmanship of the USDA Human Nutrition Research Center in Beltsville, Maryland.

Chromium is required for maintaining appropriate blood levels of glucose tolerance factor, which in turn is required for insulin to function properly. Chromium is an essential trace element necessary for the normal metabolism of glucose; its function is directly related to the normal function of insulin.

Average American Serum Chromium

Mean Cr blood levels (u/L)	Year
28 - 1,000	1948
180	1959
520	1962
170	1962
28	1960
23	1968
13	1971
10	1972
4.7 - 5.1	1973
0.73 - 1.6	1974
0.16	1978
0.43	1980
0.14	1983
0.13	1985

"The most consistent effect of marginal chromium deficiency is elevated insulin response, and the first effect of chromium supplementation is the restoration of a normal response. It appears…that if we improve glucose tolerance, restore normal insulin levels and at the same time lower cholesterol levels - particularly LDL cholesterol (the bad cholesterol) - we may reduce the risk of cardiovascular disease."

Dr. Richard J. Doisy, Ph.D., professor of biochemistry at the State University of New York, Upstate Medical Center, tested the effect of supplemental chromium on clinically normal twenty to twenty-five year olds. He found out that when healthy individuals were given chromium supplements, their pancreas did not have to produce as much insulin to manage their blood sugar levels. "This could be interpreted that even in 'normal' subjects the dietary intake of chromium is marginal."

Dr. Doisy concluded, "My contention is that probably one-fourth to one-half of the people in this nation are deficient in chromium…We have relatively high tissue levels of chromium at birth and its downhill from there on in. And the result for the health of Americans is that millions have maturity (type II) onset diabetes. And millions suffer from vascular disease."

"You tend to increase (the rate of) your chromium excretion when you're consuming excessive carbohydrates," said Dr. Doisy. "And if the diet is not providing sufficient chromium (to make up for the increase in loss), then you are going to be in negative balance."

We have known since the 1957 reports by Dr. Walter Mertz, that the deficiencies of chromium and vanadium are the primary causes of diabetes, however, the concurrent deficiencies of other essential mineral (co-factors) will "throw gasoline on the fire" of diabetes and produce all of the complications associated with the chronic form of the disease.

On August 31, 2004, Harvard investigators released the results of a 15 year study on toe nail chromium levels and their relationship to the rate of diabetes. The Harvard School of Public Health scientists analyzed the toenails of 33,000 men ranging from 40 to 75 years of age. They found that the men with the lower levels of chromium in their toenails had higher rates of heart disease and diabetes. The study was published in the September 2004 issue of *Diabetes Care*, the official journal of the American Diabetes Association.

In 1991, the University of B.C., Vancouver, Canada announced that the trace mineral vanadium could replace insulin for the control of adult onset type II diabetes.

Vanadium appears to function in a similar manner to insulin, by altering cell membrane function for the ion transport process; vanadium has a highly beneficial effect for humans with glucose tolerance problems by making cell membrane receptors more sensitive to insulin.

Vanadium inhibits cholesterol synthesis in animals and humans, this is followed by a drop in plasma cholesterol and a reduction in aortic cholesterol deposits.

Diabetic Health Program

Diet: The diabetic must give up fruit and juices and all forms of sugar including dry cereals, toaster pastries, meat sauces, pancakes, waffles, and soft drinks - even the diet drinks. Reduce or eliminate all carbohydrates, except a small amount of mixed salted nuts.

The diabetic must eat animal protein with each meal, eat several eggs each day, eat dairy including cheese, and eat several servings of vegetables each day.

Supplement adult diabetics with:

1. 90 essential nutrients

2. Chromium 400 mcg per day

3. Vanadium 800 mcg per day

4. Selenium 600 mcg per day

5. Omega-3 EFA 12 gm per day

6. Bitter melon 50 mg per day

7. Antioxidants

    Green tea - EGCG

    Grape seed extract - proanthocyanins

    Sugar-free phytonutrients

Chapter 8

"The most simplistic view of obesity is that, 'the fat person simply consumes more calories than they burn.' However, it is quite clear that obesity is not that simple. Fat people are driven to eat! Their conscious will can only override this command to eat for so long and eventually they will succumb to the command and eat, and eat, and eat."

- ***Dr. Joel D. Wallach & Dr. Ma Lan***
  Hell's Kitchen

"There was no great gathering of doctors concerned about the loss of essential minerals; there were no Senate or Congressional hearings worrying over the loss of essential minerals and as a result of disregard for the basic needs of the human body, we have the modern epidemic of disabling diseases including obesity."

- ***Dr. Joel D. Wallach & Dr. Ma Lan***
  Hell's Kitchen

"The habit of eating clay, mud or dirt is known as geophagy. Some experts lump it into the same category as pica, which is the abnormal urge to eat coins, paint, soap, or other non-food items such as (corn starch or wood ashes)."

- ***Marc Lallanilla***
  ABC News: Eating Dirt:
  It might be good for you
  October 3, 2005

Obesity in Blacks

Obesity is a problem that, to one degree or another, plagues about 40 percent of Americans. Obesity presents a "social stigma" as well as a serious health risk.

One 2002 study concluded that there are 832 million pounds of excess fat packed on American men and 1.468 billion pounds of excess fat loaded on American women, for a grand total of 2.3 billion pounds of excess fat. Obesity occurs at a greater rate in the middle aged, low socioeconomic individuals and African American women.

A report released October 14, 2003 by the Rand Corporation, found that the number of severely obese people (100 or more pounds over a healthy weight) increased from one in 200 in 1986 to one in 50 in 2000. "More than 4 million U.S. adults are in this category, says Roland Sturm," a senior economist.

On December 8, 2004, the Northwestern University Medical School of Chicago, Illinois released a report that was published in the *Journal of the American Medical Association*, the report highlighted the American obesity epidemic's effect on the Medicare system - "with current trends of increasing overweight and obesity afflicting all age groups, urgent preventative measures are required not only to lessen the burden of disease and disability associated with excess weight but also to contain future health care costs incurred by the aging population.'

The report from the Feinberg School of Medicine, "found that the annual average medicare charges for severely obese men were $6,192 more than for non-overweight men - 84 percent higher." For men, "the total average annual Medicare charges for those not overweight were $7,205, for those overweight $8,390, for those obese $10,128, and for those men who were severely obese $13,674."

For severely obese women, "the annual average Medicare charges were $5,618 more - 88 percent higher than for women of normal weight." The total average annual Medicare charges "for women in the same weight groups as men were: $6,224, $7,653, $9,612 and $12,342 (respectively)."

In 1971, 14.5 percent of Americans were obese; in 2004 the obesity rate rose to 30.9 percent; and in 2010 the rate of obesity is projected to reach 40 percent. The number of American deaths attributed to obesity is 400,000 per year and was predicted to rise significantly and become the biggest cause of preventable death by 2010.

From 1996 to 2001, 2 million American teens and young adults swelled the ranks of the clinically obese. According to the *Journal of the American Medical Association*, March 2004, the total cost for this level of obesity is a whopping $117 billion per year.

In 2005, 65 percent of Americans were deemed to be overweight and 31 percent were obese (30 pounds or more over ideal weight for height); by 2010 experts predict that 75 percent or more of Americans will be overweight and 40 percent will be obese, leaving as few as five percent in the normal or healthy weight range.

In June of 2004, Medstat, a division of the Thomson Corporation, reviewed statistics county by county in the U.S. and determined that the rate of obesity is not equally distributed. In the West and Southwest, obesity occurs at the rate of 11.4 to 15 percent; in the upper mid-West and the Plains states, obesity occurs at the rate of 19.1 to 20 percent; and in the Old South, obesity occurs at the rate of 21.1 to 27 percent.

The greatest concentration of obese people in America is found in the "heart attack, stroke and cancer belt of America."

Obesity is not a genetic disease and does not cause other diseases, however, obese people have a higher risk for several other diseases because the cause of obesity is also the same cause of the other diseases!

Obese individuals are 42 percent more likely to develop hypertension compared with 20 percent of the average sized adult population; the obese are 30 percent more likely to develop insomnia compared with 15 percent of the average sized adult population; obese individuals are 39 percent more likely to develop arthritis compared with 19 percent of the average sized member of the adult population; the obese individual is 26 percent more likely to develop depression compared with 12 percent of the average sized adult population; and obese individuals are 23 percent more likely to develop diabetes compared with 9 percent of the average sized adult population.

Obesity, typically approached medically as a disease of gluttony, increased by 95 percent between 1990 and 2000; anti-obesity drugs, diets, exercise and surgery have made 20th and 21st century doctors wealthy, however, obesity continues to cut into the bottom line of many other industries including the travel industry.

According to the Center for Disease Control, in a November 2004 article in the journal, the *American Journal of Preventive Medicine*, during the 1990s, the average American typically gained 10 pounds. This seemingly small amount of weight gain was devastating to the American Airline industry. The extra weight resulted in the airlines spending an extra $275 million to burn 350 million more gallons of jet fuel in the year 2000 alone, just to carry the extra weight of the larger passengers. The extra fuel burned also had an unexpected environmental impact, because an estimated 3.8 million extra tons of carbon dioxide were dumped into the atmosphere.

For current analysis of obesity, economists with RTI International, a non-profit think tank and the Center for Disease Control, examined two national surveys that track absences and medical information on more than 20,000 full-time employees, ages 18 to 64. Among the findings, adjusted for 2004 dollars:

* Normal-weight men miss an average of 3.0 work days per year, compared with 5.0 days for men who are 60 or more pounds over a healthy weight.

* Normal-weight women miss about 3.4 days per year, compared with 5.2 days for women who are obese, that is 30 to 60 pounds overweight, and 8.2 days for extremely obese, 100 pounds or more over a healthy weight.

* The average medical expenditure for a normal-weight man is $1,351 per year. Men who are 30 to 60 pounds overweight cost $462 more based on added medical costs and absenteeism. Extremely obese men cost $2,027 a year more.

* Average medical expenditures for normal-weight women are $1,956. Women who are 30 to 60 pounds overweight cost $1,372 more when medical costs and missed work are included. Women who weigh 60 to 100 pounds too much cost $2,485 more.

* The most obese workers (those 100 pounds too heavy) make up 3 percent of the employed population but account for 21 percent of the cost of obesity.

"One reason the medical costs for women are higher is that they are more likely to seek treatment," says lead author Eric Finklestein, a health economist for RTI International.

Obesity is a mineral deficiency disease that became an epidemic nightmare across the board in the industrialized nations shortly after they switched from wood (wood ashes are the plant minerals that are left when the carbon in the wood is burned as fuel) as the universal fuel to newer forms of energy - electricity, natural gas, propane, liquid paraphin, kerosene and heating oils.

The universal use of wood as a fuel produced a useful by-product (wood ashes - a.k.a.: plant minerals) by just daily living. The switch to fuels other than wood eliminated the traditional source of essential plant minerals for humans - the source of essential minerals that had been used by successful human cultures for tens of thousands of years disappeared between 3:00 p.m. on Monday September 4, 1882 and 1950 - a brief 70 year period. There was no great gathering of doctors concerned about the loss of essential minerals; there were no senate or congressional hearings worrying over the loss of essential minerals and as a result of disregard for the basic needs of the human body, we have the modern epidemic of disabling diseases including obesity.

The most simplistic view of obesity is that, "the fat person consumes more calories than they burn." However, it is quite clear that obesity is not that simple. Fat people are driven to eat! Their conscious will can only override this command to eat for so long and eventually they will succumb to the command to eat, and eat, and eat.

This almost psychotic urgency to eat in spite of being obese, in spite of having high blood pressure, in spite of heart disease, in spite of having diabetes, in spite of social rejection is a powerful and irresistible force.

This force that commands a fat person to eat despite all human effort to resist can only be created by one possible condition - mineral deficiencies that result in pica, a.k.a. the "munchies."

The Amish

The Old Order Amish arrived in North America in the early 1700s, about 100 years after the arrival of the first Black slaves, and yet today in the 21st century, they maintain their old ways. The Amish have rejected almost all modern conveniences including electricity, natural gas, propane, internal combustion engines and telephones.

The Amish still use horses to pull their family carriages and buggies instead of automobiles, they still use horses to power and pull their farm implements, they use kerosene or fireplaces to light homes at night, they use wood fires to cook and heat with, and in the 21st century they are still adding the wood ash byproduct of their kitchen stoves and hearth to their composts and gardens.

There are 30,000 Old Order Amish in the U.S. today, compared with almost 300 million Americans (Black and White) who have willingly and gleefully given up the old ways and transitioned their daily lives from wood as a fuel to electricity, from buggies to automobiles, from draft horses to farm tractors and from mail to telephones. The Amish are self insured rather than use HMOs or Blue Cross/Blue Shield, or the Medicare or Medicaid systems; and the Amish do not use the advanced high tech health care system that the American medical system promotes.

The rates of obesity (4%) and type II diabetes (6%) in the Amish population are only 10 percent and 50 percent of those reported by their "modern" White and Black neighbors living in the same country, but on the other side of the cultural fence.

Most casual observers believe the lower rate of obesity and diabetes in the Amish is due to a better, more wholesome diet, and the physical demands of an 18th century farm life.

We have spent a considerable amount of time living with the Amish in Lancaster County, Pennsylvania and we can assert with complete certainty and honesty that the Amish consume more sugar, more fat, more red meat, and more dairy products than anyone in North America. They are famous for Shoofly pie, mince meat pie, apple pie, sweet-potato pie, hot oatmeal with brown sugar, potatoes of every type, gravy, breads, pancakes, molasses and waffles heavy with maple syrup.

The Amish are heavy consumers of whole milk, butter and cheese; they eat pork, beef, goat and mutton three times each day; and they are big consumers of poultry and eggs - a diet heavy with animal fat, yet they have the lowest rate of obesity of any culture in America.

The carriage and draft horses do most of the physical work on an Amish farm, so what gives them a significantly lower rate of obesity and diabetes? It's the wood ashes! The wood ashes are the humble source of essential minerals that are dutifully put into their gardens every morning as humans have done since before written history. Wood ashes are like oxygen, we can't do without them (or their plant mineral replacement supplements), yet they are hidden in plain sight! They don't get any respect!

What then is Obesity?

Obesity, bottom line, is a deficiency disease - a deficiency of an entire category of essential nutrients - minerals. Certainly the symptoms and clinical presentation of the simple uncomplicated deficiencies are rarely seen anymore, as they are exacerbated or aggravated by the increased intake of sugars and carbohydrates and reduction in exercise levels.

The deficiencies of just about any or all essential minerals will result in pica, cribbing, cravings, binge-eating and the munchies in varying degrees. The deficiency of even one of the essential minerals, results in a slight increase in food cravings and the "stand in front of the open refrigerator door" behavior.

It is the intersection of multiple mineral deficiencies and the excess intake of calories (primarily carbohydrate calories) that produce obesity - not the intake of calories alone.

The deficiencies of essential minerals, also explains why women gain excess weight during a pregnancy and breastfeeding, they lose minerals to their mineral hungry, rapidly growing babies, and if the mother fails to replace minerals faster than the babies steal them, the resulting pica and munchies cause the pregnant women, new mom, and lactating mom to eat, and eat, and eat.

"Geophagy" or earth eating and pica were historically common in pregnant women; it was well documented in Black slaves coming to North America; and is still common in sub-Saharan Africa and among African American women in the rural South in 2006.

The deficiency of two or more essential minerals will provoke a significant level of pica, cravings, the munchies and binge eating. Iron and phosphorus deficiencies occurring at the same time will result in an almost, psychotic binge eating and soft drink consumption rampage that results in morbid obesity.

Approximately half of the excess calories consumed by Americans come from beverages. According to studies conducted by the University of North Carolina, liquid sources of calories account for 20 percent of the caloric intake of those aged two years and older. At least half come from sweetened beverages, such as juice and soft drinks, of which consumption has climbed 300 percent; from an average of 50 calories per day in 1977 to nearly 150 calories per day in 2001 - that's a sufficient increase in calories to produce a weight gain of 15 pounds per year!

Extra calories in beverages aren't the only problem, numerous studies of hunger and satiety, show that the brain doesn't register the calories that are imbibed in drinks as accurately as those that are eaten with a fork and chewed - the end result is that liquid calories are less satisfying and can lead to the consumption of more calories (pica, cravings, binging, the munchies, etc.).

Barry M. Popkin, director of the Interdisciplinary Obesity Program at the University of North Carolina at Chapel Hill and researchers from the University of Connecticut, the Harvard School of Public Health, Johns Hopkins University, Oregon State University, the Pennington Biomedical Research Center in Baton Rouge, Louisiana and partially funded by the manufacturers of Lipton Tea created a beverage ranking or "guidance system" to help consumers make better choices:

Water: Tap, bottled, nutrient enhanced or flavored water all rank as top choices. Water filled food and drinks - including fruit and vegetables, soups and stews, coffee and tea - count toward the nine to 13 cups required per day. Water and water based nutritional products can also provide essential minerals, including major minerals such as calcium and magnesium and trace minerals. Overhydration or "water intoxication" occurs in one out of every 1,000 ultra-indurance athletes and accounts for several deaths each year.

Coffee or tea: These two popular beverages came in second only to water based on strong evidence for health benefits of moderate consumption. Among the greatest benefits: reduced risk of type II diabetes whether or not one drinks regular or decvaffeinated; other benefits of coffee and tea drinking include a reduced risk of Parkinson's disease for men (not women). The downside of coffee and tea drinking is that they can increase risk of hypertension, increases homocysteine levels (an indicator of a folic acid deficiency), and unfiltered boiled coffee and espresso boost low density lipoprotein (LDL - bad cholesterol) levels.

Increased immunity is one of tea's benefits, others include better bone density, decreased risk of kidney stones, less tooth decay, and reduced risk of heart attacks.

Use little or no sugar. One study showed that women who drank gourmet coffee with the works consumed an extra 206 calories daily (per cup) compared with those who didn't.

Milk: In the April 2006 issue of *American Journal of Clinical Nutrition*, the Popkin team noted that, "Milk provides a small amount of bone-preserving calcium and vitamin D, milk is also an excellent source of high quality protein. Milk also appears to reduce the risk of the Metabolic Syndrome (hypertension, elevated cholesterol and triglycerides, insulin resistance and abdominal obesity) formerly known as Syndrome X. Drink a minimum of three eight ounce glasses of milk per day. Soy milk, rice milk, and cashew milk are not good substitutes for mother's, cow's, goat's or mare's milk, as they contain significant levels of sugar.

Diet drinks: Sweetened with sugar substitutes contain few calories. The dangers include carbonation which neutralizes stomach acid, which then results in a lower absorption of minerals, and phosphoric acid, which raises one's calcium requirements.

Juice, sports drinks and alcohol: In general, juices, alcohol and sports drinks are high in sugar and calories; eat fruit rather than drink fruit juice (vegetable juice is alright); limit of two alcoholic beverages per day for men, one for women (none for pregnant women); sports drinks and energy drinks tend to be devoid of nutrition and high in sugar - the exception is Rebound fx which contains time release energy sources (monosaccharides, oligosaccharides and polysaccharides), antioxidants, vitamins, electrolytes, major minerals and trace minerals.

Soft drinks: Soft drinks contain high levels of calories originating from sugar, they contain little or no nutrients and even the diet ones contain carbonation which neutralizes stomach acid and reduces the availability of minerals; they contain phosphoric acid which increases one's requirement for calcium.

The act of reducing calories from carbohydrate, fat and protein can result in weight loss, however, reducing calories alone does not solve the systemic and behavioral effects of mineral deficiencies, which explains why individuals who drop off of highly restricted diets of all types will regain the weight that they had lost; it also explains why many individuals maintain or gain weight even when they are exercising and/or they are truly cutting back on calories.

Glucose is an "all-purpose" sugar fuel that can be used as a source of energy by every cell, tissue, organ and system in the body including the brain. However, the overt intake of sugar is not necessary, as adequate levels of blood glucose can be made from dietary or stored fat and protein.

Sugars and carbohydrates are not essential sugars or essential nutrients, they are quick sources of energy, they can be fun to eat, however, they are not necessary or essential to consume, as our body actually manufactures all the blood sugars and all of the complex carbohydrates that it needs.

The increased intake of carbohydrate in the form of sugar (one half pound per person per day in 2004 compared with one pound per person per year in the 1700s) and the deficiencies of minerals are the basic root causes of obesity.

It is an interesting fact that as Asian and Latin American countries "catch up to western countries in terms of lifestyles and economics," their rates of obesity catch up with the American rate as well!

The reason that the transition from Third World cultures to industrialized cultures results in an almost immediate increase in obesity and diabetes is that they give up using wood as a fuel and lose the daily byproduct that is essential to a slim, healthy and long life - they convert to electricity, natural gas and propane for heating and cooking fuels! There are no wood ashes left to put in their gardens or for use as "culinary ashes" (plant minerals mixed in food).

Chapter 9

"At least 30,000 years ago, humans, driven by a salt hunger, began to mix wood ashes (wood ashes were used to cut the more valuble salt 3:1 to as much as 10:1 to extend its volume) with their dietary salt, add them directly to food as "culinary" ashes, and additionally mixed the balance of each days production of ashes into their gardens as a plant mineral rich fertilizer which produced greater fertility, greater survival rates of children, longer lives and stronger skeletons that survived the millennia."

- Dr. Joel D. Wallach and Dr. Ma Lan
Hell's Kitchen

"Healthy proteoglycans look like fresh Christmas trees; in osteoarthritis they are as scraggly as cast-off (Christmas) trees in February."

- Harvard Health Letter 1992

Arthritis and Osteoporosis in Blacks

April 16, 2006, orthopedic surgeons reported that, "baby boomer's love of exercise (is) catching up with them." Led by baby boomers, the generation born after World War II between 1946 and 1964, sports injuries (to weakened joints and bones) have become the No. 2 reason for a boomer's visit to a doctor's office, behind the common cold, according to a 2003 survey by National Ambulatory Medical care.

A Bureau of Labor Statistics study said, "infirmaties, associated with the athletic activities of middle-aged adults, were the source of 488 million days of restricted work in 2002."

When people sweat, they don't just sweat out water, they sweat out a "soup" that contains all of the essential nutrients found in blood. "Athletes," whether an adult weekend warrior, a jazzercise or aerobics participant, pee wee league participant, high school, university or professional athlete or a person who does physical labor in their trade or hobby sweat - that's why their joints and bones breakdown before those of non-sweating librarians.

Orthropedic surgeons report that doctors in the U.S. perform 270,000 knee replacements and 170,000 hip replacements annually.

The problem with joint replacement surgery is that the implantation of a joint prosthesis does not stop the progression of osteoporosis or arthritis systemically - only the use of a complete vitamin and mineral supplement program can have any hope of stopping the progression of the disease and reversing or curing it altogether.

Arthritis or degenerative joint disease is not a single disease, rather it is a group of diseases that have similar origins and symptoms - they cause pain, inflammation, and a restricted range of motion of the joints. There are more than 100 joint diseases, with the most common form called osteoarthritis.

A joint that has osteoarthritis is characterized by a degeneration of the cartilage, allowing the opposing bones of the joint to rub against each other. The primary symptom of osteoarthritis is pain, with inflammation appearing late in the disease. The White and the Black medical doctors of America want patients to believe that osteoarthritis is "incurable."

Arthritis and osteoporosis were rarely reported in Blacks during the slave days and only became a serious problem in the Black community after the turn of the 20th century. Today, according to the Center for Disease Control, 80 percent of Black people over the age of 50 already have arthritis and osteoporosis of one type or another and to one degree or another; and that one-third of all American adults suffer from some type of joint disease.

Neither arthritis or osteoporosis are genetic diseases, they are simple nutritional deficiency diseases. The December 2002 issue of *Time* magazine featured a cover story entitled, *The Coming Epidemic of Arthritis*.

It's almost as if we are watching the "formation of an epidemiological perfect storm." The appearance of the 76 million "baby boomers," and the exercise and fitness craze amongst them has produced a younger generation of arthritis victims. Add five decades of jogging, high impact aerobics and fast breaking sports such as football, soccer, tennis and basketball, where quick stops and sharp turns and pivots produce maximum wear and trauma to the vertebrae, ankles, knees and hips.

Despite the high rate of arthritis and osteoporosis in the Black community, there is not a single medical treatment designed to prevent or cure these diseases. The universal medical approach to arthritis and osteoporosis in both Whites and Blacks is pain management and surgery - both of which will ultimately fail.

Interestingly enough we learned 300 years ago in Europe and over 1,000 years ago in China, how to prevent and cure arthritis and osteoporosis in animals.

While medical doctors claim that, "Someday you may pop a pill and your cartilage will continue to grow, but (they claim) that's 10 years away at least." In fact, we have been able to repair and regrow cartilage, ligaments, tendons, connective tissue, bone matrix and bone for more than 300 years.

Osteoarthritis is a complex vitamin and mineral deficiency disease - calcium supplementation alone or combined with glucosamine and chondroitin sulfate, will produce some benefit for the prevention, management and even reversal of arthritis to some small degree. If you want to prevent and cure osteoarthritis 100 percent it requires the use of calcium and a minimum of 89 additional vitamin, amino acid, essential fatty acid and mineral cofactors.

Osteoporosis: Osteoporosis is a disease of all of the bones of the body including the 24 bones of the skull, face and jaw.

In November of 2001, a five year Canadian Multi-Centre Osteoporosis Study study of almost 10,000 men and women over the age of 50, showed that, "men are as likely as women to suffer from osteoporosis."

"We didn't think that men fractured," said Jonathan Adachi, a rheumatologist and professor of medicine at St. Joseph's Hospital and McMaster University. In fact we knew 100 years ago that men suffered from osteoporosis at the same rate as women; it was not until 1958, when the pharmaceutical industry learned how to manufacture estrogen, that osteoporosis became a "post menopausal women's problem."

The results turn the tables on the belief that post menopausal women are the prime victims of the condition - osteoporosis occurs at an equal rate in men.

Osteoporosis is characterized by a loss of more than 60 different minerals, particularly calcium, to varying degrees from the skeleton. Specific diseases that are manifestations of osteoporosis include periodontal disease (osteoporosis of the face and jaw), osteoarthritis, shrinking height, kidney stones, bone spurs, calcium deposits, hypertension, glaucoma, Osgood-Slaughter disease, trigeminal neuralgia, Bell's palsy, peripheral neuropathies, sciatica, compression fractures, life threatening fractures of the hips and major leg bones; degenerative disc disease often accompanies ankylosing spondylitis or the grafting together of bone spurs and calcium deposits on adjacent vertebrae.

Arthritis: The human skeletal system contains 143 different joints which act as hinges, levers, and shock absorbers, and "permit us to stand, walk run, kneel, jump, dance, sit, grasp, push, pull, shake hands, scrach our heads, eat, and otherwise perform the thousands of motions, that get us through the day."

There are three basic types of joints, all of which are susceptible to arthritis and osteoporosis:

Synarthroidal joints - skull: immovable joints.

Amphiarthroidal joints - sacroiliac: slightly movable joints.

Diarthroidal joints - synovial joints: hinge joints - elbow.
    ball and socket - hip; saddle joints - base of thumb; gliding joints - hands and feet

    There is a basic anatomy common to all joints;

Joint capsule - a resilient, tendon-like, water-tight, fluid-filled "sack" that surrounds the joint and helps to hold the adjacent bones in proximation and proper alignment.

Synovium - the inner lining of the joint capsule, that produces synovial fluid to lubricate as well as nourish the joint cartilage.

Cartilage - typically covers the ends of bones, absorbs shock, creates a slippery surface, allowing the ends of the bones to "glide" painlessly over each other during movement.

Ligaments - heavy connective tissue bands (flat or round) or "straps" that connect one bone to another.

Tendons - heavy connective tissue bands (flat or round) or "straps" that originate in the muscle and insert into the bone.

Bursae - sacs filled with synovial fluid that cushion ligaments and tendons and reduce friction as they move over joints.

Collagen - a protein that is banded together into cables or ropes to form tendons, ligaments, cartilage, bone matrix, and other connective tissue structures.

Proteoglycans - are large molecules that consist of proteins and sugar. Cartilage is made up of water, collagen and proteoglycans.

Glucosamine sulfate - is an important building block of the
    proteoglycans. Glucosamine is required to make glycosaminoglycans
    - proteins that bind water in the cartilage matrix. Glucosamine is also
    a stimulant of cartilage growth.

Chondroitin sulfate - acts as a "liquid magnet." A long chain of repeating
    sugars, chondroitin helps attract fluid into the proteoglycan molecule.
    Cartilage has no blood supply, so all of the nourishment for
    cartilage comes with the liquid that ebbs and flows into the joint
    as pressure to the joints comes and goes. Without this fluid cartilage,
    becomes malnourished, dry, thinner and begins to break
    down. Stimulates production of proteoglycans, glycosaminoglycans
    and collagen - all building blocks of cartilage.

Osteoarthritis Compared With Rheumatoid Arthritis

Osteoarthritis	Rheumatoid Arthritis
Historically began after age 40	Appears between 25 and 50
Has a gradual progression	Comes & goes suddenly, without warning
Redness, warmth & swelling rare	Redness, warmth, & swelling is universal
Clinical effects worse in weight bearing joints	Affects most joints; clinical effects worse in digits
does not cause systemic disease	Overall feeling of illness, fatigue, weight loss & fever
Caused by nutritional deficiencies	caused by an infection with *Mycoplasma synoviae*

There are several forms of arthritis: generally speaking, arthritis refers to a degenerative disease of the cartilage, bone, ligaments, tendons of the joints, disc between the vertebrae, and bone matrix. Noise, crackling, crepitation, pain, swelling and a loss of range of motion characterize arthritis.

Osteoarthritis - Medical doctors typically believed that osteoarthritis was a disease of old age; however, they now know that osteoarthritis, the most common of almost 100 forms of arthritis, begins its methodical, relentless, at first painless course while one is a toddler - there are few minerals in apple juice, cold cereals, peanut butter and jelly sandwiches or macaroni and cheese.

Osteoarthritis is not an autoimmune disease, it is not a genetically transmitted disease, but rather osteoarthritis is one of many manifestations of osteoporosis and is caused by a shopping list of nutritional deficiencies.

Initially, one won't believe anything has gone wrong, until one reaches their 20s, 30s, 40s or 50s and begin to hear joint noises, feel twinges or notice low levels of pain and sometimes swelling - by then the damage has already been done and even the best of medical therapies can't do much more than reduce pain, reduce inflammation or surgically replace the joints with prosthesis, while the cartilage and bones of the afflicted joints and bones continue to degenerate.

Vioxx, a very popular analgesic (COX-2 inhibitor anti-inflammatory and pain reliever) and anti-inflammatory drug that claimed to be safer than aspirin or ibuprofen, was produced by Merck and approved by the FDA. For the four years that Vioxx was on the market, there were 139,000 heart attacks and strokes that were attributed to the drug; and depending on whose data you use, 55,000 to 85,000 of these affected people died.

The FDA never removed the drug from the market, rather Merck "voluntarily" removed Vioxx from the market because there was $27 billion worth of law suits by the fourth year on the market - they could never sell enough to pay off the anticipated court awards.

In 1998, the Consumer Product Safety Commission examined emergency room visits, and they discovered that sports-related injuries to baby boomers had risen by 33 percent since 1991, and created $18.7 billion in medical costs.

July 11, 2002, the *New England Journal of Medicine*, published an article that stated, "Arthroscopic Knee Surgery for arthritis is a worthless procedure."

In a type of study, only rarely conducted, some subjects received the standard arthroscopic surgery of their knee, while others underwent a "sham" surgery where the skin was incised but the joint itself was not actually operated on.

At every examination over the following two years, those individuals that had received the sham surgery could painlessly climb stairs and walk faster on average than those who received the complete arthroscopic surgery.

So, why do orthopedic surgeons continue to use the failed procedure? In 2001, the income generated for surgeons by this one failed procedure was $1.5 billion, however, it was not illegal - so, why would surgeons give it up? And the surgeons continue to use the "useless" surgery.

Rheumatoid arthritis - Rheumatoid arthritis is a systemic, infectious disease, caused an infection with *Mycoplasma synoviae*. The most visible changes characteristic of rheumatoid arthritis are swollen joints and crippling stiffness with a reduction in the range of motion, especially in the small joints of the hands and feet. "People who are jogging one day," says Dr. Stanley Cohen of Dallas' St. Paul Medical center, "can't get out of bed two weeks later." In chronic cases of rheumatoid arthritis, there are usually severe anatomical and dysfunctional changes, oftentimes rendering the affected joints useless.

Approximately 75 percent of those infected with rheumatoid arthritis also have osteoarthritis. The *Mycoplasma* organism is an interesting bug in that it initially and preferentially attacks and infects the respiratory system of rats, pigs, non-human primates and humans. The infection tends to be manifested as a chronic and persistant bronchitis that just won't go away; when the organisms invade the circulatory system they lodge in the synovial capsule of the joints and produce the classic rheumatoid arthritis.

Mycoplasma synoviae has features of a virus in that it uses the host's DNA and RNA to duplicate; and, it has the weaknesses of bacteria, in that antibiotics will almost always kill it.

To eliminate the acute phase of rheumatoid arthritis, tetracycline or minocycline can be used at the low acne dose that a teenager would use for one entire year along with the nutritional treatment for osteoarthritis.

After one year, the antibiotic may be discontinued, however, the nutritional support must be continued forever to avoid a reoccurance of the osteoarthritis.

The characteristic deformities of the fingers that come with chronic rheumatoid arthritis can sometimes be overcome without surgery by the use of the nutritional approach.

Non-medical Treatment of Arthritis & Osteoporosis for Adults

1. 90 Essential nutrients
2. 2,500 mg of available (liquid) colloidal chelate calcium
3. Glucosamine sulfate (1,000 - 2,000 mg per day)
4. Chondroitin sulfate (800 - 1,600 mg per day)
5. Collagen (2,500 mg per day)
6. Omega-3 essential fatty acids (12 gm per day)
7. Peppermint Oil, Tea Tree Oil, Eucalyptus Oil
8. Antioxidants

   Green tea

   grape seed extract,

   exotic fruit juices

9. Topical analgesia (pain relief) - CM Cream

Chapter 10

"$30 billion War on Cancer a bust?"

- Steve Sternberg
USA Today May 29, 1997

"It's not the amount of meat in your diet that increases risk of colo-rectal, breast and protate cancer, its how you cook the meat that counts."

- Dr. Joel D. Wallach & Dr. Ma Lan
Dead Doctors Don't Lie, 1993

"Until now, the benefits of green tea might have seemed a little like, well, snake oil. Now the evidence is overwhelming that there's something to it."

- Lester Mitscher, Chemist
University of Kansas, 1998

Cancer in Blacks

"Despite 26 years of work and $30 billion spent, the U.S. government's 'War on Cancer' has failed to reduce death rates from the disease substancially," according to an analysis published in the May 29, 1997 issue of the *New England Journal of Medicine*.

United States Cancer Incidence

Dates	1900	1962	1971	2005
Total Cases	25,000	520,000	635,000	1,368,200
Prostate	N/A	31,000	35,000	231,230
Breast	N/A	63,000	69,600	217,440
Lung	N/A	45,000	80,000	186,550
Colon/rectum	N/A	72,000	75,000	146,940
Uterus	N/A	N/A	N/A	51,000

"The effect of new treatments for cancer on morbidity has been largely disappointing," said John Bailer and Heather Gornick from the University of Chicago. "The most promising approach to the control of cancer is a national commitment to prevention," he continued.

In the 1993 audiocassette tape, *Dead Doctors Don't Lie*, Wallach quoted a study that said, "An anti-cancer diet had been found." The September 15, 1993 study was sponsored by the National Cancer Institute, it stated that it was "the first hard evidence that some antioxidant substances can provide a 'protective' effect against cancer."

The study showed that daily doses of beta carotene, vitamin E and selenium dramatically reduced the risk of dying from cancer for thousands of farmers in a rural region of China.

Other dietary supplements, including vitamin C, retinol, zinc. riboflavin, molybdenum and niacin, had no statistically significant effect on cancer deaths after five years.

However, in a group of 29,000 middle-aged Chinese adults between the ages of 40 and 69, those who took the combination of beta carotene, vitamin E and selenium for five years, "the results were striking: 13 percent fewer deaths from all cancers; 21 percent reduction in deaths from stomach cancer; and a nine percent decrease in deaths from all causes."

In 1994, a study of 50,000 men and in January 21, 1999, a study of 90,000 women disputed the popular belief that a high fiber diet protects against colon cancer. "Fiber intake has no effect on the risk (of colon cancer)," according to researchers for the Nurses Health Study, published in the *New England Journal of Medicine*. The theory that fiber reduces the risk of colon cancer, stems from a faulty 1960's observation that colon cancer, a leading killer in the West, was uncommon in tribal Africa, where they consumed whole grains.

On March 10, 1999, the *Journal of the American Medical Association*, the Harvard Nurse's Health Study of 90,000 women, showed that, "eating a low fat-diet does not reduce the risk of breast cancer. In a comparison of those women consuming less than 20 percent of their calories as fat versus those who ate more than 50 percent of their calories as fat showed that there was no difference in the rate of breast cancer."

"I'm convinced by the results," says lead author Michelle Holmes of Brigham and Women's Hospital in Boston; she continued, "It will have to be up to the public and the scientific community to make their own conclusion."

Lung Cancer

Smoking is a significant health hazard. In 1995, the Brown and Williamson documents showed that the tobacco industry knew of the health risk produced by their products. Approximately 10 percent of the world's deaths are the direct result of tobacco use.

The World Health Organization states that the annual number of premature deaths caused by tobacco use will rise to 10 million by the year 2005. Over 500 million people currently, including the 200 million currently under the age of 20, will die from tobacco related disease, and 100 million of these will be classed as middle age. World-wide, 1.1 billion people smoke, and 330 million of them are Chinese.

Six million children between the ages of 13 and 19 are addicted smokers, and over 140,000 children under the age of 13 are addicted smokers.

Smoking among Blacks is significantly higher than the smoking rate in Whites.

According to the National Academy of Sciences report "*Marijuana and Health*" smoking marijuana also increases the risk of cancer. Marijuana smoke has 50 percent more carcinogenic hydrocarbons than cigarette smoke.

There are more than 2,000 chemical substances generated by tobacco smoke.

The "gas phase" contains carbon monoxide, carbon dioxide, ammonia, nitrosamines, nitrogen oxide, hydrogen cyanide, sulfurs, nitriles, ketones, alcohols and acrolein.

The tars from tobacco contain highly dangerous carcinogenic hydrocarbons, which include nitrosamines, benzo(a)pyrenes, anthracenes, acridines, quinolines, benzenes, naphthols, naphthalenes, cresols, and insecticides (DDT), as well as a few radioactive compounds such as potassium-40 and radium 226.

U.S. Deaths: War vs. Smoking

World War I	116,708
World War II	407,316
Korean War	54,246
Vietnam War	58,151
Smoking (annually)	603,700
Second Hand Smoke/year	55,000

On January 26, 2006, Christopher Haiman, an assistant professor of preventative medicine at the University of California, reported a study of more than 180,000 people, half of whom were minorities, in *The New England Journal of Medicine*, that, "Blacks who smoke up to a pack (of cigarettes) per day are far more likely than Whites who smoke similar amounts to develop lung cancer." The racial differences disappeared when smokers puffed one and one half packs or more each day. Even though the study was not designed to look at the possibility of a genetic link, Haiman couldn't resist saying, "the findings suggest (Black) genes may be one of the factors that explain the phenomenon."

On February 8, 2006, "A surprise finding that low-fat diets don't reduce the rate of heart disease, stroke, breast cancer, or colo-rectal cancer, or even result in greater weight loss," was published in the Journal of the *American Medical Association*.

Cancer, the second leading cause of death in the United States, was expected to kill 564,800 Americans in 1998, one out of four of America's deaths due to disease. Cancer "kills more people annually than AIDS, accidents, and homicide combined." In 1996 cancer accounted for the deaths of 469,406 White Americans (23.5 percent of total White deaths) and 60,766 Black American deaths (21.5 percent of Black deaths). After a more-than-10-year trend of increasing age-related mortality continuing throughout the 1980s, "(b)etween 1991 and

1995 the national cancer death rate fell 2.6 percent." Age-adjusted mortality rates for African Americans - initially lower than Whites, but began increasing and surpassing Whites from the mid-1950s onwards - demonstrated similar trends, reaching a high point of 182.0 deaths per 100,000 resident population in 1990, which was 38.4 percent higher than the White rate, declining to 171.6 deaths per 100,000 population by 1995, which was still 35.1 percent higher than the White death rate.

Between 1979 and 1990, Ki Moon Bang observed: "Blacks experience 10 percent higher cancer incidence and 30 percent higher mortality than Whites."

The American Cancer Society (ACS) noted in 1998 that "(b)etween 1990 and 1994, mortality rates fell 0.3 percent per year for Whites and 0.7 percent per year for African Americans." However, the Black/White racial mortality rate ratios, 1.3 in 1980 and increasing to 1.4 in 1990, remained at the higher level in 1995, and the slight drop in cancer mortality in 1996 was not generally considered statistically significant by the NCHS.

Of all racial or ethnic groups in the United States, Black Americans continue to have the highest age-adjusted cancer incidence and mortality rates for all types of cancer. The ACS noted:

Overall, African Americans are more likely to develop cancer than Whites. In 1994, the incidence rate for African Americans was 454 per 100,000 and for Whites, 394 per 100,000. Between 1990 and 1994, cancer incidence rates increased 1.2 percent per year in African Americans and decreased 0.8 percent per year in Whites.

Cancer incidence is at least 50 percent higher in African Americans for multiple myeloma, cancers of the esophagus, cervix (uterus), larynx, prostate, stomach, liver, and pancreas than for Whites. Additionally, Blacks demonstrate a higher incidence rate for cancers of the lung and bronchus, urinary bladder, and leukemia.

Due to the higher age-adjusted mortality rates previously quoted, "African Americans are about 30 percent more likely to die of cancer than Whites." Blacks have at least a 50 percent greater risk than Whites of dying of multiple myeloma and cancers of the esophagus, cervix (uterus), liver, and pancreas. Much of this differential negative outcome results from the five year relative survival rate for African Americans, which "was 12 percent below that of non-minorities (1973 - 1981)" and is now 44 percent compared to 60 percent for Whites - a 16 percent differential - between 1989 and 1993.

As Claudia Baquet and Carrie Hunter noted in *Cancer Prevention and Control*

(1995): "African Americans experienced substantially higher age-adjusted incidence and mortality rates and lower 5-year survival rates for cancers of the oral cavity and pharynx, esophagus, liver, pancreas, lung and bronchus, cervix uteri, and prostate than their White counterparts." Also, "(A)lthough African American patients exhibited lower overall incidence rates than did Whites for cancers of the colon and rectum, breast, and corpus uteri, the mortality rates among the African Americans for these cancers were comparable to or exceeded those for Whites." As the ACS noted, "Much of this difference in survival can be attributed to African Americans being diagnosed at a later stage of disease."

A significant proportion of cancers, including lung, prostate, colon and rectum, and female breast, cervical and uterine cancers, are diagnosed more often at localized stages in Whites than in Blacks. Examining survival trends, Bang points out: "Survival rate is much better in cases of localized cancer than regional cancer." And according to the ACS, "Most of these sites represent cancers for which screening tests are available; and early detection and timely treatment could increase survival." Truly, for Black Americans, the delays in detection and thus later stage at diagnosis, often followed by more delay and differences in treatment, far override biological/constitutional factors for catastrophic outcomes. The Secretary's Task Force revealed:

Much of the scientific literature to date supports a hypothesis that the differences in cancer survival between non-minorities and Blacks are attributable to social or environmental factors rather than inherent genetic or biological deficits. Emerging theory suggests that distribution of resources…can affect cancer outcome, e.g., survival.

Although lifestyle factors such as cigarette smoking, alcohol consumption, eating habits, occupational/environmental exposure to toxins, lead, asbestos, lack of screening, genetic/biological factors, and cultural values and taboos, and belief systems regarding health care are important; socioeconomic status/resource distribution: "Factors such as lack of health (education), health insurance or transportation can impede access to health care and can lead to late diagnosis and poorer survival," according to the ACS. To make matters worse, "Studies have shown that poor and medically underserved populations receive fewer cancer prevention services," according to George Alexander, past chief, Special Population Studies Branch of the NCI.

Breast Cancer

Risk of Developing Breast Cancer by Age

By age 25: 1 in 19,608	By age 60: 1 in 24	By age 30: 1 in 2,525
By age 65: 1 in 17	By age 35: 1 in 622	By age 70: 1 in 14
By age 40: 1 in 217	By age 75: 1 in 11	By age 45: 1 in 93
By age 80: 1 in 10	By age 50: 1 in 50	By age 85: 1 in 9
By age 55: 1 in 33	> age 85: 1 in 8	

On November 18, 1998, Dr. Wei Zheng of the University of South Carolina, reported that "cooking meat at high temperature, by frying or grilling, has long been known to produce a chemical compound called heterocyclic amines that are known to cause cancer."

"Charred meat has a high level of heterocyclic amines," said Zheng. This is also true of fish and chicken cooked at high temperatures. Women in the study were ranked according to how they cooked their meat, fish or poultry; a score of three for those who ate their meat cooked rare or medium; and a score of nine for those who ate their meat cooked well done or burnt.

Among women who preferred all meat very well done, with doneness scores of nine, there was a 462 percent greater chance of having breast cancer than for women who ate their meat cooked rare or medium."

Breast Self Examination

With minimal instruction, every woman can effectively perform breast self-examination. Patients actually find approximately 90 percent of breast cancers, either accidently or by self-examination. Less thn 40 percent of women regularly perform breast self-exmination. Breast self-examination should be performed monthy by both men and women.

Monthly breast examinations should be performed within a few days after the menstrual period begins as the breasts are not swollen or tender at that time. Following menopause, one should pick a particular date each month to examine the breasts:

1. Stand topless in front of a mirror and lean forward. Look for changes in size or shape of breasts, discharge, or pulling inward of nipples, and for changes in skin tones and texture.

2. Place hands behind the head and repeat observations.

3. Push down on hips with both hands and repeat observations.

4. Lie on your back and examine each breast; gently but firmly palpate or feel for masses.

5. Examine each armpit in a similar manner, gently but firmly feeling for lumps.

6. Squeeze nipple, look for discharge, changes in shape, size or skin of nipple.

Screening mammograms do not prolong life amongst women between the ages of 40 to 49. These women are now being told that there is no role for mammographic screening in this age group. In February 1993, the NCI hosted an international workshop that concluded: "The randomized trials of women ages 40 to 49 are consistant in showing no statistically significant benefit in mortality after 10 to 12 year follow-up ... no reduction in mortality from breast cancer that can be attributed to screening."

Phytoestrogens

There is a medical dogma that says older Japanese women have a lower incidence of breast cancer than American women because of their significant consumption of soy products, compared with American women. This dogma has propelled the soy industry in America to dizzying sales heights.

Soy has two phytoestrogens, genistein and daidzem. They were initially considered to be weak estrogens because they bound weakly to the alpha Estrogen receptor. It is now realized that the soy phytoestrogens are strong sources of estrogen-like sterols because they bind tenaciously to the beta Estrogen Receptor. Animal studies have revealed that soy products can stimulate the growth of estrogen receptor positive breast cancer cells implanted into "nude" mice.

Extracts of vitex, dong quai, American ginseng, and cohosh (all contain phytoestrogens) all bind estrogen receptors in exactly the same way as estrogens produced naturally in the human.

Prostate Cancer

2005 Incidence of Prostate Cancer per 100,000

USA African American	137
USA White	101
USA Japanese-American	47
Zimbabwe Blacks	29
Uganda Blacks	28
USA Chinese-American	20

In 1987, Dr. Thomas A. Stamey, Stanford University urologist, was amongst the first to suggest that the level of prostate-specific antigen (PSA), a protein produced in the prostate gland, might be useful in the early detection of prostate cancer. Since then, millions of men over the age of 50 have relied on the PSA test to screen for protate cancer.

In October of 2004, Stamey made headlines again when he declared that, "The (PSA) test is not a reliable predictor of (prostate) cancer."

Based on an analysis of more than 1,300 prostates removed over the past 20 years, Stamey reported in the October 2004 issue of the *Journal of Urology*, that, "the PSA test is currently predictive of cancer in only 2 percent of cases."

Stamey now says, "A higher PSA level may most often reflect a harmless age-related increase in prostate size."

Studies have shown that 80 percent or more of men over age 70 die with - but not from - prostate cancer.

While the standard medical methods of preventing and treating cancer in America had not changed substantially for more than 100 years (surgery, chemotherapy and radiation), there are ancient therapies and veterinary therapies, that can actually prevent and cure cancer.

On April 1912, in *Popular Mechanics Magazine*, Profesor A. von Wasserman, of Berlin, Germany, declared that he had "discovered a chemical substance (selenium) that will cure cancer in mice." He went on to say, "(the trace mineral) selenium has a selective action on cancer cells and not on healthy tissue," and that, "the cancer in mice is so similar to that in humans, that it is believed an important advance had been made toward the cure of that veritable scourge (cancer, in humans)."

On Decmber 1996, Dr. Larry Clark, of the University of Arizona, School of Medicine, "found that a modest dose (200 mcg) of selenium supplement reduced overall cancer incidence by 42 percent, further, taking selenium slashed cancer death rates by half."

Clark's randomized double-blind study (the "gold standard" of medical research) "followed 1,312 older people ....for an average of seven years. Half took 200 mcg of selenium the others took a placebo."

Clark's final analysis showed that, "taking selenium slashed the occurrence of prostate cancer by 69 percent, colorectal cancer by 64 percent, and lung cancer, 39 percent."

Wallach petitioned the FDA to obtain claims for the cancer preventing-benefits of selenium and was successful in getting the following claims: "This product contains selenium, a trace mineral that has been shown to reduce the risk of certain cancers," and "this product contains selenium, a trace mineral that can produce certain anti-cancer substances in the body"

Colon Cancer

On October 1, 1998, a study of 90,000 women in the Harvard Nurses' Health Study, was reported in the journal, *Annals of Internal Medicine*; the report showed that, "Women who take multivitamins for at least 15 years may cut their risk of colon cancer by 75 percent." Edward Giovannucci, a researcher at Brigham and Women's Hospital in Boston, continued, "The study went on to say that women who took in 400 mcg of folic acid had substancially fewer colon cancers than women who took in only 200 mcg per day."

There are no drugs that will reduce one's risk of colon cancer by one percent.

Leukemia

On November 5, 1998, researchers from the Memorial Sloan Kettering Cancer Center in New York said, "Arsenic may prove a life saver against one type of leukemia." Their study involved 12 seriously ill patients suffering from acute promyelocytic leukemia, an often fatal type of leukemia that originates in the blood and bone marrow.

"We now know that arsenic (trioxide) can safely bring patients with APL into remission, which may ultimately give them a second chance at life," said Dr. Raymond Worrell Jr., a leukemia specialist at Sloan-Kettering and senior author of the study, which was published in the *New England Journal of Medicine*.

Chinese researchers were the first to report success with arsenic as a treatment for APL in the journal *Blood*, in 1997. In China, those APL patients treated with arsenic remained in "remission" for as long as 10 years without a recurrence.

"Based on highly sensitive molecular tests, treatment with arsenic trioxide appears to exceed the effectiveness of any single drug to treat APL," said Dr. Steven Soignet, the lead author of the study, "it is strikingly effective."

Green Tea

In China and Japan, many epidemiological studies have found that people who drink a few cups of tea each day have a lower risk of cancer than Americans, especially Black Americans. In 1992, it was reported that mice given green tea and then exposed to chemical carcinogens and ultraviolet light developed an astonishingly smaller number of tumors than mice that were not given green tea. The green tea fed mice developed 90 percent fewer tumors than those not getting the green tea.

Additional studies have shown that, "even after cancer is already diagnosed, the catechins or EGCGs in green tea can block the enzyme that tumors employ to grow new capillaries which are required for new tumor growth" according to Jerzy Jankun, a tumor biologist at the Medical College of Ohio.

Green tea contains antioxidants called catechins (EGCG) that are 100 times more powerful than vitamin C in protecting against free radical damage to DNA; and 25 times more effective than vitamin E in protecting DNA from free radical damage.

The University of Colorado released a report indicating that one serving each day of the antioxidants found in dark berries can reduce the risk of colon cancer by 60 to 80 percent.

Certain juices, including orange juice, cranberry juice, and certain exotic fruit juices such as pomegranate, noni, aloe, mangosteen and fruit/vegetable juice blends provide high levels of cancer protective antioxidants as indicated by high ORAC value ratings.

ORAC value or Oxygen Reactive Absorption Capacity measures the capability of an antioxidant to neutralize free radical damage.

Certain proteins, angiostatin and endostatin, found in shark cartilage, hyaluronic acid, collagen, gelatin, etc., have been shown to prevent or inhibit the formation of capillaries that are necessary to support metastasis (spread of cancer).

To grow into a large cancer mass, cancer cells must become vascularized

- a process known as angiogenesis. Many substances reduce or inhibit angiogenesis.

The Anti-Cancer Diet (prevention/treatment)

Eat roasted, boiled and stewed meats, fish and poultry, eat four eggs poached or soft scrambled in butter each day; eat several servings of tomatoes, onions and green leafy vegetables daily.

Supplement with:

1. 90 essential nutrients
2. Selenium 1,000 mcg/day
3. Antioxidants
   Green tea
   Grape seed extract
   Tomato extract
   Noni
   Mangosteen
   Aloe
4. Angiostatin & Endostatin

Give up fried foods, do not eat or cook in margarine, do not use oils to cook with, do not eat meat cooked well done, do not eat burnt fats; supplement daily with a complete multiple vitamin-mineral supplement containing the 90 essential nutrients, consume a wide variety of fruit and vegetable based antioxidants, consume the equivalent of four cups of green per day, and supplement with an extra 400 to 1,000 mcg of selenium per day.

Limit alcohol consumption to no more than one drink per day.

Statistically, this diet and nutritional supplement program can reduce your risk of cancer between 39 percent and 462 percent.

Chapter 11

"It takes a little bit of sugar to get the medicine to go down."

- Mary Popins

"Some (Black) households, however, had their own methods. Some families wore cotton bags holding camphor or moth balls around their necks to ward off the threat. Others drank violet-leaf tea, inhaled salt water up the nose, or carried hot coals sprinkled with sulphur or brown sugar through the house to avert the danger."

- Kirsty Duncan
Hunting the 1918 Flu
2003

Slave Quarter Cures: Materia Medica

The Black slaves, excluded from their master's healthcare systems, took the best plant medicines that the Native Americans had, added the medicines from their Arab, Spanish, Dutch and English captors and tormentors, and brought with them their own African "medicines" to create a body of slave medicine or "Slave Quarter Cures." These cures had to be cheap, real cheap, because the Black slaves were financially incapable of paying for the state of the art English health care.

Asafetida Pouches: These little pouches contained the aromatic Asafetida herb, also known as "Asafizzit" or "devil's dung," from India. The plant was cut off at the root and a foul smelling (it is one of the few herbs that is more pungent than garlic), aromatic sap exuded from the cut surface. The sap droplets hardened into rock-like hard beads; it was ground into a powder and mixed with flour.

One teaspoon of the Asafetida powder-flour mix was placed between two squares of gingham, calico or plain cotton cloth 2 inches by 2 inches, that were then sewn together to form a pouch or bag.

The Asafetida pouch or bag was hung by a string around the neck of children and young adults or pinned to their shirt and used in particular to protect children from the common infectious childhood diseases. These pouches were to be worn by all children from birth to age 12. This simple, but effective slave quarter approach protected children and young adults from epidemics and the common childhood diseases that are commonly vaccinated against in modern times.

Because of the foul smell, children often times "lost" their Asafetida pouch. Lost patches were promptly replaced. Southern Black grandmothers constantly produced these pouches as they sat and rocked on their porch and had one on the ready in the event that a child did not have one on.

Asafetida powder was often mixed with gin and taken as a remedy for worms.

According to Dr. Yah Yah, a 19th century New Orleans Voodooist, violets were excellent for avoiding or curing any illness or disease. To gain the benefits, place some violets in a red flannel pouch, tie the top shut, attach a cotton string and wear the bag around your neck for protection - change the violets in the bag every seven weeks.

During the 1918 "Spanish" flu, Black families still resorted to the old ways that had saved Blacks from epidemics, pandemics and plagues during the 17th century. Some families wore cotton bags holding camphor or moth balls around their necks to ward off the threat. Others drank violet-leaf tea, inhaled salt water up the nose, or carried hot coals sprinkled with sulphur or brown sugar through the house to avert danger.

Poultices of goose-grease, bran, and lard and turpentine and compresses of fir-tree stills (pine needle distillate), mutton tallow, and mustard were among the concoctions applied to the chests of the sick. Drinks of of warm milk, ginger, sugar, pepper, and baking soda soothed the ill.

Wood Ashes: A world-wide by-product of daily living prior to the use of coal (Industrial Revolution 1741) and electricity (1882), wood ashes (plant minerals) were the slave's historical source of essential minerals. It was used as a fertilizer for garden vegetables, grains, fruit trees and nut trees; it was also used as "culinary ashes" that were mixed into their food as a condiment; and was used to cut costly table salt at a rate of 10 parts wood ashes to one part salt.

U.S. Patent No. 1 was awarded in 1790, for the production and use of wood ash as fertilizer. "Potash fever" roared through the new American country as the demand for the wood ash fertilizer and culinary ashes skyrocketed; trees were burned by the millions of tons for the ash destined for domestic use as well as for export to England.

A good description of how wood ashes are used as fertilizer in primitive societies is found the the book, *Hunza Land*, by Dr. Allen E. Banik:

"...the Hunza soil is almost a manufactured soil. Every solitary thing that can serve as food for vegetables, field crops and fruit trees is diligently collected, stored and distributed in rationed equality over every square foot of hundreds of terraces. Sunken compost pits are conveniently located, and into them go ashes from cooking and heating fires, inedible parts of vegetables, pulverized animal bones, dead leaves, rotten wood and the collected manure of animals."

A typical recipe from the 18th century that included culinary ashes, "potash" or "pearl ashes" was found in Amelia Simmons' cookbook, *American Cookery*, 1796:

Simmons' Honey Cake

6 pounds flour	1 oz ginger
2 pounds honey	orange peel (orange zest)
1 pound sugar	2 tsp pearl ahes (potash or white ahes)
2 oz cinnamon	6 eggs

Dissolve the pearl ash (white wood ash) in milk, put the whole together, moisten with milk, bake 20 minutes.

"Pearl ashes" or "potash" are specifically the wood ashes that came from underneath the cast iron cooking pot. Pearl ashes and potash were whiter than the surrounding ashes because the heat reflected downward from the bottom of the cooking pot burned more of the carbon, thereby producing whiter ashes - no one wanted gray or black bread or cake.

Herbs: Herbs are plant medicines. The slave's knowledge of herbs came from their African culture and from the herbal traditions of their various tormentors, task masters and allies, including Europeans, Arabs, East Indians and Native Americans. Herbs were commonly used as plant medicines to treat a great variety of diseases.

Voodoo: Folk voodoo magic, which has its origins in African magic and religion, appeared in the New World between the sixteenth and nineteenth centuries on the slave ships. In an effort to avoid persecution for their pagan belief system, slaves blended their gods and spiritual beliefs into a mix of Catholicism and Christianity to appease their masters. This hybridization of beliefs resulted in the creation of several spiritual practices. In Brazil it produced Macumba and Candomble; in Cuba it gave rise to Santeria and Nyannego; in Jamaica to Bongoism and African Cumina (also known as Maroon Dance); in Trinidad to Shango; in Haiti to Voudoun (Voodoo); and in the United States to Hoodoo.

South American Indian beliefs, along with the Spiritism of Allan Kardec, popular in the 19th century, played key roles in the formation of Macumba in Brazil; Jewish, Christian and pagan folklore of the European immigrants to the U.S., mixed with the traditional herbs of the Native American shamans, produced Hoodoo folk magic.

Name Magic

In *The African Presence in Carribean Literature*, Edward Kamau Braithwaite, says: "People feel a name is so important that a change in his name could transform a person's life." Faith in the secret power of the name is significant in Hoodoo magic. It is the reason why Hoodoo doctors adopt animal names such as, Dr. Crow or Dr. Snake, they assumed the name of the bird, reptile or beast from which they derived their power. For a Hoodoo doctor, picking a new name is a way of shaping their personal destiny. Likewise, blues musicians such as Muddy Waters, Lightnin' Hopkins and Howlin' Wolf took on their names as a sign of magical transformation.

"Anything may be conjure and nothing may be conjure...."

- *Zora Neale Hurston*
Mules and Men, 1935

"Sour, hour, vinegar-V!
Keep this sickness off of me!"

- *Voodoo vinegar charm*
Times-Picayune, New Orleans
October 20, 1918 (peak of Spanish Flu Pandemic)

Essential Oils:

A common 17th - 21st century home remedy approach used by poor rural Blacks and poor Black and White city dwellers for many diseases was the "turpentine and sugar" remedy. They boiled or steamed the needles, twigs, wood and bark of coniferous trees including the spruce, fir, pine and cedar to obtain a "distillate" of the sap and pitch held within the plant or "fir spill." The slaves would put several drops of the resulting "turpentine" or "essential oils" on sugar and consume the mix several times each day for several weeks. This basic approach to essential oil therapy was used by the Black slaves and Native Americans for many diseases including sore throat, respiratory infections, influenza, sinusitis, toothache, headache, arthritis, osteoporosis, pain, for disinfecting wounds and as a general fall and spring "tonic."

Essential oils of evergreen trees or "turpentine" was used daily in many Black households. Four drops of sugar each morning before leaving the house or seven drops on the feet each morning before going to school. It was thought to be important to use only seven drops; four on the sole of one foot and three on the sole of the other foot; the number seven was felt to enhance the healing and cleansing power of the "turpentine."

Applying the "turpentine" to the soles of the feet in this manner was believed to protect the body from catching disease encountered when exposed to infected strangers. Applying "turpentine" to the soles "made it so people can't cross you." In other words, the person using the "turpentine" on their feet was protected from people trying to put a bad spell or curse on them and was protected from evil that might "cross" their path.

While African Americans valued education and opportunity to go to school, there was considerable fear of illnesses that might be contracted while at school. And there was considerable concern that one's body be free of disease and fully cleansed before returning to school in the fall.

To achieve "cleansing," fir tree or spruce tree "turpentine" or essential oils were mixed with castor oil and given by mouth two days prior to going to school at the end of summer. If the mixture was vomited up or if diarrhea did not ensue, the treatment was repeated until it stayed down and diarrhea followed. Depending on the household, this "cleansing" was repeated weekly or at a minimum twice each year. In every household castor oil was given weekly. Wealthier Negroes were able to afford a slice of fresh orange to chase the dose of castor oil.

The castor oil/turpentine "cleanse" was not a tasty ritual, however, the lack of access to the White medical system and the knowledge that when one got sick you either got well or died, motivated the women of the house to firmly insist that all members of the household submit to the castor oil/turpentine purge to ward off illness.

Slave Quarter Cures

Essential oils are aromatic volatile lipids distilled from shrubs, flowers, trees, bark, roots, bushes and seeds. Simple vegetable oils are easily oxidized and rapidly become rancid and transformed into dangerous trans-fatty acids. Essential oils can't become "rancid," they are not "greasy" and contain potent aromatic antimicrobials.

The following list includes many of the essential oils or "turpentines" ultimately used by Black healers, root doctors, conjurers and home remedies for common "Slave Quarter Cures."

Angelica (*Angelica archangelica*)

Beginnings: Angelica originated in Syria and then transplanted to France and Belgium. Known as the "Holy Spirit root' or the "oil of angels" by Europeans; Angelica's healing powers were believed to be so strong that it was believed to be of divine origin. During the time of Paracelsus, the essential oil of angelica was known to protect against the plague. During the European plague of 1660 angelica stems were chewed to repel infection.

Description: Two similar oils are either distilled or solvent-extracted into solutes; one is derived from the seeds and the other from the roots. Key constituents:
  Lemonene (60-70%)
  Alpha Pinene (5-8%)
  Alpha and Beta Phellandrene (3-6%)

Therapeutic Properties: Angelica has been used for a female tonic, bruises, colic, coughs, respiratory infections, indigestion, menopause, dysmenorrhea, PMS, anorexia and rheumatic discomfort.

Routes of Application; The essential oils of angelica can be applied by inhalation and massage. It mixes well with patchouli, vetiver, clary sage and most citrus oils.

Caution: Consult physician before use if pregnant; avoid use if diabetic; because angelica contains bergopten, it can be photo-sensitizing and should not be applied to skin that will be exposed to direct sunlight or UV light within three to five days.

Anise (*Pimpinella anisum*)

Beginnings: Anise originated in Turkey.

Description: The essential oils are extracted by steam distillation from the seeds. Key constituents:
- Trans-Anethol (85-95%)
- Methyl Chavicol (2-4%)

Therapeutic properties: Anise is an antiseptic, antispasmodic, diuretic and stimulant.

Basil (*Ocimum basilicum*)

Beginnings: Basil was commonly used in baths and as a massage oil by Greek nobles - they particularly liked its fragrant aroma. The name basil is derived from the Greek word for king - basileus; in Ayurvedic medicine it is called tulsi. It is considered a holy herb in India, sacred to the gods Krishna and Vishnu. The Egyptians used basil as an offering to their gods and combined with essences of myrrh and frankincense it was used to embalm bodies for their passage into the "after life." The 16th century herbalist, John Gerard said, "Basil's scent taketh away sorrowfulness.

Description: Basil is a native plant of Africa, Egypt, Madagascar and the Seychelles and in modern times it is commonly grown as a culinary herb in Europe. It typically is a compact bush that grows up to three feet in height and is characterized by small white to pink flowers. The oil is distilled from the leaves; it is pale greenish-yellow in color with "sweet green overtones." Key ingredients:
- Methylchavicol (estragol) (40-80%)
- Linalol (10-50%)
- 1,8 Cineole (1-7%)
- Eugenol (1-10%)

Therapeutic properties: Basil is used as a nerve tonic; can be used to lift fatigue, anxiety and depression. Basil is commonly used for relieving the symptoms of bronchitis, colds, fever, gout, increases circulation and calms indigestion. Basil is characterized by having high levels of linalool or fenchol; it is primarily used for its antiseptic properties; basil high in methyl chavicol is more anti-inflammatory than antiseptic; and basil with high levels of eugenol has both anti-inflammatory and antiseptic properties. Basil mixed with thyme is used topically as an antiseptic.

Routes of application: Basil can be applied medicinally through inhalation, baths and massage. It has both hot and cold properties and has an invigorating effect. Basil blends well with bergamot, black pepper, cedarwood, Roman chamomile, clary sage, coriander, cypress, eucalyptus, fennel, geranium, ginger, grapefruit, juniper, lavender, lemon, marjoram, niaouli, orange, oregano, palmarosa, pine, rosemary, sage, tea tree and thyme.

Cautions: Basil should not be used for therapeutic purposes in pregnant women; overdoses can cause sudden and severe depression.

Bay (*Pimenta racemosa*)

Beginnings: Roman emperors commonly wore bay laurel leaves (Roman laurel *Laurus nobilis*) as a sign of wealth and power and to repel evil spirits. Greek priestesses chewed bay leaves for their soporific effect; after meals bay was chewed as a breath freshener. Historically the bay leaf was distilled with rum in the West Indies, which gave rise to "bay rum," a classic hair tonic and body rub for colds, flu, bronchitis and muscle aches.

Description: Bay is commonly used as a culinary herb. Bay grows as an evergreen bush, shrub, tree or hedge that can reach 25 feet in height and is characterized by clusters of yellowish-green flowers that bloom in the spring. A spicy, highly aromatic oil, is extracted from the leaves and berries; the essential oil is a yellowish-brown color.

Therapeutic properties: Bay is a general tonic, pulmonary antiseptic, and is commonly to relieve bronchitis, colds and flu. It can be used to promote healthy digestion and restful sleep. Bay oil can be used topically to relieve rheumatic aches and pains.

Routes of application: Bay is used as an inhalant, and as an additive to bathes and massage. Bay is commonly used in perfumes and exotic bath essences. Bay blends well with bergamot, black pepper, cardamom, cinnamon, clove, coriander, frankincense, geranium, ginger, lavender, grapefruit, lemon, mandarin, nutmeg, orange, petitgrain, rosemary, sandalwood and ylang-ylang.

Benzoin (*Styrax benzoin*)

Beginnings: The gum of the benzoin tree was first used in Asia in incense to repel evil spirits. The Arabic name for benzoin, *luban jawi*, means "incense of Java"; European traders shortened the name to banjawi, then later changed it to "Benjamin" and then finally to benzoin. The tincture is used in friar's balsam and as a "fixative" in perfume.

Description: The benzoin tree is cultivated in Borneo, Java, Malaysia, Sumatra, and Thailand. Similar to the rubber tree, its gum is extracted from the bark by making a deep incision in he trunk. The gum is dark and is characterized by reddish-brown streaks. The pigments contain oils that produce a vanilla-like aroma.

Therapeutic properties: Benzoin is commonly used for urinary infections. Benzoin has a warming, relaxing property; it is useful as a chest rub for treating bronchitis, coughs and colds. Benzoin is effective for treating skin problems and gout.

Routes of application: Benzoin can be used in inhalants, massage oils and in cough medicines. Benzoin produces an energizing oil which can be used in one of two forms; a simple tincture or as a compound (the tincture is the safest form of benzoin).

Bergamot (*Citrus bergamia*)

Beginnings: Bergamot originated in Morocco; its use as an essential oil started in Italy after Christopher Columbus brought bergamot to Bergamo in northern Italy from the Canary islands. It was reintroduced to Italy in 1600 from Pergamum, now called Bergama, Turkey. Today, as much as 90% of the world's supply of bergamot is produced in Reggio di Calabria, Italy. It is also a major cash crop of the Ivory Coast, Morocco, Tunisia and Algeria.

Description: The small bergamot tree produces a small, green, bitter fruit that is related to the orange. The essential oils of bergamot are extracted from the fresh peel of the ripe fruit. The oil is emerald green and smells spicier than lemon oil. Bergamot is used as the flavoring for Earl Grey tea. Key constituents:
    Limonene (30-45%)
    Linaly Acetate (22-36%)
    Linalol (3-15%)
    Gamma-Terpinene (6-10%)
    Beta-Pinene (5.5-9.5%)

Therapeutic properties: Bergamot has a strong uplifting and refreshing action. It has antiseptic properties and is commonly used for infections of the mouth, sore throat and skin. Bergamot is used to reduce fever and relieve bronchitis and indigestion.

Routes of application: Bergamot mixes well with most essential oils including black pepper, clary sage, cypress, frankincense, geranium, helichrysum, jasmine, lavender, mandarin, nutmeg, orange, ormenis flower, rosemary, sandalwood, vetiver and ylang-ylang; and is a common additive to perfumes.

Cautions: In concentrations above one percent bergamot can irritate the skin. While bergamot is commonly added to commercial "tanning" products to stimulate the production of melanin, one should never attempt to make their own tanning agents.

Birch (*Betula lenta, B. aleghaniensis*)

Beginnings: The birch tree originated from Scandinavia, Canada and northern Maine. The essential oil of birch is steam distilled from the wood. The North American birch is a large tree with a fragrant inner bark; it is the original source of the "wintergreen" essential oil used for chewing gum, candy and breath mints.

Description: Key ingredients:
  Methyl salicylate (> 90%)

Therapeutic properties: Birch has analgesic, antispasmodic, anti-inflammatory, and liver tonic properties; it is used to relieve arthritis pain, rheumatism, inflammation, muscular pain, fibromyalgia, tendonitis, cystitis, eczema, acne, urinary infections, gout, gallstones, edema, high blood pressure, osteoporosis and cramps. The active ingredient, methyl salicylate, is similar in action to that of commercial aspirin as an anti-inflammatory and analgesic.

Routes of application: Birch essential oil can be applied neat to the bottom of the feet or diluted with an "extender" oil; it can be diluted at three to five drops in a Tblsp of bath oil and added to a "hand hot" bath or used as a massage oil. Birch oil blends well with basil, cypress, geranium, juniper berries, lavender, lemongrass, marjoram, peppermint and Roman chamomile.

Cautions: Pregnant women should consult their physician before use.

Black Pepper (*Piper nigrum*)

Beginnings: Black pepper originated in Madagascar, Egypt and India. Black pepper was used in India over 4,000 years ago. Black pepper was used by the Egyptians in their art of mummification (black pepper was found in the nostrils and abdomen of the mummy of Ramses II). Indian monks ate several black peppercorns each day to maintain their stamina and energy.

Description: Black pepper is a climbing woody vine. The vine clings to trees for support and shade; it is characterized by small white flowers that produce red berries. The essential oils of black pepper are steam distilled from the berries. Key constituents:
    Beta Caryophyllene (25-35%)
    Limonene (8-12%)
    Sabinene (8-10%)
    Alpha and Beta Pinenes (10-15%)

Therapeutic properties: The essential oils of black pepper are used to relieve toothache, as an expectorant, enhances digestion, has analgesic properties and reduces fever.

Routes of application: Black pepper oil is classically applied to the bottom of the feet; massage; add to base oil for safe application. Black pepper oil mixes well with bergamot, clary sage, clove coriander, cumin, fennel, frankincense, geranium, ginger, grapefruit, juniper, lavender, lemon, lemongrass, lime, mandarin, marjoram, myrrh, orange, nutmeg, palmarosa, patchouli, rosemary, sage, sandalwood, spikenard, tea tree, valerian, vetiver, ylang-ylang and other spice oils.

Cautions: If pregnant consult physician before use.

Cajeput (*Melaleuca leucadendra*)

Begginings: In Malaysia and other Indonesian islands, cajaput was used for respiratory infections, headaches, rheumatism, toothache, skin conditions, throat infections and sore muscles. Cajeput is the Malaysian word for white tree.

Description: Key constituents:
    Eucalyptol (50-65%)
    Alpha-Terpineol (7-13%)
    Limonene (3-8%)
    Alpha Pinene (1-3%)

Therapeutic properties: Cajeput is traditionally used to relieve arthritis, acne, respiratory infections, asthma, bronchitis, urinary complaints, coughs, cystitis, stiff joints, toothache, hay fever, bursitis, headaches, insect bites, intestinal problems, laryngitis, dysentery, psoriasis, rheumatism, sinusitis, oily skin, sore throat and viral infections.

Routes of application: Inhale, diffuse or rub on the bottom of the feet. Cajeput mixes well with wintergreen/birch, eucalyptus, juniper berries, and peppermint.

Cautions: Pregnant women should consult physician before use.

Calamus (*Acorus calamus*)

Beginnings: Calamus was an herb traditionally used in Egypt and India to help improve mental focus, wisdom and sexuality. In China, calamus was used to aid in the recovery from stroke. Historically Native Americans would hold a piece of calamus root in their mouth while running long distances.

Description: Essential oils of calamus are extracted from the plant root by steam distillation. Key constituents:
- Alpha and Beta-Asarones (16-22%)
- Shyobunone (5-10%)
- Shyobunone Isomeres (7-13%)
- Calamuscenone (6-12%)
- Preisocalamendial (5-9%)

Therapeutic properties: Singers use calamus to numb their throat so they can clear the phlegm and keep singing; calamus can be used to reduce the desire for tobacco; deodorize feet, asthma, bronchitis, colic, memory loss, stroke and depression.

Routes of application: Inhale, massage, foot rub.

Cardamom (*Ellettaria cardamomum*)

Beginnings: Cardamom is a relative of ginger root; it is a native to the Middle and Far East; it is used traditionally in Turkish coffee and East Indian Chai tea to impart a warm spicy flavor and aroma. East Indians have traditionally considered the cardamom aroma warmly romantic and a potent aphrodisiac. The essential oil was first distilled in 1544 by Valerius Cordus, following a Portuguese explorer's procuring them from the southwest Indian coast.

Description: Perennial rush-like herb with blade-like leaves; it produces small yellow flowers with violet tips that produce a seed-bearing fruit. Key constituents:
- Alpha Terpinyl Acetate (45-55%)
- 1,8 Cineol (Eucalyptol) (16-24%)

Linalol (4-7%)
Linalyl Acetate (3-7%)
Limonene (1-3%)

Therapeutic properties: The oil of cardamom is antiparalytic, antispasmodic, antibacterial, expectorant, anti-infectious and a vermafuge. The oil of cardamom has been used to relieve paralysis, arthritis, rheumatism, cardiac disorders, seizures, spasms, pulmonary disease, indigestion, intestinal maladies and a wide variety of urinary tract inflammations, anorexia, coughs, debility, bad breath, fatigue, headaches, heartburn, nausea, sciatica, dysmenorrheal, insect bites and general infections.

Routes of application: Diffuse, rub on the bottom of the feet, chest, stomach, solar plexus and thighs. The oil of cardamom blends well with bay, bergamot, black pepper, cedarwood, cinnamon, cistus, clove, coriander, fennel, ginger, grapefruit, jasmine, lemon, lemongrass, *Litsea cubeba*, mandarin, neroli, orange, palmarosa, patchouli, petitgrain, rose, sandalwood, vetiver and ylang-ylang.

Caution: Pregnant women should consult their physician before use.

Carnation (*Dianthus caryophyllus*)

Beginnings: This variety of carnation is commonly referred to as "pinks" because of the color of the flowers. The name is thought to have been derived from the fact that the flower was woven into ancient garlands and crowns - hence carnation.

Description: The carnation was first described in Egypt and France. The plant is a perennial herb, with long, narrow, gray-green leaves growing from the stem. The pink flowers have many petals that sport ragged edges. Where the petals join the center of the flower there are dark pink to purple flecks. The essential oils are extracted from the flower heads. It takes 500 kilograms of flowers to make 1 kg of "concrete" that yields 100 grams of carnation absolute. Key constituents:

Eugenol
B-Caryophyllene
Caryophyllene Oxide

Therapeutic properties: Carnation essential oils have calmative, sedative, neurotonic and soporific properties. It is used primarily in aroma-psychology, such as emotional problems, stress, feelings of detachment, overactive mind, inability to communicate, emotional solitude and feelings of neglect.

Routes of application: Carnation blends well with rose maroc, rose otto, cardamom, clary sage, clove, coriander, hyacinth, jasmine, lemon, black pepper, bergamot, lemon, Roman chamomile, orange, neroli, vetiver, ylang-ylang and yuzu.

Cedarwood (*Cedrus deodora, C. atlantica, Juniperus virginiana*)

Beginnings: Cedarwood oil, like sandalwood oil, was used by the Egyptians for embalming solutions. Cedarwood was historically and is also currently used as an antiseptic and as an ingredient in cosmetics. The original cedarwood oil came from the Lebanese cedar, however, it now comes from the red cedar. Bible references include: Leviticus 14:4 *"Then shall the priest command to take for him that is to be cleansed two birds alive and clean, and cedarwood, and scarlet, and hyssop."* Leviticus 14:6 *"As for the living bird, he shall take it, and the cedarwood, and the scarlet, and the hyssop, and shall dip them and the living bird in the blood of the bird (that was) killed over the running water."* Leviticus 14:49 *"And he shall take to cleanse the house two birds, and cedarwood, and scarlet, and hyssop."*

Description: The cedarwood tree is an evergreen that grows to 50 to 100 foot tall and can live for more than 1000 years. The cedarwood oil comes primarily from North Africa and the United States. The clear syrup-like oil is steam distilled from cedarwood unfit for furniture manufacturing; the scent of cedarwood oil is the same as the scent from wooden pencils. Key constituents:
   Alpha-Himachalene (10-20%)
   Beta-Himachalene (35-55%)
   Gamma-Himachalene (8-15%)
   Delta-Cadinene (2-6%)

Therapeutic properties: Typically cedarwood is used for respiratory problems including bronchitis and catarrh; for skin problems including acne, alopecia, dandruff and eczema; and as a diuretic and urinary disinfectant.

Routes of application: Can be administered as an inhalant and topically as a massage oil; can increase sexual response. Cedarwood oil blends well with bay, bergamot, cardamom, clary sage, cypress, eucalyptus, frankincense, geranium, grapefruit, juniper berries, lavender, marjoram, orange, neroli, palmarosa, petitgrain, rosemary, rose oils, sandalwood and ylang-ylang.

Cautions: Pregnant women should contact their physician before use. Cedarwood can produce skin irritation in high concentrations.

Chamomile (*Anthemis nobilis;* German -*Matricaria recutita*)

Beginnings: The Egyptians looked at chamomile as a sacred flower and used it to connect with the sun god. Chamomile was used in various religious ceremonies and used medicinally for seizures and reducing fevers.

Description: Chamomile is found growing wild and is cultivated throughout Europe and North Africa. Chamomile is characterized by fine feathery leaves with small white or yellow-centered daisy-like flowers. The chamomile fragrance is so apple-like, that the Spanish call it manzanilla, or "little apple" and the Greeks refer to it as "earth apples." The pale blue oil is extracted by steam distillation from the flowers and has an apple-like aroma. Chamomile blends well with rose, geranium and lavender oils. Key constituents:
  Chamazulene (2-5%)
  Bisabolol Oxide A (32-42%)
  Trans-Beta-Farnesene (18-26%)
  Bisbolol Oxide B (3-6%)
  Bisbolone Oxide A (3-6%)
  Cis Spiro Ether (4-8%)

Therapeutic properties: Chamomile is prized for its anti-inflammatory and sedative properties. It is typically used for earache, allergies, anemia, burns, dermatitis, diarrhea, fever, indigestion, insomnia, dysmenorrhea, menopause, rheumatism, toothache, inflammation, acne, chilblains, muscle spasms and ulcers.

Routes of application: Chamomile is used as an infusion; the oil can be used orally, in the bath, and as hair preparations. Can be diluted and used for childhood ailments. It blends well with bergamot, Roman chamomile, lavender, cypress, frankincense, geranium, marjoram, lemon, grapefruit, naiouli, patchouli, pine, ravensara, rosemary and tea tree.

Chamomile (Roman) (*Chamaemelum nobile*)

Beginnings: Plant originated in Egypt and Utah. Roman chamomile was used traditionally to relieve skin conditions. For centuries mothers have used chamomile to sedate crying children.

Description: The essential oil of Roman chamomile is steam distilled from the flowers. A very gentle aromatherapy essential oil. Key constituents:
  Isobutyl Angelate + Isamyl Methacrylate (30-45%)
  Isoamyl Angelate (12-22%)
  Methyl Allyl Angelate (6-10%)

Isobutyl n-butyrate (2-9%)
2-Methyl Butyl Angelate (3-7%)

ORAC value (Oxygen Radical Absorbance Capacity) 2,446

Therapeutic properties: Calming for preanesthesia and tension, antispasmodic, anti-inflammatory, antiparasitic, relieve earache, reduce fever, soothe stomach ache and indigestion, relieve toothaches and teething pain, relieves allergies, supports skin regeneration, bruises, cuts, depression, insomnia, muscle tension, restless legs, dermatitis, acne, eczema and rashes.

Routes of application: Diffuse, inhale, massage and apply to feet, ankles and wrists; Roman chamomile blends well with lavender, geranium, lemon, tea tree, eucalyptus, palmarosa, grapefruit, rose, neroli, jasmine, clary sage.

Cinnamon (*Cinnamomum zeylanicum, C. verum*)

Beginnings: Cinnamon oil was mixed with just about all ancient Chinese remedies. Cinnamon is one of the oldest spices known to man; it is mentioned in the Old Testament; and it was used liberally in ancient Greece, Rome and Egypt. The word cinnamon is derived from the Greek word kinnamon which translates to tube or pipe which describes the bark when used as a spice.

Description: Cinnamon is a large, subtropical evergreen tree with a fragrant bark that can be harvested twice a year for 30 years; it is widely grown in the Far East, Asia, the East Indies and China. Cinnamon has a distinct hot pepper-like taste and aroma; the twigs and leaves are distilled to produce a pungent, bitter-sweet aromatic oil; the oil is a dark yellow-brown color; cinnamon oil is oftentimes used in perfumes. Key constituents:
Trans-Cinnamaldehyde (40-50%)
Eugenol (20-30%)
Beta-Carophyllene (3-8%)
Linalol (3-7%)

ORAC value - 103,448

Therapeutic properties: Cinnamon can be used to relieve fatigue and depression; it is used as a general tonic and as a tonic for the respiratory and digestive systems; the oil is particularly useful for coughs, colds, flu, stomach ache and diarrhea. Cinnamon oil is frequently used as an aphrodisiac and for impotence.

Routes of application: Can be administered as an inhalant or a massage oil. Cinnamon can be burned to prevent the spread of flu virus; cinnamon bark and oils are added to pot pourri; can be used as a massage oil or compress to relieve muscle spasm. It blends well with clove, nutmeg, ylang-ylang, mandarin, orange, lemon, grapefruit, *Litsea cubeba*, rose maroc, bay, bergamot, carnation, coriander, cardamom, frankincense, geranium, ginger, lemongrass, marjoram, patchouli, petitgrain and yuzu.

Cautions: Cinnamon should be used as a diluted oil in low concentrations or under professional supervision. Pregnant women should contact their physician before use.

Citronella (*Cymbopogon nardus*)

Beginnings: Citronella originated from Sri Lanka, Philippines and Egypt. Numerous cultures have used citronella oil to eliminate intestinal parasites, relieve indigestion and dysmenorrhea, headaches, respiratory infections, neuralgia, fatigue, insomnia, oily skin and used as an insecticide.

Description: This tropical grass releases its strong fragrance when broken or crushed. It was recorded that in 332 B.C., Alexander the Great, while riding an elephant along the Egyptian border "became intoxicated when he inhaled the fragrance of nard (the old name for citronella) as it was crushed under foot." The oil of citronella is steam distilled from the leaves. Key constituents:
- Geraniol (18-30%)
- Limonene (5-10%)
- Trans-Methyl Isoeugenol (4-10%)
- Geranyl Acetate (5-10%)
- Borneol (3-8%)

Therapeutic properties: Antibacterial, insect-repellant, antifungal, anti-inflammatory, antiseptic, antispasmodic, deodorant and insecticidal. The oil of citronella can be used as an attractant in fish bait, however, a primary use was and is to keep away mosquitoes, ticks, fleas and other insects.

Routes of application: Diffuse, inhale, massage and topical application to the bottom of the feet. Citronella oil blends well with bergamot, cedarwood, geranium, lemon, orange and pine.

Clary Sage (Clear eye) (*Salvia sclarea*)

Beginnings: The name Salvia is taken from the Latin word for "good health." It is used to flavor cheap wines in an effort to give them the taste of Muscatel; it is used in the manufacturing process of vermouths and liqueurs; in Europe it is commonly used as a substitute for hops in fermenting beer; the seeds are used in folk medicine for conditions of the eye - thus the name "clear eye."

Description: Clary sage is a biennial plant that grows up to three feet high; it is characterized by long hairy leaves, it has lilac-pink flowers that sit atop long thin stems. The oil is steam distilled from the flowering tops. Key constituents:

    Linalol   (7-24%)
    Linalyl Acetate (56-78%)
    Germacrene D (2-12%)
    Sclareol   (0.4-3%)
    Geranyl Acetate

Therapeutic properties: Clary sage has antiseptic, calmative, tonic, emmenagogue, anti-infectious, antispasmodic, antisudorific, aphrodisiac, nerve tonic, nervine and estrogen-like properties; it is typically used for muscular fatigue, dysmenorrhea, calming, stress, depression, cramps and excessive perspiration.

Routes of application: Diffuse or apply topically to the bottoms of the feet, ankles and wrists. Clary sage blends well with geranium, lemon, grapefruit, lavender, sandalwood, cypress, mandarin, jasmine, juniper, rose, bergamot, bay, black pepper, Roman chamomile, coriander, lime, patchouli, tea tree (it blends well with almost all flower absolutes in small doses).

Cautions: Pregnant women should consult their physician before use.

Clove (*Syzygium aromaticum, Eugenia caryophyllata*)

Beginnings: Clove originated from Madagascar and the Spice Islands. Clove was used in ancient China as a medicine. To fragrance their mouth, courtiers would put clove buds in their mouth when speaking to the emperor. The people on the island of Ternate were free of epidemics until the 16th century when Dutch conquerors invaded the island and destroyed the clove groves cultivated on the island. European doctors historically breathed through clove-filled leather beaks to ward off the plague. It is steam distilled from the buds and small twigs and stems.

Description: Clove buds are the unripe flower buds of a short, slender evergreen tree that bears buds for at least 100 years. Key constituents:

  Eugenol (75-87%)
  Eugenol Acetate (8-15%)
  Beta-Carophyllene (2-7%)

ORAC value 10,786,875

Therapeutic properties: Clove essential oils are highly antimicrobial, antiseptic, analgesic, bactericidal, antioxidant, hemostatic and anti-inflammatory. Historically used as a home remedy and by the dental industry for relieving toothache. According to Dr. Jean Valnet, clove oil can prevent contagious diseases, relieve arthritis, bronchitis, cholera, cystitis, dental infection, amoebic dysentery, diarrhea, tuberculosis, acne, fatigue, thyroid dysfunction, bad breath, headache, hypertension, insect bites, nausea, neuritis, dermatitis, rheumatism, sinusitis, skin cancer, chronic skin disease, bacterial colitis, sores, viral hepatitis, warts and lymphoma.

Route of application: Diffuse, inhale or apply topically diluted with a carrier oil; add one or two drops in four fluid ounces of water and use as a gargle. Apply undiluted to palms of hands, bottom of feet, and on gums and teeth. Blends well with bay, basil, bergamot, cinnamon, clary sage, grapefruit, geranium, grapefruit, ginger, jasmine, lavender, lemon, nutmeg, mandarin, orange, palmarosa, peppermint, Roman chamomile, rose, rosemary and ylang-ylang.

Caution: If pregnant consult physician before use; do not use undiluted clove oil directly on an infant's skin or gums.

Comfrey (Symphytum officinale)

Beginnings: Comfrey was a favorite of Nicholas Culpepper, the 17th century English herbalist - "Comfrey helpeth those that spit blood or maketh a bloody urine." The root was boiled in water or wine and the extract consumed for all kinds of internal maladies, "ulcers of the lungs" and increase blood flow.

Description: Comfrey commonly grows wild along wet or swampy waterways. Comfrey is characterized by hairy and fleshy leaves that can irritate the skin of susceptible individual. The stem grows to three feet in height and displays a purplish flower. The leaves and roots are used in herbal decoctions, while the oil is extracted from the stalks and leaves.

Therapeutic properties: Comfrey contains allantoin, a phytochemical that can stimulate cell repair following injuries; comfrey oil is of particular use for the treatment of wounds and skin disorders including eczema, psoriasis, stretch marks, dysmenorrhea and menopausal symptoms.

Routes of application: Massage oils and compresses.

Coriander (*Coriandrum sativum*)

Beginnings: The coriander plant originated in Russia and India. Coriander seeds were found in the ancient Egyptian tombs of Ramses II and Tutankhamun. Coriander seeds are used to flavor Chartreuse and Benedictine liqueurs that are produced by French monks.

Description: Coriander oil is steam distilled from the seeds. Key constituents:
- Linalol (65-78%)
- Alpha-Pinene (3-7%)
- Camphor (4-6%)
- Gamma-Terpinene (2-7%)
- Limonene (2-5%)
- Geranyl Acetate (1-3.5%)
- Geraniol (0.5-3%)

Therapeutic properties: Coriander oil is used to relieve arthritis, diarrhea, respiratory infections, indigestion, digestive spasms, poor circulation, diabetes, supports pancreatic function, rheumatism, gout, infections, measles, headaches, nausea, muscular aches, pain, neuralgia, acne, psoriasis, dermatitis, PMS and stress.

Routes of application: Primarily applied topically; it blends well with bergamot, clary sage, black pepper, cardamom, cinnamon, clove, cypress, frankincense, geranium, ginger, grapefruit, jasmine, lemon, neroli, nutmeg, orange, palmarosa, petitgrain, pine, ravensara, sandalwood, vetiver and ylang-ylang.

Caution: Coriander oil can be strongly sedative. If pregnant consult physician before use.

Cypress (*Cupressus sempervirens*)

Beginnings: Egyptians used cypress oil for medicinal purposes and the wood to decorate their stone coffins. The tree gave its name to the island of Cyprus. The cross of Jesus is believed to have been made of cypress. The French traditionally plant the trees in grave yards.

Description: A tall conical evergreen tree that originated in Asia, and became commonly grown throughout the Mediterranean, including Algeria and France. The essence is made by distilling the leaves, twigs and cones of the tree. The oil is clear and pale yellow or green; it has a spicy and refreshing fragrance similar to pine needles. Key constituents:

Alpha-Pinene (40-65%)
Beta-Pinene (0.5-3%)
Delta-3-Carene (12-25%)
Limonene (1.8-5%)
Cedrol (0.8-7%)
Myrcene (1-3.5%)
Manoyle Oxide
Iso-pimaradiene
Karahanaenone

Therapeutic properties: Cypress is highly regarded for its astringent and antiseptic properties. Cypress oil is commonly used as a sedative, muscular tonic, for circulatory problems, colds, coughs, flu, hemorrhoids, varicose veins, whooping cough, dysmenorrhea and menopausal problems. It is often used as an astringent for oily skin.

Routes of application: Massage, bath and inhalation are common routes of administration. Cypress oil can be used as a compress for swelling or rheumatism. It blends well with bergamot, cedarwood, clary sage, eucalyptus, frankincense, geranium, jasmine, lemon, lavender, orange, lime, pine, mandarin, marjoram, ravensara, Roman chamomile, rosemary, sandalwood and tea tree.

Cautions: Cypress oil should not be used for people who suffer from hypertension.

Eucalyptus (*Eucalyptus globulus*)

Beginnings: Eucalyptus is one of the tallest trees in the world. The tree originated in Australia and transplanted to Tasmania, China, United States, Brazil and the Mediterranean. There are about 200 or more species of eucalyptus trees. The Australian Aborigines are considered to be the first people to use eucalyptus oil medicinally. Eucalyptus oil was first distilled in Australia in 1788 by the Surgeon General of the colony, Dr. John White. The tree is fast growing and requires large volumes of water which has allowed it to convert swamp land into usable farm land. Because this process eliminated the breeding ground of the malaria mosquito, the trees took on the reputation during the 1800s of eliminating "miasma" or "fever" when the etiology and epidemiology of malaria was not yet known. Thus the name - "fever tree."

Description: The silvery, pale blue-green leaves produce a pale- yellow oil. The oil has a cool camphorous aroma. The fresh leaves produce a high yield of a highly

potent oil that is used widely in aroma therapy programs. Key constituents:
    1,8 Cineole (58-80%)
    Alpha Pinene (10-22%)
    Limonene (1-8%)
    Para-Cymene (1-5%)
    Trans-Pinocarveol (1-5%)
    Aromadendrene (1-5%)
    Globulol (0.5-1.5%)

ORAC value 24,157

Therapeutic properties: The primary constituent of eucalyptus oil is the highly antiseptic eucalyptol. The oil is highly regarded for use in asthma, bronchitis, flu, sinusitis, clear a stuffy head, cystitis, skin infections, rheumatism and sores; it is also used to reduce fever and as a diuretic.

Routes of application: Baths, diffuse, inhalation, humidifier, rubs and massages. The oil has a general cooling effect on the body. Eucalyptus oil blends well with cypress, geranium, German chamomile, ginger, grapefruit, juniper, lavender, lemon, lemongrass, melissa, peppermint, pine, Roman chamomile, rosemary, sandalwood and thyme.

Caution: Do not take internally; if pregnant consult with physician.

Fennel (*Foeniculum vulgare*)

Beginnings: Ancient Greeks and Romans used fennel seeds to give them strength and long life, repel evil spirits, kill fleas and to freshen their breath. Pliny lists 22 remedies that contained fennel. The Greek name for fennel was marathrion (derived from maraino) which translates to "to grow thin."

Description: Fennel is a perennial/biennial European plant that grows by the sea; they have delicate bright green feathery leaves; there are tufts of yellow flowers; it is often referred to as "licorice" plant or anise because it tastes and smells like licorice. The oil is steam distilled from crushed seeds. The fresh leaves are used as a culinary herb for fish dishes; fennel seeds, which smell and taste like anise seed are used in the making of licorice. Key constituents:
    Trans-Anethol (60-80%)
    Fenchone + Linalol (12-16%)
    Alpha-Pinene (3-5%)
    Methyl Chavicol (2-5%)

Therapeutic properties: Fennel seeds are used as a diuretic and a laxative; they have estrogen-like properties; they are used in the treatment of colic, constipation, indigestion, kidney stones, menopausal symptoms, nausea and obesity. It is used as a carminative, emmenagogue, phyto-estrogen, galactagogue, depurative, diuretic, stimulant, regenerative, anti-spasmodic, antiseptic, antibiotic, vermafuge and expectorant. Fennel seeds can be used to increase milk production for breastfeeding.

Routes of application: Massage, the oil is used for indigestion and flatulence; it is an ingredient of gripe water and is commonly defused as a tea. Fennel blends well with juniper, geranium, lavender, bergamot, black pepper, cardamom, cypress, ginger, grapefruit, lemon, marjoram, niaouli, pine, ravensara, rosemary, sandalwood and ylang-ylang.

Cautions: People with seizure disorders and estrogen sensitive cancer should avoid the use of fennel oil; pregnant women should consult their physician before use.

Frankincense (*Boswellia thurifera*)

Beginnings: Frankincense (also known as olibanum) and myrrh were the first tree resins used as incense by the Egyptians. They were burned to cleanse the air of sick rooms and during religious ceremonies to fend off evil spirits. Frankincense and myrrh were considered to be as valuable as gem stones. Frank incense and myrrh were given as gifts to the Christ child by the three Magi or Wise Men. The Christ child was born in a barn filled with animal manure, animal urine, flies and animals. The child mortality rate was very high 2000 years ago and the choice of the anti-bacterial and the anti-viral resins of frankincense and myrrh were the perfect and appropriate gifts. The resin comes from a small tree grown in Arabia, Africa and China. It was first brought to Europe in the late 17th century.

Description: To harvest the resin, a deep cut is made into the tree trunk, the resin flows from the bark and forms into teardrop shaped nuggets that harden on contact with the air. The oil is spicy with camphor tones that become lemon-like when mixed with myrrh. Key constituents:
    Alpha-Pinene (28-49%)
    Limonene (10-16%)
    Sabinene (3-7%)
    Myrcene (8-12%)
    Beta Caryophyllene (3-7%)

Alpha Thuyene (4-8%)
Paracymene (2-5%)

Therapeutic properties: The aroma has an uplifting effect with enhancement of concentration; it acts as an expectorant and is useful for bronchitis, coughs, colds, and laryngitis; frankincense is used as an astringent for the skin and is thought to reduce wrinkles.

Routes of application: Inhalation, baths and massage. Inhale to loosen catarrh or relax with several drops in the bath. It blends well with basil, bergamot, clary sage, cypress, geranium, grapefruit, lavender, lemon, orange, mandarin, myrrh, neroli, palmarosa, patchouli, pine, rose maroc, rose otto, sandalwood, vetiver and ylang-ylang.

Geranium (*Pelargonium adorantissimum, P. graveoloens*)

Beginnings: The geranium originated in Africa and was not brought to Europe until 1690. It was used in the ancient days for tumors, burns and wounds.
Description: Geranium plants are widely cultivated throughout Europe; the plant grows to two feet in height. There are 700 species of geranium, most of which are grown for their flowers. The pelargoniums in particular produce a rich lemony and sweet yellow-green essential oil. The oil is distilled from the leaves, stalks and flowers. Key constituents:
Citronellol + Nerol (35-50%)
Citronnellyl Formate (9-15%)
Geraniol (5-10%)
6,9-Guaiadene (4-8%)
Isomenthone (4-8%)

Therapeutic properties: Geranium oils are used for relieving tension and depression; they are antispasmodic, stimulates adrenal, anti-tumor, astringent, hemostatic, antibacterial, and antifungal; they are used to support skin health, they are used for chilblains, circulatory problems and superficial wounds.

Routes of application: Geranium is used frequently in the perfume industry; as an essential oil, it can be used as a massage and inhaled. Geranium blends well with all other oils, including lemon, grapefruit, lavender, rosemary, Roman chamomile, peppermint, clove, clary sage, ginger, palmarosa, ylang-ylang, sandalwood, mandarin, juniper, cypress, bergamot, black pepper, fennel, frankincense, orange, rose maroc, rose otto and jasmine.

Caution: If pregnant consult physician.

Ginger (*Zingiber officinale*)

Beginnings: The ginger plant was originally native to China. Ginger was historically used to combat the effects of motion sickness and has been revered for its gentle stimulating effect. Women in the West African country of Senegal weave belts of ginger root fiber to restore their impotent mate's sexual prowess. It is used to make ginger ale, ginger beer, ginger wine and ginger candy.

Description: The ginger plant is a perennial herb growing to more than four feet high. Long lance-shaped leaves protrude from a central stem; the yellow flowers grow from the top of the stalk. Ginger essential oils are steam distilled from the roots. Digestive tonic, sexual tonic, reduces pain and expectorant.
Key constituents:
>Zingibene + Alpha-Selinene (25-40%)
>Beta-Sesquiphellandrene + Delta-Cadinene (7-14%)
>Beta-Phellandrena + 1,8 Cineol + Limonene (8-15%)
>AR Curcumene (5-11%)

Therapeutic properties: Ginger root is traditionally used to relieve arthritis, rheumatism, indigestion, digestive disorders, motion sickness, alcoholism, loss of appetite, chills, respiratory infections, congestion, coughs, muscular aches and pains, nausea, sinusitis sore throats and sprains.

Routes of application: Diffuse or apply topically. Ginger root or the essential oils are commonly added to food. Ginger essential oils mix well with all spice oils, bergamot, cedarwood, all citrus oils, clove, coriander, *Eucalyptus radiata*, frankincense, geranium, grapefruit, jasmine, juniper, lemon, lime, mandarin, myrtle, neroli, palmarosa, patchouli, rose maroc, rosemary, sandalwood, spearmint, vetiver and ylang-ylang.

Caution: Pregnant women should consult their physician before use; avoid direct sun exposure after use; repeated use can produce contact sensitivity on skin.

Goldenrod (*Solidago canadensis*)

Beginnings: Goldenrod originated in Canada. The genus name, Solidago, is derived from the Latin solide, which translates to "to make whole." During the Boston Tea Party, after English tea was thrown into the harbor, American colonist drank goldenrod tea, which they called "Liberty Tea."

Description: Goldenrod oils are steam distilled. The general action is diuretic, anti-inflammatory, liver tonic, macrolytic, stimulant and tonic.

Key constituents:
- Germacrene D (22-35%0
- Alpha-Pinene (10-18%)
- Myrcene (8-15%)
- Sabinene (5-11%)
- Limonene (6-12%)

Therapeutic properties: Goldenrod oil helps to thin mucus secretions, asthma, relieves candida infestations and relieves congested mucus; it promotes urination, cleans out the kidney, relieves hypertension, reduces inflammation and reduces the risk of infection.

Routes of application: Diffuse or apply topically; can be used as a wash or compress for wounds, headaches, arthritis and rheumatism, as a gargle, sore throat, laryngitis and thrush.

Grapefruit (*Citrus paradise*)

Beginnings: The grapefruit tree was introduced into the West Indies from China by a Captain Shaddock and the fruit was locally known as the "Shaddoc" fruit. In 1809 the seeds traveled with Spanish settlers to the United States, however, it was not grown commercially until 1880. Grapefruit is now grown in the USA, South Africa, Israel and Brazil and is actually a hybrid between *C. maxima* and *C. sinensis*.

Description: Grapefruit oils are mechanically cold pressed from the fresh skin.
Key constituents:
- Limonene (88-95%)
- Myrcene (1-4%)

Therapeutic properties: Grapefruit oil is antiseptic, disinfectant, detoxifying and diuretic, fat-dissolving properties, skin cleansing for oily skin, antidepressant, emotionally uplifting, agent for drug withdrawal, eating disorders, fatigue, jet lag, liver disorders, migraine headaches, PMS, stress and cleansing effect on the lymphatic and vascular system.

Routes of application: Diffuse, apply topically and take orally. Grapefruit oil mixes well with essential oils of basil, bergamot, cedarwood, chamomile, cypress, frankincense, geranium, juniper, lavender, peppermint, rosemary, rosewood and ylang-ylang.

Caution: Pregnant women should consult physician before use.

Helichrysum (*Helichrysm italicum, H. angustifolium*)

Beginnings: Helichrysum originated in France, Hungary, Yugoslavia and Corsica. Helichrysum has been used to encourage regeneration of tissue and nerves, improving circulation and various skin conditions. This everlasting flower is also called everlast and immortelle.

Description: Helichrysum is an evergreen herb that reaches 20 inches in height, it has long stems, off of which grow many thin, needle-like, velvety leaflets. At the top of each stem is a clump of about 30 tiny flower heads that are covered in bright yellow scales. There are more than 500 varieties of helichrysum; the oil is extracted from the flowers by steam distillation. Key Constituents:
    Neryl Acetate (25-35%)
    Gamma Curcuneme (9-15%)
    Limonene (8-13%)
    Neryl Propionate (3-7%)
    Alpha Pinene (3-8%)
    Beta-Caryophyllene (1-5%)
    Linalol (1-4%)
    Nerol (2-5%)

ORAC value 17,420

Therapeutic properties: The essential oil of helichrysum has anticoagulant, anesthetic, dissolves hematomas, mucolytic, expectorant and antispasmodic properties; it stimulates the liver, reduces scar tissue and skin pigments; it balances blood pressure and detoxifies chemicals and various toxins from the body; stems bleeding, relieves hearing loss, pain, arteriosclerosis, atherosclerosis, hypertension, congestive heart failure, cardiac arrhythmias, thrombosis, embolism, liver disorders, phlebitis, sciatica, sinus infection and skin disorders including eczema, dermatitis and psoriasis.

Routes of application: Diffuse and apply topically around outside of ear, temple, forehead, back of neck or affected area. It blends well with bergamot, black pepper, cedarwood, German chamomile, clary sage, cypress, frankincense, geranium, grapefruit, juniper, lavender, lemon, mandarin, naiouli, oregano, palmarosa, ravensara, pine, rosemary, sage, tea tree, thyme, rose maroc, rose otto, ylang-ylang, vetiver and eucalyptus.

Caution: Pregnant women should consult with their physician.

Hyacinth (*Hyacinthus orientalis*)

Beginnings: Named by Linnaeus after Hyacinthus, a Spartan youth beloved by Apollo and Zephyrus. In modern times the countries of origin are Holland, France and Egypt.

Description: It is a perennial herbaceous bulbous plant, with narrow, slender light to dark green leaves and large flower heads with bell shaped white, pink or blue flowers. Key constituents:
- Benzyl alcohol
- Troxo cinnamly alcohol
- Benzaldehyde
- Phenylethyl-Alcohol

Therapeutic properties: It has powerful hypnotic, sedative, antidepressant and antiseptic properties. It is used in aroma-psychology, emotional crisis, as a sedative, to relieve stress and tension, calming, mental fatigue, sorrow and feelings of distress.

Routes of application: It blends well with rose maroc, rose otto, lemon, bergamot, grapefruit, *Litsea cubeba*, neroli, ylang-ylang, frankincense, orange, cypress, sandalwood, petitgrain and geranium.

Hyssop (*Hyssopus officinalis*)

Beginnings: Hyssop is mentioned as part of sacrifice ceremonies in the Old Testament. Ancient alchemist used the powdered leaves and roots as a vermafuge. Small quantities were mixed with honey or crushed figs as a mild laxative.

Description: The essential oil is extracted from the leaves and flowers; it is used in perfumes and liqueurs (i.e. - Chartreuse). The plant is characterized by long stalks and blue flowers. Key constituents:
- Beta Pinene (13.5-23%)
- Sabinene (2-3%)
- Pinochamphone (5.5-17.5%)
- Iso-Pinochamphone (34.5-50%)
- Gemacrene D (2-3%)
- Limonene (1-4%)

Therapeutic properties: Hyssop is typically used for skin disorders, supporting the cardiovascular system, including blood pressure problems; bronchitis, coughs and colds.

Routes of application: Hyssop oil is applied through massage and inhalation; it is commonly mixed with cough syrups.
Cautions: Do not use during pregnancy; use only small amounts.

Jasmine (*Jasminum officinale, J. grandiflorum*)

Beginnings: Used commonly by Arabs, Indians and Chinese as perfume and for scenting tea. Jasmine was brought to Europe from Iran in the 16th century. The 17th century herbalist Nicholas Culpepper recommended rubbing the essential oil into "hard contracted limbs to ease muscle cramps." Jasmine has been nicknamed "queen of the night" and "moonlight of the grove."

Description: The *Jasminum grandiflora* species is a small bush that originated in the East Indies and Egypt; it is grown in southern France, Spain, Algeria, Morocco, India and Egypt. Jasmine produces tiny white flowers with a "honey-sweet" floral bouquet with fruity undertones. A deep red essential oil is produced by enfleurage; the essential oil is one of the more expensive ingredients of the perfume industry - the production of one pound of jasmine oil requires 1,000 pounds (3.6 million unpacked jasmine flowers) of jasmine blossoms. Key constituents:

    Benzyl Acetate (18-28%)
    Benzyl Benzoate (14-21%)
    Linalol (3-8%)
    Phytol (6-12%)
    Isophytol (3-7%)
    Squalene (3-7%)

Therapeutic properties: Jasmine is commonly used as a mood enhancer for individuals with anxiety and depression; it is used as an aphrodisiac for both frigidity and impotence; it is used for dysmenorrhea.

Routes of applications: Inhalation, bath and massage will all produce the warming and relaxing properties of jasmine. It blends well with bay, rose maroc, rose otto, neroli, sandalwood, palmarosa, geranium, lemon, clove, grapefruit, clary sage, bergamot, mandarin, orange, patchouli, petitgrain, ylang-ylang, coriander and ginger.

Juniper (*Juniperus communis*)

Beginnings: Grown in North America, Asia, Africa and Europe; juniper is a small shrub with aromatic needles and berries; it was burned as an incense for religious ceremonies and to "ward off the plague" and small pox. The juniper berries are used in the manufacturing process of gin. Bible references include: Job 30:45 *"Who cut up mallows by the bushes, and juniper roots for their meat."*

Description: Juniper is an evergreen bush with rough thick branches, needle-like leaves, small yellow flowers and bluish-purple berries. The pale yellow essential oil is distilled from the berries (a different essence is obtained from the twigs - cade oil, which is used in veterinary medicine). Key constituents:

    Alpha-pinene (20-40%)
    Sabinene (3-18%)
    Myrcene (1-6%)
    Camphor (10-18%)
    Limonene (3-8%)
    Bornyl Acetate (12-20%)
    Terpinene-4-ol (3-8%)

ORAC value 2,517

Therapeutic properties: Juniper is used as an antiseptic, astringent, digestive stimulant, diuretic and a urinary antiseptic including for cystitis, acne, colic, coughs, dermatitis, eczema, flatulence, rheumatism, promotes excretion of uric acid and the healing of skin ulcers. It blends well with rosemary, geranium, lavender, lemon, grapefruit, sandalwood, cypress, clary sage, pine, frankincense, vetiver, cedarwood, sage, mandarin, eucalyptus, bergamot, fennel and rose otto.

Routes of application: Inhalation, baths and massage.

Labrador tea (Ledum) (*Ledum groenlandicum*)

Beginnings: Labrador tea is a plant native of North America; it is a strongly aromatic herb that has been used for centuries as a home remedy. The native peoples of Eastern Canada used this herb for a tea, as a general tonic and to relieve a wide range of kidney diseases. Labrador tea has been used by the Native American people to prevent and cure scurvy for more than 5000 years. The Cree nation uses Labrador tea to reduce fevers and relieve cold symptoms.

Description: Labrador tea is a plant native of North America; the oil is steam distilled from the leaves. Key constituents:

    Limonene (20-35%)
    Cis- and Trans-Paramenth 1(7) 8 Diene 8-ol (12-17%)
    Cis- and Trans-Paramenthatriene 1,3,8 (8-15%)

Therapeutic properties: Anti-inflammatory, antitumoral, relieves insomnia, relieves prostate infection and congestion, antibacterial, diuretic, hepatoprotectant, hepatitis, cirrhosis, fatty liver, cough, flu, hoarseness and decongestant.

Routes of application: Diffuse or apply topically diluted one dop to one teaspoon of carrier oil.

Lavender (*Lavendula officinalis, L. angustifolia*)

Beginnings: The name lavender is derived from the Roman lavera and the Latin lavandus, which is translated "to wash." Lavender was a revered essential oil that the Romans used in their daily baths; the Romans and the Greeks burned lavender sprigs to perfume their dwellings as well as to defend against the plague. Lavender was introduced into Europe by the Romans. Historically it was used as an antidote against the bites of the funnel web spider, black widow spider and certain snakes (i.e. - vipers and adders).

Description: Lavender is a woody herb that sports long narrow leaves; as the name implies lavender is characterized by purple-blue "lavender" flowers on tall spikes. The lavender oils are steam-distilled from the dried plant; the oil is clear to pale yellow in color with a strong aroma. Key constituents:
 Linalyl Acetate (24-45%)
 Linalol (25-38%)
 Cis-beta-Ocimene (4-10%)
 Trans-beta- Ocimene (1.5-6%)
 Terpinene-4-ol (2-6%)

ORAC value 3,669

Therapeutic properties: Lavender has sedative and tonic effects; it is used to "balance" the nervous system, insomnia, migraines, it is antiseptic, skin conditions including acne, stretch marks, burns, sun burn, dandruff, hair loss, infections of the respiratory system, digestive tract, reduces hypertension, PMS, menopausal symptoms, nausea, phlebitis and the urinary system. Lavender oil can be used to cleanse and disinfect cuts, bruises and skin irritations.

Routes of application: Lavender can be applied through inhalation, baths, room dispersers and massage. Cold wraps, warm towel wraps applied to the chest or forehead can be used as a soothing relaxation to end a long stressful day. It blends well with Roman chamomile, German chamomile, lemon, geranium, eucalyptus, thyme, rosemary, tea tree, peppermint, grapefruit, clary sage, palmarosa, mandarin, juniper, cypress, pine, black pepper, marjoram, cedarwood, bergamot, lemongrass and ravensara.

Lemon (*Citrus limonum*)

Beginnings: The name lemon is derived from the Persian or Arabic, limun, which is thought to have come from the Indian Sanskrit. The lemon tree is thought to have come from the northeast of India and brought to Europe through Arabia. The tree was introduced into California in 1887. Lemons were used by 18th century British sailors to prevent and cure scurvy, purify the ships drinking water and as an antiseptic to clean wounds, bruises and insect bites.

Description: The lemon fruit grows on a classic citrus tree which has whitish-pink blossoms and bright yellow fruit the size of a hen's egg. Lemon is grown in orchards in just about all Mediterranean countries, Brazil, the United States, Argentina, Israel and Africa. The pale yellow essential oil is mechanically expressed from the skin (petitgrain essential oil is derived from small spines on the branches of the lemon tree). The lemon essential oil is used in perfumes; the oil can have a short shelf life and will deteriorate if not stored properly.

Key constituents:
- Limonene (59 -73%)
- Gamma-Terpinene 96-12%)
- Beta-Pinene (7-16%)
- Alpha-Pinene (1.5-3%)
- Sabinene (1.5-3%)

Therapeutic properties: Lemon oil is astringent and antiseptic and is typically used to cleanse and disinfect the skin, boils, shingles, herpes and warts; it can be used for reducing elevated blood pressure, colds, indigestion, fever, asthma, anemia, parasites, malaria, sore throat, varicose veins and gallstones. The vaporized essential oils of lemon can kill *Meningococcus* bacteria in 15 minutes, typhoid bacilli in one hour, *Staphylococcus aureus* in two hours and Pneumococcus bacteria within three hours. Even a 0.2% solution of lemon oil can kill diphtheria bacteria in 20 minutes and inactivate tuberculosis bacteria.

Routes of application: Inhalation, diffuse, baths and massage are typical methods of delivery. Lemon oil combines well with all essential oils including chamomile, *Eucalyptus radiata*, fennel, frankincense, geranium, juniper berries, peppermint, sandalwood and ylang-ylang.

Lemongrass (*Cymbopogon citratus*)

Beginnings: A sweet scented grass that was initially used as an insect repellant and to season food in India, Africa, the Seychelles, Indonesia and Sri Lanka.

Description: lemongrass is a tall-stemmed, grass-like tropical plant growing to four feet in height. Its essential oil is steam-distilled from fresh cut grass and has a lemon-like aroma that is prized for "citrus" soaps, perfumes and skin cleansers. Citral, a primary constituent of lemongrass, is a cleansing antiseptic, deodorant and the dried grass was burned to "clear the mind." Key constituents:

    Citral
    Citronellal
    N-Decylic Aldehyde
    Dipentene
    Farucsol
    Geranial (35-45%)
    Geraniol (5-10%)
    Neral (25-40%)
    Trans-beta-Caryophyllene (2-6%)

ORAC value 17,765

Therapeutic properties: Lemongrass oil is typically used for skin conditions, sore throats, athlete's foot, cardiac tonic, digestive support, insect repellant, respiratory conditions (colds, coughs, bronchitis) and headache.

Routes of application: Typically lemongrass oil is applied via inhalation and massage; lemongrass oil blends well with basil, bergamot, black pepper, cedarwood, clary sage, coriander, cypress, fennel, geranium, ginger, grapefruit, lavender, lemon, marjoram, orange, patchouli, palmarosa, rosemary, tea tree, thyme linalol, vetiver, ylang-ylang.

Litsea Cubeba (May-Chang Oil) (*Litsea citrate*)

Beginnings: The countries of origin include China and Java. The name cubeba comes from the small round fruit that resemble those on the climbing shrub *Piper cubeba*, a native plant of Java.

Description: Litsea is a shrub-like tree reaching 30 feet in height; it belongs to the laurel family; slender branches produce lance-shaped leaves, white flowers and small green fruit the size of a peppercorn. The oil is steam distilled from the ripe fruit. Key constituents:

    Citral
    Neral
    Geranial

Linalool

Therapeutic properties: Litsea is used as a calmative, anti-infectious, antibiotic, stimulant, vulnerary, antiseptic, stomachic and antidepressant. It is used therapeutically for nervousness, a general tonic, relaxing skin care, acne, indigestion, depression, anxiety, stress, poor appetite, anorexia, cleansing, tissue toning and for eliminating cellulite.

Routes of application: It blends well with bay, basil, black pepper, cardamom, cedarwood, clary sage, coriander, cypress, *Eucalyptus citriodora*, *Eucalyptus radiata*, frankincense, geranium, ginger, grapefruit, juniper, marjoram, orange, patchouli, palmarosa, petitgrain, Roman chamomile, rosemary, sandalwood, tea tree, thyme, vetiver and ylang-ylang.

Mandarin (*Citrus reticulata*)

Beginnings: The Mandarin orange originated in China, Madagascar and Italy - the fruit was a traditional part of the northern Chinese diet, especially a favorite with the aristocracy.

Description: The plant is a small evergreen tree with white, highly scented flowers that produce a small flattened-round, loose-skinned orange fruit. The essential oil is mechanically extracted by the cold press method from the fresh skin of the fruit. Key constituents:
- Citral
- Citronellal
- Limonene (65-75%)
- Gamma-Terpinene (16-22%)
- Geraniol
- Alpha-Pinene (2-3%)
- Beta-Pinene (1.2-2%)
- Myrcene (1.5-2%)

Therapeutic properties: The essential oil of Mandarin acts as a weak antispasmodic, digestive tonic, antiseptic, antifungal, stimulates the gallbladder, acne, digestive problems, edema, insomnia, intestinal problems, oily skin, scars, liver spots, age spots, tones the skin, stretch marks, relieves nervous tension and restlessness.

Route of application: Diffuse and can be applied topically. Mandarin essential oil blends well with basil, black pepper, cinnamon, clove, frankincense, jasmine, juniper, lavender, myrrh, neroli, nutmeg, palmarosa, patchouli, petitgrain, citrus oils, Roman chamomile, sandalwood, ylang-ylang and spice oils.

Caution: Pregnant women should consult their physician before using Mandarin oil. Do not use on skin before exposure to the sun.

Manuka (*Leptospermum scoparium*)

Beginnings: All parts of the manuka plant have been used by the Maori people from New Zealand as an important part of their folk medicine. When Captain Cook and his crew landed in New Zealand, they used the manuka leaves for making tea. Cook wrote in his ship's log, "It has a very agreeable bitter taste and flavor when (the leaves) are recent but losses some of both when they are dried." Cook's men learned that if they brewed the tea too strong, it caused them to regurgitate. Manuka was the original "tea tree."

Description: The manuka plant is a narrow shrub or small tree with a rich red wood; small, dark, pointed, concave leaves; and small pink or red flowers. The essential oil is steam distilled from the leaves and branch tips. Key constituents:
>   Beta-Caryphyllen
>   Geraniol
>   Geranial
>   Linalol
>   Alpha-Pinene
>   Geranuylacetate

Therapeutic properties: Manuka essential oil has antibiotic, antifungal, antiseptic, anti-infectious, analgesic and vulnerary properties; and it is used to treat athlete's foot, ringworm, thrush, skin infections, colds, flu, sore throat, rheumatism, muscular pain, urinary infections, intestinal infections, burns and wounds.

Route of application: Blends well with basil, bergamot, black pepper, Roman chamomile, German chamomile, clary sage, cypress, eucalyptus, geranium, grapefruit, lavender, lemon, marjoram, orange, patchouli, peppermint, petitgrain, pine, ravensara, rosemary, sage, sandalwood, tea tree, thyme, *Litsea cubeba* and yuzu.

Marjoram (*Origanum marjorana, Majorana hortensis*)

Beginnings: The Greeks cultivated marjoram for their perfumes and medicinal herbal preparations. Marjoram was known as the "herb of happiness" to the Romans and "Joy of the Mountains" to the Greeks. It was grown as a potted plant by the ancient Egyptians; it was used in unguents and perfumes. Greek women used oils infused with marjoram on their heads as a relaxant. It was used in 16th century Europe, on the floors of rooms to produce a pleasant odor as you walked.

Description: A widely used culinary herb that is now grown world-wide. The amber essential oil is steam-distilled from the fresh and dried leaves and flowers; its "warm and spicy" oil is commonly used in male fragrances. Key constituents:
>Terpinene-4-ol (25-35%)
>Gamma-Terpinene (12-20%)
>Linalol +Cis-4-Thujanol (3-8%)
>Alpha-Terpinene (6-13%)
>Alpha-Terpineol (2-6%)
>Sabinene (2-6%)

Therapeutic properties: The essential oil is a warming agent that is used to relieve muscle spasm and cramps, anxiety, insomnia, arthritis, rheumatism, antibacterial, asthma, bronchitis, respiratory infections, fungal and viral infections, ringworm, shingles, circulatory conditions, regulates blood pressure and edema, constipation, headaches, anxiety, dysmenorrhea, muscular strains, bruises, burns, sunburn, cuts, neuralgia and as a nerve tonic.

Routes of application: Inhalation and massage; it blends well with bergamot, lavender and rosemary. Marjoram oil can be steam-inhaled and rubbed into the sinuses and temples; it blends well with Bergamot, cedarwood, chamomile, cypress, lavender, nutmeg, orange, rosemary, rosewood and ylang-ylang.

Cautions: Do not use marjoram oil in the first trimester of pregnancy. High doses of the oil can produce a narcotic-like depressing effect, including a sexual depressant.

Melaleuca alternifolia (*Melaleuca alternifolia*)

Beginnings: The legendary melaleuca tree originated in Australia. The essential oil of melaleuca (Tea tree oil) is steam distilled from the leaves. The antibacterial, antimicrobial and antiseptic properties of the essential oils were discovered by the Aboriginal people of Australia.

Description: Key constituents:
>Gama Terpinene (10-28%)
>Alpha-Terpinene (5-13%)
>1,8 Cineole (Eucalyptol) (0-15%)
>Alpha-Terpineol (1.5-8%)
>Para-Cymene (0.5-12%)

Terpinenol-4 (30-45%)
Limonene (0.5-4%)
Aromadendrene (trace-7%)
Delta-Cadinene (trace-8%)
Alpha Pinene (1-6%)

Monoterpenes: alpha pinene, beta-pinene, myrcene; Sesquiterpenes; Monoterpene alcohols (45-50%); Terpene oxides.

Therapeutic properties: Anti-infection, antibacterial (active against wide spectrum of gram positive and gram negative bacteria), antifungal, antiviral, antiparasitic, antiseptic, anti-inflammatory, immunostimulant, cardiotonic, venous decongestant, relieves phlebitis, neurotonic, analgesic, athlete's foot, bronchitis, respiratory infections, gingivitis, receding gums, pyorrhea, skin problems (acne, burns, candida, cold sores, shingles, ingrown toenails, warts and wounds), sore throat, sunburn, tonsillitis and vaginal yeast infections.

Routes of application: Diffuse or apply topically. Melaleuca oils blend well with all citrus oils, cypress, *Eucalyptus radiata, E. globulus,* clary sage, juniper, pine, marjoram, oregano, peppermint, ravensara, thyme. lavender, rosemary, basil, bergamot, black pepper, Roman chamomile, German chamomile, thyme.

Caution: Pregnant women should consult their physician before use.

Melaleuca ericifolia (*Melaleuca ericifolia; a.k.a. Australian Rosalina*)

Beginnings: The *Melaleuca ericifolia* tree originated in Australia.

Description: Key constituents:
Alpha-Pinene (5-10%)
1,8 Cineol + Beta Phellandrene (18-28%)
Alpha-Terpineol (1-5%)
Para-Cymene (1-6%)
Linalol (34-45%)
Aromadendrene (2-6%)

Therapeutic properties: Relieves respiratory diseases (bronchitis, asthma, colds, etc.), cystitis and sinus infections.

Routes of application: Diffuse or apply topically on temples, wrists, throat, face or chest; blends well with basil, bergamot, black pepper, lavender, rosemary, lemon, Roman chamomile, German chamomile, *Eucalyptus globulus, E. radiata,* clary sage, juniper, cypress, pine, marjoram, oregano, peppermint, ravensara, thyme. Dilute four to eight drops of essential oil in 30 ml of a carrier oil for massage.

Caution: Pregnant women should consult their physician before use.

Melaleuca quinquenervia (Niaouli) *(Melaleuca quinquenervia)*

Beginnings: The Niaouli tree originated in Australia; the essential oils are steam distilled from the leaves and limbs.

Description: Fragrance is "sweet and delicate." Key constituents:
- Limonene + 1,8 Cineole (55-70%)
- Alpha-Pinene (7-15%)
- Beta-Pinene (2-6%)
- Viridiflorol (2-6%)

Therapeutic properties: This essential oil has androgen-like properties, a general tonic, anti-inflammatory, anti-infection, antibacterial, antiviral and antiparasitic (amoeba and blood parasites); relieves respiratory problems (allergies, colds, bronchitis, etc.), urinary tract problems and hemorrhoids.

Route of application: Diffuse, steam, compress, vapor, rub or apply topically; basil, bergamot, black pepper, lavender, rosemary, lemon, Roman chamomile, German chamomile, *Eucalyptus globulus, E. radiata*, clary sage, juniper, cypress, pine, marjoram, oregano, peppermint, ravensara, thyme.

Caution: Pregnant women should consult their physician before use.

Melissa (Lemon balm) *(Melisa officinalis)*

Beginnings: The Greeks and Arabs widely used melissa in their daily lives; Paracelsus, the 16th century physician, claimed that melissa was "the elixir of life." The 17th century herbalist Gerard said that Melissa "maketh the heart merry, joyful, strengtheneth the vital spirits."

Description: Melissa is a plant native to Europe and later cultivated in the United States (Idaho and Utah); it is commonly known as "sweet balm" or "lemon balm." Melissa was the primary ingredient in Carmelite water, a combination of alcohol and essential oil distilled in France since 1611 by the Carmelite monks. Melissa is a bushy perennial of the mint family. The highly aromatic oil is distilled from the leaves, it smells like lemon. Key constituents:
- Geranial (25-35%)
- Neral (18-28%)

Beta Caryophyllene (12-19%)

Therapeutic properties: It has been classically used as an uplifting and calming "cure" for "melancholia"; it has tonic and anti-spasmotic properties; it is used for relieving allergies, hypertension, colds, cold sores, chicken pox, diarrhea, cholera, hypertension, dysmenorrhea, migraine and stress headaches, insomnia, insect bites, nausea and palpitations.

Routes of application: Inhalation, baths and massage.
Blends well with essential oils of geranium, Roman chamomile, rose, neroli, petitgrain, frankincense, lavender, floral and citrus (typically used alone).

Mountain Savory (*Satureja Montana*)

Beginnings: The mountain savory originated in France. The essential oils are steam distilled from the flowering plant.

Description: Key constituents:
    Carvacrol (22-35%)
    Thymol (14-24%)
    Gamma-Terpinene (8-15%)
    Carvacrol Methyl Ether (4-9%)
    Beta-Caryophyllene (3-7%)

ORAC value 113,071

Therapeutic properties: Mountain savory contains significant anti-infection properties, general tonic, relieves acute pain, relieves circulatory problems, antiseptic, stimulates healing, traditionally used to treat abscesses, burns and wounds.

Routes of application: Diffuse or apply topically mixed with a massage oil.
Caution: Pregnant women should consult their physician before use.

Myrrh (*Commiphora myrrha*)

Beginnings: The Egyptians and the Greeks viewed myrrh as a valuable commodity; it was used as their Kyphi incense to worship their gods, perform rituals, and it was commonly used in cosmetics, perfumes and herbal therapies. Myrrh was combined with frankincense for embalming purposes by the Egyptians. It is thought to be one of the substances used by the Queen of Sheba for her seduction of King Solomon. Myrrh and frankincense were given as gifts to the Christ child by the three wise men because of their antiseptic properties -

remember, the Christ child was born in a stable full of animals, manure, urine, flies, bacteria and viruses. Genesis 37:25 "And they sat down to eat bread: and they lifted up their eyes and looked, and behold, a company of Ishmelites came from Gilead with their camels bearing spicery and balm and myrrh, going to carry it down to Egypt." Genesis 43:11 "And their father Israel said unto them, If it must be so now, do this; take of the best fruits in the land in your vessels, and carry down the man a present, a little balm, and a little honey, spices and myrrh, nuts, and almonds." Exodus 30:23 "Take thou also unto thee principal spices, of pure myrrh five hundred shekels, and of sweet cinnamon half so much, even two hundred and fifty shekels, and of sweet calamus two hundred and fifty shekels."

Description: A small, thorny, shrub-like tree, myrrh is native to Arabia, Somalia, Ethiopia and most North African countries. The resin is steam distilled to extract a dense, viscous yellow essential oil. The oil has a warm spicy aroma.
Key constituents:
    Lindestrene (30-45%)
    Curzerene (17-25%)
    Furanoendesma-1,3-diene (4-8%)
    Methoxyfuronogermacrene (5-9%)
    Beta-and Gamma-Elemenes (3-6%)

Therapeutic properties: Myrrh has anti-inflammatory and expectorant properties; it is typically used to relieve bronchitis, catarrh, coughs, colds, skin diseases, indigestion and infections of the mouth and throat.

Routes of application: Inhalation and massage. Myrrh is still used widely today in pharmaceuticals, herbal preparations and in perfumes. Myrrh blends well with frankincense, bergamot, patchouli, sandalwood, cypress, juniper, geranium, lavender, lemon, palmarosa, tea tree, *Eucalyptus radiata*, rosemary, Roman chamomile, grapefruit, pine, vetiver, ylang-ylang, all spice oils, camphor and lavender.

Caution: Pregnant women should consult their physician before use.

Myrtle (*Myrtus communis*)

Beginnings: The myrtle tree originated in Tunisia and Morocco. Nehemiah 8:15 "And that they should publish and proclaim in all their cities, and in Jerusalem, saying, Go forth unto the mount, and fetch olive branches, and pine branches, and myrtle branches, and palm branches, and branches of thick trees, to make booths, as it is written." Isaiah 41:19 "I will plant in the wilderness the cedar, the shittah tree, and the myrtle, and the oil tree; I will set in the desert the fir tree, and the pine, and the box tree together." Isaiah 55:13 "Instead of the thorn shall come up the fir tree, and instead of the brier shall come up the myrtle tree: and it shall be to the Lord for a name, for an everlasting sign that shall not be cut off."

Description: The essential oils of myrtle are steam distilled from the leaves. Key constituents:
    Alpha Pinene (45-60%)
    1,8 Cineol (Eucalyptol) (17-27%)
    Limonene (5-11%)
    Linalol (2-5%)

Therapeutic properties: Expectorant, anti-infectious, liver stimulant, prostate decongestant, mild antispasmodic, tonic for the skin (acne, blemishes, oily skin, psoriasis, etc.), thyroid and ovaries. Relieves bronchitis, coughs, decongestant, hypothyroidism, insomnia, sinus infections, asthma, cystitis, diarrhea, dysentery, indigestion, hemorrhoids; particularly useful for children with respiratory complaints and coughs.

Routes of application: Diffuse, humidifier, topical. Blends well with bergamot, lavender, lemon, lemongrass, *Melaleuca alternifolia*, rosewood, rosemary, spearmint and thyme.

Neroli (bitter orange) (*Citrus aurantium*)

Beginnings: The use of neroli was first recorded by the Egyptians and Romans. In 1680, neroli was named after the Prince of Nerola, Flavio Orsini from Italy. He went to great effort to ensure a steady supply of the essential oil to scent the bath water and the gloves of his wife Anna-Maria de la Tremoille Orsini, Princess of Nerola - she brought the neroli fragrance into fashion with the Italian aristocracy.

Description: Neroli is commonly known as orange blossom; it is produced from the white blossoms of the bitter orange tree which was first discovered in China. Bitter orange is cultivated in orchards in Egypt, Morocco, Algeria, the United States, Italy and southern France. The pale yellow oil is expensive to produce - it takes one ton of blossoms to produce two pounds of oil. The oil is distilled from the blossoms still in the bud stage. Key constituents:

    Linalol (28-44%)

Limonene (9-18%)
Beta-Pinene (7-17%)
Linalyl Acetate (3-15%)
Trans-Ocimene (3-8%)
Alpha Terpineol (2.5-5%)
Trans-Nerolidol (1-5%)
Myrcene (1-4%)

Therapeutic properties: Used commonly as a sedative and anti-depressant; neroli is used to relieve anxiety, hysteria, insomnia, dysmenorrhea, PMS, shock, palpitations, circulatory problems, skin problems, hemorrhoids, anti-infectious, antibacterial, antiparasitic, relieves hypertension, digestive problems and menopausal symptoms.

Routes of application: Inhalation, baths, topical and massage. Blends well with cedarwood, coriander, frankincense, mandarin, geranium, ginger, jasmine, lavender, lemon, orange, rose, ylang-ylang, yuzu and sandalwood.

Nutmeg (*Myristica fragrans*)

Beginnings: Nutmeg originated in Tunisia and Indonesia. This spicy essential oil was traditionally used to increase muscle and joint circulation.

Description: The essential oil of nutmeg is steam distilled from the fruit and seeds. Key constituents:
Sabinene (14-29%)
Beta-Pinene (13-18%)
Alpha-Pinene (15-28%)
Limonene (2-7%)
Gamma-Terpinene (2-6%)
Terpinene-4-ol (2-6%)
Myristicine (5-12%)

Therapeutic Properties: The essential oil of nutmeg is antiseptic, antiparasitic, analgesic, relieves PMS and dysmenorrhea, rheumatism, circulatory and nervous system tonic, relieves fatigue and supports the immune system; it improves appetite and digestion. The essential oil of nutmeg has adrenal cortex-like properties, relieves frigidity, impotence, gout, nausea and peripheral neuropathies.

Routes of application: Apply topically diluted with extender oil. Nutmeg blends well with cinnamon, clove, cypress, frankincense, lemon, *Melaleuca alterifolia*, Melissa, orange, patchouli, rosemary oils.

Caution: Pregnant women should consult their physician before use; individuals with seizure disorders should avoid the use of nutmeg oil.

Orange (*Citrus sinensis, C. aurantium*)

Beginnings: China was the birth place of the orange tree. The orange tree was transplanted to the Mediterranean from China and Asia by the Saracens during the Crusades; it is now grown in Sicily, Israel, Spain and the United States - the essential oil has different medicinal characteristics depending on the country of origin. The fragrant oil was used for culinary, cosmetic and medicinal purposes.

Description: The sweet and bitter oils are extracted mechanically by pressing the fresh orange peel. The oil ranges from yellow to brown in color and will ignite at a low temperature of 75 F. Key constituents:
  Limonene (85-96%)
  Myrcene (0.5-3%)

ORAC value 18,898

Therapeutic properties: Orange oil is used as a tonic for anxiety and depression, relieves jaundice, scurvy, heartburn, angina, palpitations, cardiac spasm, lowers cholesterol, mouth ulcers, edema, insomnia, chronic bronchitis, respiratory infections, colds, prolapse of the uterus and the anus, hemorrhoids, indigestion and constipation and oral ulcers. The essential oil is rich in vitamin C.

Routes of application: Baths and massage. Orange oil is used widely in the packaged food (chocolate-orange candies) and cosmetic industries. Blends well with bay, bergamot, black pepper, cinnamon, clove, coriander, cypress, frankincense, geranium, grapefruit, jasmine, juniper, lavender, lemon, *Litsea cubeba*, marjoram, neroli, nutmeg, patchouli, petitgrain, sandalwood, rosewood, vetiver and ylang-ylang.

Cautions: Pregnant women should consult their physician before use; the user of orange oil topically should avoid direct sunlight or UV light for at least 72 hours; limit bath applications to four drops per bath as excess orange oil can irritate sensitive skin.

Oregano (*Origanum compactum*)

Beginnings: Oregano originated in Utah, Turkey and France.

Description: A densely branched perennial herb growing to 20 inches. Oregano

essential oils are steam distilled from the oval leaves and pink flowers of the plant. Key Constituents:
> Carvacrol (60-75%)
> Gamma-Terpinene (3.5-8.5%)
> Para-Cymene (5.5-9%)
> Beta Caryophyllene (2-5%)
> Myrcene (1-3%)
> Thymol (0-5%)

ORAC value 153,007

Therapeutic properties: Potent anti-infectious essential oil for respiratory infections, gastroenteritis, genital infections, nerve tonic, blood and lymphatic tonic; it has a broad spectrum antiseptic property against bacteria, mycobacteria (tuberculosis), fungus, yeast, viruses and parasites; it is a general tonic and will stimulate the immune system; relieves asthma, bronchitis, pulmonary tuberculosis, rheumatism and whooping cough, digestive problems and pneumonia.

Routes of application: Oil of oregano can be applied topically to the bottom of the feet without dilution; dilute with extender oil when applied to other parts of the body. Oregano oil blends well with essential oils of bay, basil, bergamot, cypress, eucalyptus, fennel, geranium, lemon, lemongrass, *Litsea cubeba*, myrtle, orange, petitegrain, pine, Roman chamomile, rosemary and thyme.

Caution: high phenol content can irritate the skin, therefore dilute with extender oils at the rate of one drop oregano oil to 50 drops of a massage oil; avoid contact with all mucus membranes; pregnant women should consult physician before use. It is a good idea to test skin for sensitivity.

Palmarosa (*Cymbopogon martini*)

Beginnings: Palmarosa grass originated in India and Conoros. Historically was called "Turkish geranium oil" or "East Indian geranium oil." Because the high geranil content produces a rose-like odor, palmarosa is often used to adulterate rose essential oil.

Description: Palmarosa is related to lemongrass; the oil is steam distilled from the leaves. Key constituents:
> Geraniol (70-85%)
> Geranyl Acetate (6-10%)
> Linalol (3-7%)

Therapeutic properties: Antimicrobial, antibacterial, antifungal, antiviral, cardiotonic and uterine tonic; used to relieve yeast infections including candida, beneficial for the cardiovascular system, circulation, digestion, infection, nervous system, skin conditions, athlete's foot and rashes.

Routes of application: Apply topically; palmarosa oil blends well with basil, fennel, geranium, lemongrass, myrtle, pine, rosemary and thyme.

Caution: Pregnant women should consult their physician before use.

Parsley (*Petroselinum sativum*)

Beginnings: There was a medieval belief that parsley could only be grown in the gardens of honest men and women. Parsley was chewed to "repel the devil."

Description: Parsley was a native plant of Asia Minor, it is now cultivated commercially and in home gardens around the world. The oil is extracted by distillation from the ripe parsley seeds and leaves. Parsley is used for culinary and herbal medicinal purposes. Key constituents:
p-mentha-1,3,8-triene (6-60%)
Myristicin (7-33%)
Parsley Apiol (trace-18%)
Elemicin (0.2-3%)

Therapeutic properties: Parsley is used as a diuretic, for kidney diseases, urinary infections and relieving edema. Parsley is considered to contain high levels of vitamin A and iron and is used to promote healthy hair, skin, teeth, eyes, relieve anemia, support liver function, "clears" toxins, calms the nervous system and relieves symptoms of dysmenorrhea and menopause.

Routes of application: Massage is a common way to deliver the essential oil. Parsley oil blends well with fennel, lemon and rosemary oils.

Patchouli (*Pogostemon patchouli, P. cablin*)

Beginnings: Alongside of rose, jasmine, sandalwood and basil, patchouli was a favorite essential oil used in India; shawls and blankets were impregnated with the oil. It was historically used as an aphrodisiac and was reintroduced as an aphrodisiac in herbal preparations in the 1960s. The word patchouli comes from the south Indian Tamil language, patch, meaning "green" and ilai meaning "leaf."

Description: The essential oil is extracted by steam distillation from the dried and fermented leaves of the small, hairy perennial shrub. The oil is characterized by an intense, woody, sweet-spicy balsamic aroma. The oil gains in quality over time. Key constituents:

    Patchoulol (25-35%)
    Alpha-Bulnesene (14-20%)
    Alpha-Guaiene + Seychellene (15-25%)
    Alpha-Patchoulene (5-9%)

Therapeutic properties: Patchouli has significant astringent and diuretic properties and is used to enhance scalp and skin health, relieves wrinkles, dandruff, acne, eczema, hemorrhoids and reduces scars. The oil is a general tonic and is traditionally used to relieve anxiety and depression.

Routes of application: Inhalation, massage and baths. Small quantities have a stimulating effect while larger doses have a sedative effect. Blends well with bergamot, clary sage, frankincense, geranium, ginger, lavender, lemongrass, myrrh, pine, rosewood and sandalwood.

Peppermint (*Mentha piperata*)

Beginnings: The Egyptians originally used peppermint to flavor wine and food and it was historically said to be an aphrodisiac. According to Greek mythology the genus Mentha takes its name from the nymph Minthe, who was seduced by Pluto and turned into a plant by his jealous wife, who stomped Minthe into the ground. Pluto turned her into the herb, knowing that Minthe would then be appreciated by many people for thousands of years. Culpepper, the 17th century herbalist, stated that peppermint was "the herb most useful for complaints of the stomach, such as wind and vomiting, for which there are few remedies of greater efficiency."

Description: The leaves of the peppermint plant are shorter and broader than spearmint and are characterized by large spikes of purple flowers. Peppermint is a British classic herb that was spread around the world during their colonial reign. The colorless peppermint oil is distilled from the partially dried leaves and stems. It is commonly used in beverages, ice cream, sauces and jellies, liqueurs, medicines, toothpastes and mouth washes, cleaners, cosmetics, tobacco, desserts and chewing gums. Key constituents:

    Menthol (34-44%)
    Menthone (12-20%)
    Menthofurane (4-9%)
    1,8 Cineol (Euclyptol) (2-5%)

Pulegone (2-5%)
Menthyl Acetate (4-10%)

Therapeutic properties: Peppermint and peppermint oil is used to relieve indigestion, heart burn, varicose veins, hemorrhoids, hot flashes, dysmenorrhea, congestion, skin disorders, itching of ringworm, herpes blisters, scabies, poison oak and poison ivy, muscle spasm, arthritis, rheumatism, colds, throat infections, flu, flatulence, headaches, nausea, toothache and sunburn.

Routes of application: Inhalation, tea, baths and massage. It blends well with basil, pine, lemon, geranium, rosemary, tea tree, lavender, eucalyptus, grapefruit, juniper, cypress, black pepper, niaouli and ravensara.

Cautions: For skin complaints, use peppermint oil in concentrations of less than one percent as higher doses can cause skin irritation; pregnant women should use mint tea for nausea instead of the purified essential oil.

Petitgrain (*Citrus aurantium, C. amara, C. brigaradier*)

Beginnings: The petitgrain comes from the word for little fruit or little grains. In 1694 the essential oil was distilled from the small unripe fruit called orangettes, which are seeds or kernels.

Description: The essential oil is steam distilled from the tips of the fresh leaves, small twigs and in very high quality oil the small unripe green fruit is used. Key constituents:
Linalyl Acetate
Linalol
Geranyl Acetate
Nerol
Terpineol
Nerolidol

Therapeutic properties: The essential oil is antispasmodic, antidepressant, stimulant, tonic, calmative, anti-infectious, antiseptic and has nervine properties; it is used in the treatment of nervous conditions, acne, insomnia, depression, general debility, anxiety, stress-related conditions, indigestion and skin disorders.

Routes of application: The essential oil of petitgrain blends well with rosemary, clove, cedarwood, cypress, *Eucalyptus citriodora*, frankincense, geranium, jasmine, juniper, lavender, lemon, mandarin, marjoram, neroli, orange, palmarosa, patchouli, rose maroc, rose otto, sandalwood, ylang-ylang and yuzu.

Pine (*Pinus sylvestris, P. palustris, P. abies*)

Beginnings: The pine, also known as the "Scottish pine." This tree is cultivated for wood, cellulose, tar, pitch, turpentine and essential oils. The Scandinavians had traditionally used pine oils or "turpentine" in their saunas and steam baths for their refreshing and antiseptic qualities.

An ancient Egyptian cookbook describes the use of "pine nuts" as a highly nutritious food.

Description: The pine grows wild and is cultivated throughout Europe, North America and the former USSR. Pine oil comes from the heartwood of the tree, however, the finest quality of pine oil is distilled from the pine needles. The clear thick oil is characterized by a fresh aroma with a resinous woody undertone.

Key constituents:
- Alpha Pinene (55-70%)
- Beta Pinene (3-8%)
- Limonene (5-10%)
- Delta 3 Carene (6-12%)
- Sylvestrene
- Pumilone
- Dipentene
- Cadinene

Therapeutic properties: Acts as an antiseptic and adrenal tonic; pine oils are especially useful for the relief of respiratory complaints including bronchitis, catarrh, colds, coughs, flu and sinusitis; cystitis and urinary infections; and arthritis, fibromyalgia and aches and pains.

Routes of application: Inhalation, baths and massage. Pine oil is commonly used in balms, body rubs, soaps, bath oils and as a shoe deodorizer and disinfectant. The essential oil of pine blends well with bergamot, cedarwood, clary sage, cypress, *Eucalyptus radiata*, frankincense, grapefruit, juniper, lavender, lemon, marjoram, *Melaleuca alternifolia*, peppermint, ravensara, rosemary, sandalwood and thyme.

Ravensara (*Ravensara aromatica*)

Beginnings: The ravensara plant originated in Madagascar; the essential oils are referred to by the people of Madagascar as "the oil that heals." The bark of the tree is used as an ingredient in the production of a local rum; the seeds are known as Madagascan nutmeg are used in cooking and African folk medicine.

Description: The tree is characterized by a pungent aromatic dark, smooth evergreen leaves. It produces flowers and seeds which are used as cooking spices. The essential oil is steam distilled from the leaves and branches. Key constituents:

    Limonene + Eucalyptol (50-65%)
    Sabinene (6-12%)
    Alpha-Terpineol (5-11%)
    Alpha-Pinene (4-9%)
    Beta-Pinene (1-5%)

Monoterpenes- Alpha and Beta-pinene; Sesquiterpenes; Monoterpenols; Terpene esters; terpenyle acetate; Terpene oxides; 1,8 cineole.

Therapeutic properties: The oils of ravensara are anti-infectious, antiviral, antibacterial, expectorant, antimicrobial; it acts as a tonic for the nervous and respiratory system; relieves bronchitis, asthma, cystitis, burns, cholera, herpes, infectious mononucleosis, insomnia, muscle fatigue, rhinopharyngitis, shingles, sinusitis and viral hepatitis; disinfects and stimulates healing of cuts, scrapes and wounds.

Routes of application: Diffuse or apply topically. Ravensara blends well with bay, bergamot, black pepper, cardamom, cedarwood, clary sage, cypress, eucalyptus, geranium, frankincense, ginger, grapefruit, lavender, mandarin, marjoram, lemon, palmarosa, pine, rosemary, sandalwood, tea tree and thyme.

Caution: Pregnant women should consult their physician before use.

Rose (Maroc/*Rosa centifolia,* Otto/ *R. damascena*)

Beginnings: The word rose comes from the Greek "roden" which translates to red - the original rose is thought to have been crimson. In ancient myth, the rose sprang from the blood of Adonis or Venus. The rose and rose oils have been revered before the beginnings of the Roman Empire; the rose was used in garlands, scented bathes, perfumes and for ostentatious public events. Rosebushes were brought to Bulgaria by Turkish merchants; traditionally, the rose bush was grown as a dense hedge as a living fence around wheat and bean fields, between rows of trees and home gardens. The first recorded commercial distillery was started in 1612 in Shiraz, Persia (Iran).

Description: The Damascena rose is cultivated in Bulgaria, where the flowers are picked at dawn and the yellow-brown oil is extracted by enfleurage within 24 hours. It takes five tons of rose flowers to produce two pounds of rose oil.

The Centifolia rose is cultivated in France, Algeria, Morocco and Egypt. The essential oil from the rose is the least toxic of all of the oils. Key constituents:
- Geraniol (12-28%)
- Citronellol (34-44%)
- Farnesol
- Methyl Eugenol
- Nerol (6-9%)
- Phenylethylic Alcohol (0-2%)

Therapeutic properties: Rose oil is revered as an aphrodisiac, mood enhancer, general tonic, relieves circulatory problems, constipation, headaches, mental fatigue, skin disorders, dysmenorrheal and menopausal problems. The Bulgarian *Rosa damascene* (high in citronellol) is significantly different from the Moroccan *Rosa centifolia* (high in phenyl ethanol) - they are characterized by different colors, aromas and therapeutic properties.

Routes of application: Baths, inhalation and massage. Rose essential oil blends well with jasmine, neroli, geranium, lavender, clary sage, sandalwood, lemon, Roman chamomile, mandarin, ylang-ylang, petitgrain, vetiver, bergamot and patchouli.

Caution: Pregnant women should consult with their physician before use.

Rosemary (*Rosmarinus officinalis*)

Beginnings: The Egyptians were the first culture to actively use rosemary. The popularity of rosemary soon moved into 1000 B.C. Greece and Rome who used the essential oils to symbolize love and death. During outbreaks of the plague, rosemary was burned in public places and worn as garlands around the neck as an antiseptic. Rosemary was an original ingredient of the "Marseilles Vinegar" a.k.a. "Four Thieves Vinegar" used by grave robbers and bandits to protect themselves during the 15th century plague. The name of the plant is derived from the Latin words for "dew of the sea" (ros + marinus). All ancient healers used rosemary, including the 16th century Swiss physician and alchemist, Paracelsus.

Description: Rosemary is a small shrub that grows to three foot in height; it is characterized by grey-green needle-like leaves, pale blue-white flowers. The clear oil is steam-distilled from the flowers and leaves and has a "warm woody aroma." Key constituents:
- 1,8 Cineol (Eucalyptol) (38-55%)

Alpha-Pinene (9-14%)
　　　Beta-Pinene (4-9%)
　　　Camphor (5-15%)
　　　Camphene (2.5-6%)
　　　Borneol (1.5-5%)
　　　Limonene (1-4%)

ORAC value 3,309

Therapeutic properties: Rosemary oil is revered as a stimulant for the circulation, memory; it can relieve rheumatism, myalgia, hepatitis, PMS, hypertension, alopecia, colds, cold sores, canker sores, bronchitis, burns, dandruff, indigestion, diarrhea, flatulence, asthma and headaches.

Routes of application: Baths and massage. Rosemary oil can be inhaled from a handkerchief for headaches and to clear sinuses. The oil of rosemary blends well with the oils of basil, bergamot, black pepper, cedarwood, cypress, *Eucalyptus radiata*, frankincense, geranium, juniper, lavender, lemon, *Litsea cubeba*, mandarin, marjoram, naiouli, oregano, peppermint, pine and ravensara oils.

Cautions: Use in low concentrations as high doses have reportedly caused seizures. Do not use in the first trimester of pregnancy or in individuals who have high blood pressure.

Rosewood (*Aniba rosaeodora*)
Beginnings: The rosewood tree originates from Brazil; the essential oil is steam distilled from the wood.

Description: Key constituents:
　　　Linalol (70-90%)
　　　Alpha-Terpineol (2-7%)
　　　Alpha-Copaene (Trace-3%)
　　　1,8 Cineole (Eucalyptol) (Trace-3%)
　　　Geraniol (0.5-2.5%)

Therapeutic properties: Anti-infectious, antibacterial, antiviral, antiparasitic, antifungal; relieves acne, candida, depression, eczema, oral infections, skin problems and vaginitis.

Routes of application: Diffuse or apply topically.

Cautions: Pregnant women should consult their physician before use.

Sage (*Salvia officinalis, S. sclarea* - Clary sage)

Beginnings: Sage is considered to be a sacred herb by many cultures; it was used to enhance female fertility; and the Chinese have used sage as a medicinal herb for thousands of years.

Description: There are many varieties of common sage, they are all shrubby herbs characterized by rough wrinkled leaves. The essential oil is distilled from the leaves and has a potent, fresh and spicy aroma with a mild camphor overtone. Key constituents:

    Alpha-Thuyone (18-4350
    Beta-Thuyone (3-8.5%)
    1,8 Cineole (Eucalyptol) (5.5-13%)
    Camphor (4.5-24.5%)
    Camphene (1.5-7%)
    Alpha-Pinene (1-6.5%)
    Alpha-Humulene (0-12%)

Monoterpenes: Alpha-thujene, Alpha-pinene, camphene, myrcene, limonenc; Sesquiterpenes; Hydrocarbons; Esters; Phenols: thymol; Oxides (15%): 1,8 cineole; Monoterpenones (20-70%): alpha thujone (12-33%), beta-thujone (2-14%), camphor (1-26%); Aldehydes; Coumarins.

Therapeutic properties: Sage oil is a general tonic; it is used to relieve dysmenorrhea, arthritis, aches, infections, sore throat and edema. Clary sage is used for its sedative and euphoric effects; it is used to relieve insomnia, anxiety and depression. Its aroma is more floral than that of the common sage.

Routes of application: Bath and massage. Sage oil blends well with bergamot, lavender, lemon, peppermint, lemongrass, pine and rosemary.

Cautions: In high doses sage can produce significant stimulation and should be avoided by those with seizure disorders. All varieties of sage should be avoided during the first trimester of pregnancy.

Sandalwood (*Santalum album*)

Beginnings: Sandalwood was first used by the Chinese, Indians and Egyptians 4,000 years ago. It was used for perfumes for more than 2,000 years, cosmetics and furniture. Religious pilgrims used sandalwood essential oils to cover themselves during worship.

Description: The sandalwood tree is an evergreen that grows to thirty feet in

height. It is cultivated in Indonesia, Southeast Asia and in eastern India. The young sandalwood tree grows as a parasite on other trees for the first seven years after germination, the oil is not distilled from the roots and the heartwood until the tree is at least 30 years old. The syrupy, balsamic oil is extracted from coarsely chipped and powdered heartwood and root wood by steam distillation.
Key constituents:
- Alpha-Santalol (47-55%)
- Beta-Santalol (19-23%)
- Sesquiterpinol Santalol
- Santenonol
- Teresantalal
- Borneol
- Santalene

Therapeutic properties: Sandalwood is used to relieve depression and tension; it is an expectorant, aphrodisiac and anti-spasmodic and is commonly used to relieve bronchitis, coughs, nausea, cystitis and skin conditions.

Routes of application: Inhalation and massage. Sandalwood oil blends well with black pepper, clary sage, clove, palmarosa, petitgrain, cypress, frankincense, lemon, myrrh, orange, patchouli, Roman chamomile, spruce, ylang-ylang, neroli and rose oils.

Spearmint (*Mentha spicata*)

Beginnings: The spearmint plant originated in Utah. Spearmint oil is steam distilled from the leaves.

Description: Key constituents:
- Carvone (45-55%)
- Cis-Dihydrocarvone (5-10%)
- Limonene (15-25%)

ORAC value 5,398

Therapeutic properties: Relieves bronchitis, candida, cystitis and hypertension; it is an anti-inflammatory, calming agent, astringent, antiseptic, mucolytic, stimulates gallbladder and relieves dysmenorrhea. Spearmint oil is a tonic for the respiratory and nervous systems; it stimulates appetite and can help relieve halitosis, depression, indigestion, dry skin, eczema, headaches, nausea, sore gums, vaginitis and obesity.

Routes of application: Diffuse or apply topically. Spearmint oil blends well with basil, lavender, peppermint and rosemary.

Caution: Pregnant women should consult their physician before use.

Spikenard (*Nardostachys jatamansi*)

Beginnings: Spikenard originated in India and was historically used as a perfume, and as a medicinal oil. The oil is extracted from the roots by steam distillation. Song of Solomon 1:12 "While the king sitteth at his table, my spikenard sendeth forth the smell thereof" Song of Solomon 4:13 "Thy plants an orchard of pomegranates, with pleasant fruits; camphire with spikenard." Song of Solomon 4:14 "Spikenard and saffron; calamus and cinnamon, with all trees of frankincense; myrrh and aloes, with all the chief spices." John 12 "Then took Mary a pound of ointment of spikenard, very costly, and anointed the feet of Jesus."

Description: Spikenard is a perennial herb that produces a straight stem, green leaves, and small pinkish-mauve bell-shaped flowers. The essential oil is steam distilled from the plant roots. Key constituents:

- Calarene (22-35%)
- Beta-Ionene (4-8%)
- Beta-Maaliene (4-9%)
- Aristoladiene (3-7%)
- Valeranone
- Jonon
- Tetramethyloxatricycloclecanol
- Methylthymyl-Ether
- 1,8-Cineole

Therapeutic properties: The oil is antibacterial, antifungal, anti-inflammatory, deodorant, relaxing and a skin tonic; it relieves allergies, candida, indigestion, insomnia, dysmenorrhea, migraine, nausea, rashes, bacterial infections, stress, rapid heart rate (tachycardia) and tension.

Routes of application: Apply to the abdomen or topically to affected area. Blends well with lavender, lemon, clary sage, clove, juniper, cypress, geranium, rose maroc, neroli, frankincense, myrrh, patchouli, pine and vetiver.

Caution: If pregnant consult physician before use.

Spruce (*Picea mariana*)

Beginning: The spruce originated in Canada; the essential oil or "turpentine" is steam distilled from the needles and twigs. The Lakota Native Americans used spruce oils and smoke to facilitate prayers to the Great Spirit.

Description: Key constituents:
- Bornyl Acetate (18-28%)
- Camphene (17-25%)
- Alpha Pinene (12-19%)
- Beta Pinene (4-8%)
- Delta-3-Carene (5-10%)
- Limonene (2-7%)
- Santene (1-5%)
- Tricyclene (1-5%)

Therapeutic properties: Spruce oil is used to relieve arthritis, rheumatism, bone pain; it acts as a general glandular tonic, relieves candida, hyperthyroidism and prostatitis.

Routes of application: Diffuse or apply topically. Spruce essential oil blends well with wintergreen, birch, *Eucalyptus radiata,* frankincense, helichrysum and ravensara.

Caution: Pregnant women should consult their physician before use.

Tagetes (*Tagetes glanulifera*)

Beginnings: Historically used as an insecticide. It was hung in doorways, stuffed in mattresses and worn as garlands to repel mosquitoes, flies and ticks. The essential oil has been used to kill maggots in open wounds.

Description: Tagetes is a weed that grows up to six feet tall; it has deep green divided leaves and large numbers of yellow-orange flowers that resemble daisy heads. The essential oil is steam distilled from the leaves, stalks and flowers, preferably harvested when the seeds are just beginning to develop. Key constituents:
- Ocimenes
- Dihydro Tageton
- Dihydrotagetone
- Thymol

Therapeutic properties: The essential oil of tagetes has anti-infectious, antifungal, antibiotic, antispasmodic, emmenagogue, mucolytic, antiparasitic and antiseptic properties; it is used to treat athlete's foot, corns, calluses, bunions, catarrh, coughs, chest infections, parasitic infestations and fungal infestations.

Routes of application: The essential oil of tagetes blends well with bergamot, clary sage, lemon and lavender.

Cautions: Pregnant women should consult their doctor before using this oil; not to be used in children under the age of 16 years; it may cause skin irritation on sensitive skin; may cause photosensitivity.

Tansy (Blue) (*Tanacetum annuum*)

Beginnings: The tansy plant originated in Morocco and France; the essential oil is steam distilled from the leaves and flowers.

Description: Key Constituents:
Camphor (10-17%)
Sabinene (10-17%)
Beta-Pinene (5-10%)
Myrcene (7-13%)
Alpha-Phellandrene (5-10%)
Para-Cymene (3-8%)
Chamazulene (3-6%)

Therapeutic properties: Blue tansy is anti-inflammatory, relieves pain, relieves pruritits, sedates the nervous system, has antihistamine, hypotensive and hormone-like activities.

Routes of application: Topical and diffuse.

Cautions: Pregnant women should consult their physician before use.

Tarragon (*Artemisia dracunculus*)

Beginnings: The tarragon plant originates in Slovenia and France. Tarragon was traditionally used in Europe as an antimicrobial and antiseptic. The essential oil is steam distilled from the leaves.

Description: Key constituents:
Methyl Chavicol (Estragole) (68-80%)
Trans-Beta Ocimene (6-12%)
Cis-Beta-Ocimene (6-12%)
Limonene (2-6%)

Therapeutic properties: Relieves colitis, hiccups, intestinal spasm, parasites, rheumatic pain and sciatica; used for genital and urinary tract infections, nausea, PMS, dysmenorrhea, nerve tonic and wound healing.

Routes of application: Topically diluted with carrier oil; blends well with chamomile, clary sage, fir, juniper, lavender, pine, rosewood, orange and tangerine oils.

Cautions: Pregnant women should consult physician before use.

Tea Tree (*Melaleuca alternifolia*) See Melaleuca.

Beginnings: The antiseptic properties of tea tree oil were appreciated by the Australian Aborigines centuries ago; they used tea tree oil medicinally for treating sunburn, ringworm and athletes foot; tea tree oil was used to treat snake bite. In World War II, cutters and producers of tea tree oil were exempt from military service until a plentiful supply of tea tree oil was stocked; the essential oil was issued to each soldier and sailor for them to treat tropical infections and wounds.

Description: The tea tree, also known as the swamp tree and the "paper bark" tree, is a native plant of Australia and Tasmania; it produces white hanging flowers on a long spike. The pale green essential oil is extracted from the twigs and leaves and has a strong aromatic camphorous odor similar to eucalyptus.

Key constituents:
- Gamma Terpinene (10-28%)
- Alpha-Terpinene (5-13%)
- 1,8 Cineole (Eucalyptol) (0-15%)
- Alpha-Terpineol (1.5-8%)
- Para-Cymene (0.5-12%)
- Terpineol -4 (30-45%)
- Limonene (0.5-4%)
- Aromadendrene (trace-7%)
- Delta-Cadinene (trace-8%)
- Alpha Pinene (1-6%)

Therapeutic properties: Tea tree oil is a potent all-purpose disinfectant and antiseptic and is commonly used to relieve flea infestations, respiratory problems, bronchitis, laryngitis, skin conditions, athlete's foot, burns, cold sores, mouth ulcers, verrucas, thrush and warts.

Routes of application: Inhalation, topical, mouth wash and baths. Tea tree oil blends well with basil, bergamot, black pepper, lavender, rosemary, lemon, Roman chamomile, German chamomile, *Eucalyptus globulus*, *Eucalyptus radiata*, clary sage, juniper, cypress, pine, marjoram, oregano, peppermint, ravensera and thyme.

Cautions: Oxidized tea tree oil smells like melted rubber.

Thyme (*Thymus vulgaris*)

Beginnings: The ancient Egyptian embalmers mixed thyme oil in their embalming fluids. The Greeks drank an herbal infusion of thyme leaves after large banquets to aid digestion. Nicholas Culpepper claimed that thyme was "a great lung strengthener and a remedy for shortness of breath." Rudyard Kipling wrote, ""wind-bit thyme that smells like the perfume of the dawn in paradise."

Description: Thyme is a low-growing wild herb characterized by dark green leaves, woody stalks and small pink flowers. Thyme is cultivated widely throughout the Mediterranean, Algeria, Yugoslavia and Egypt for culinary and pharmaceutical uses. The essential oil is extracted from the whole plant by steam-distillation and has a pungent, sweet herbaceous aroma. The first steam distillation produces a red essential oil, the second distillation process produces a clear oil. Key constituents:

    Thymol (37-55%)
    Para-Cymene (14-28%)
    Gamma-Terpinene (4-11%)
    Linalol (3-6.5%)
    Carvacrol (0.5-5.5%)
    Myrcine (1-2.8%)

ORAC value 159,590

Therapeutic properties: Thyme is used to relieve fatigue and anxiety, rheumatic aches, asthma, pertussis, laryngitis, tonsillitis, bronchitis, colitis, cystitis, dermatitis, psoriasis, sciatica, and vaginal yeast infections; relieves insomnia, depression, indigestion, headaches, obesity, skin conditions and as an antiseptic to treat viral infections, coughs and a wide variety of respiratory infections.

Routes of application: Inhalation, compresses, salves, baths and massage; blends well with bergamot, citrus oils, cedarwood, cypress, eucalyptus, geranium, juniper, *Melaleuca alternifolia*, oregano, pine, rosemary, grapefruit, clary sage, lemon, and tea tree oils.

Cautions: Pregnant women should consult with their physician before use; undiluted thyme essential oil can irritate the skin.

Tsuga (*Tsuga Canadensis*)

Beginnings: This plant originated in Canada; the essential oil is steam distilled from the needles and twigs of a conifer evergreen tree commercially marketed as "hemlock."

Description: Key constituents:
- Alpha-and Beta-Pinenes (18-25%)
- Camphene (12-18%)
- Limonene + Beta Phellandrene (3-7%)
- Bornyl Acetate (28-38%)
- Tricyclene (4-8%)
- Myrcene (1-3%)

Therapeutic properties: The essential oil is analgesic, antirheumatic, astringent, tonic; relieves coughs, respiratory problems, kidney problems, skin problems, urinary tract infections and venereal infections.

Routes of application: Diffuse, massage and apply topically; dilute one drop of oil with one teaspoon of carrier oil.

Cautions: Pregnant women should consult with their physician before use; repeated use in a short period of time can produce sensitivity.

Valerian (*Valeriana officinalis*)

Beginnings: This herb originated in Belgium, Croatia and France; the essential oil is steam distilled from the root.

Description: The tall thin stalk produces a small round flower head of tiny, white-pink flowers. An essential oil that smells more "woodsy" is produced from the Japanese "kesso root" and from the Indian valerian (*V. wallichi*). Key constituents:
- Bornyl Acetate (32-44%)
- Camphene + Alpha-Fenchene (24-34%)
- Alpha-Pinene (4-8%)
- Beta-Pinene (2-6%)
- Isobicycolgermacrenol (3-6%)
- Myrtenyl Acetate (1-5%)

Therapeutic properties: Relieves insomnia, nervous indigestion, migraine, restlessness, stress, hypothermia and tension; it has sedative and tranquilizing properties.

Routes of application: Diffuse, inhale, massage or apply topically; blends well with cedarwood, lavender, mandarin, patchouli, petitgrain, pine and rosemary.

Cautions: Pregnant women should consult their physician before use.

Vetiver (vetivert) (*Vetiveria zizanioides*)

Beginnings: Originated in Haiti and India; it is steam distilled from the root. In India the roots are woven into fans and screens called "tatties" for doors, windows and floors to give rooms a good fragrance and repel insects.

Description: Vetiver grows as a clump of thin grass-like leaves. The roots are spindly but intensely aromatic; many claim the essential oil smells like "dirt." Key constituents:
- Alpha Vetivone (3-6%)
- Beta Vetivone (3-6%)
- Khusenol (6-11%)
- Isovalencenol (11-15%)
- Nootkatone (2-5%)
- Khusimone (3-6%)

Therapeutic properties: Vetiver oil is antiseptic, antispasmodic, calming, rubifacient, sedative, stimulant and tonic for the circulatory system and bone marrow; relieves acne, anxiety, arthritis pain, cuts, depression, insomnia and oily skin.

Route of application: Diffuse, massage or apply topically; blends well with bergamot, black pepper, clary sage, *Eucalyptus citriodora*, geranium, ginger, grapefruit, jasmine, lavender, lemon, lemongrss, *Litsea cubeba*, mandarin, melissa, orange, patchouli, rose, sandalwood, ylang-ylang and yuzu oils.

Cautions: Pregnant women should consult their physician before use.

Vitex (chaste tree) (*Vitex negundo*)

Beginnings: This tree originated in Turkey; the essential oil is steam distilled from the inner bark, small branches and leaves of the chaste tree.

Description: Key constituents:
- Beta-Caryophyllene (38-48%)
- Limonene + 1,8 Cineole (3-7%)
- Sabinene (10-15%)
- Caryophyllene Oxide (5-10%)

Longifolene + Alpha-Gurjunene (5-10%)

Therapeutic properties: Relieves symptoms of Parkinson's disease and neurological disease.

Routes of application: Diffuse or apply topically diluted with base oils; rub two to three drops in palms, cup over nose and inhale; mix two to four drops with one teaspoon of salt and add to warm bath water.

Cautions: pregnant women should consult their physician before use.

Wintergreen (*Gaultheria procumbens*)

Beginnings: The tree originated in China; the essential oil is steam distilled from the leaves. Wintergreen leaves and bark were used to replace tea as a drink during the American Civil War.

Description: Key constituents:
Methyl Salicylate (90+%)

Therapeutic properties: The essential oil is antispasmodic, anti-inflammatory and a liver tonic. Wintergreen essential oils have been used to relieve arthritis, rheumatism, inflammation, fibromyalgia, pain of tendonitis, high blood pressure and muscle spasms and cramps; Wintergreen essential oil has been used to relieve cystitis, urinary bladder infections, acne, gout, gallstones, edema, eczema, dermatitis, osteoporosis and ulcers.

Routes of application: Apply topically to the bottom of the feet; dilute with an extender oil at three to five drops of wintergreen oil to one Tblsp - add blend to a hand hot bath. Wintergreen oil blends well with basil, birch, cypress, geranium, juniper, lavender, lemongrass, marjoram, peppermint and Roman chamomile oils.

Caution: Pregnant women should consult their physician before use.

Yarrow (*Achillea millefolium*)

Beginning: The yarrow originated in Utah. The legendary Greek hero, Achilles, used yarrow to cure his wounds; the Chinese believe that the fragrance of yarrow allows the meeting of heaven and earth in the Yin and Yang tradition.

Description: The essential oil of yarrow is steam distilled from the flowering top. Key constituents:
Chamazulene (12-19%)

Trans-Beta-Caryophyllene (4-8%)
Germacrene D (4-8%)
Camphor (4-9%)
Sabinene (3-7%)
Beta-Pinene (3-7%)
1,8 Cineol (Eucalyptol) (2-6%)

Therapeutic properties: The essential oil of yarrow is anti-inflammatory, relieves indigestion, scar tissue and enhances wound healing. Yarrow essential oil is a potent decongestant of the prostate gland, balances hormones, relieves acne, dysmenorrhea, anorexia, bladder and kidney weakness, cellulite, respiratory infections, stimulates digestion, eczema, gastritis, gout, alopecia, headaches, hemorrhoids, high blood pressure, menopausal symptoms, neuritis, neuralgia, urinary infections, arthritis, rheumatism, sprains, thrombosis, ulcers, varicose veins, vaginitis and ulcers.

Routes of application: Diffuse or apply topically.

Caution: Pregnant women should consult their physician before use.

Ylang-Ylang (*Cananga odorata*)

Beginnings: Ylang-Ylang is a tropical tree that was historically used to treat malaria, insect bites and infections. The name Ylang-Ylang translates to "flower of flowers" and is known as the "perfume tree," it was used to cover the honeymoon bed of newlyweds. It was revered for its antiseptic, tonic and aphrodisiac properties. The oil extracted from the flowers was mixed with coconut oil to perfume and condition the skin and hair.

Description: Ylang-Ylang is a native of Indonesia, Commores and the Philippines and reaches a height of 60 feet. The yellow flowers are freshly picked in the early morning and the oil is extracted by steam-distillation; the second pass distillation oil is known as "cananga." Key constituents:

Germacrene D (15-20%)
Alpha Farnesene (8-12%)
Benzyl Acetate (9-15%)
Benzyl Benzoate (3-6%)
Linalol (6-10%)
Methyl Paracresol (5-9%)
Isoeugenol (3-5%)
Cinnamyl acetate (3-5%)

Therapeutic properties: Ylang-Ylang essential oil is antispasmodic. Typically Ylang-Ylang is used to relieve anxiety, depression, insomnia, hypertension, irregular heart beat, skin conditions and frigidity.

Routes of application: Baths, diffuse and massage. The Ylang-Ylang oil blends well with bergamot, clary sage, *Eucalyptus citriodora*, ginger, grapefruit, jasmine, lemon, *Litsea cubeba*, mandarin, melissa, neroli, palmarosa, patchouli, petitgrain, Roman chamomile, rose, sandalwood and vetiver oils.

Cautions: Pregnant women should consult their physician before use; high concentrations can produce headache and nausea.

Yuzu (*Citrus junos*)

Beginnings: Yuzu was first noted in China in 237 B.C. by Pu-Wei in his book, *Spring and Summer Annals*. The tree is still cultivated in north-central China, however, it is grown more extensively in Japan in modern times. The tree was introduced into Japan 1,000 years ago. Yuzu is cold resistant and is therefore able to be grown in areas unavailable to other citrus varieties. In Japan the rind, juice and fruit are used widely as flavorings in vinegars, soups, seafood dishes, sauces, pickles and salads. It is used by Shinto priests for purification before prayer. It is used as an ingredient for a soft drink popular in South America.

Description: The yuzu is an evergreen, spring fruit tree growing up to 15 feet in height with white flowers and yellow-green fruit. The fruit is low in mass for its size, it has a thick, pithy skin and minimal juice. The essential oil is cold pressed from the rind of the fruit. Key ingredients:
- Limonene
- Y-Terpinene
- B-Phellandrene
- Mycene
- Linalol
- A-Pinene
- Terpinolene

Therapeutic properties: The yuzu essential oil has tonic, stimulant, antibiotic, anti-infectious, antiputrescent, diuretic, antiviral, calmative, nervine, sedative, antiseptic, analgesic and antifungal properties; yuzu is used as a general tonic, antiseptic, and to treat nervous tension, stress, anxiety, cystitis, constipation, cleansing, nervous stomach, cramps, neuralgia, post-viral symptoms and convalescence from chronic diseases.

Routes of application: Yuzu blends well with basil, bay, bergamot, black pepper, cardamom, cedarwood, clary sage, clove, coriander, cypress, *Eucalyptus citriodora*, ginger, jasmine, lavender, marjoram, orange, lemon, patchouli, palmarosa, petitgrain, pine, Roman chamomile, ravensara, rose, rosemary, sandalwood, vetiver and ylang-ylang.

Bibliography

Afrika, L. O.: Afrikan Holistic Health. A & B Publishing Group. Brooklyn, New York. 1983.

Anon: Essential Oils: Desk Reference. Second Ed. Essential Science Publishing. USA. 2002

Aqel, M.B.: Relaxant effect of the volatile oil of Rosmarinus officinalis on tracheal smooth muscle. J Ethnopharmacol. 1991: 33 (1-2). 57- 62.

Aruna, K. and Sivaramakrishnan, V.M.: Anticarcinogenic Effects of the Essential Oils from Cumin, Poppy and Basil. Food Chem. Toxicol. 1992:30 (11). 953-956.

Bassett, I.B., et al: A comparative study of tea-tree oil versus benzoylperoxide in the treatment of acne. Med J Aust. 1990:153 (8). 455-8.

Benencia, F. et al.: Antiviral activity of sandalwood oil against herpes simplex viruses-1 and 2. Phytomedicine. 1999:6 (2). 119-123.

Branch, T.: Parting the Waters. Simon & Schuster. New York. 1989.

Branch, T.: Pillar of Fire. Simon & Schuster. New York. 1999.

Branch, T.: At Canaan's Edge. Simon & Schuster. New York. 2006.

Byrd, W. M. and Clayton, L. A.: An American Health Dilemma: A Medical History of African Americans and the Problems of Race: Beginnings to 1900. Vol. I. Routledge. New York. 2000.

Byrd, W. M. and Clayton, L. A.: An American Health Dilemma: Race, Medicine, and Health Care in the United States 1900 - 2000. Vol. II. Routledge. New York. 2000.

Carson, C.F. et al.: Antimicrobial activity of the major components of the essential oil of *Melaleuca alternifolia*. J. Appl. Bacteriol. 1995:78(3). 264-269.

Diamond, J.: Guns, Germs, and Steel. W. W. Norton & Company. New York. 1997.

Dolara, P. et al: Analgesic effects of myrrh. Nature. 1996. Jan 4: 379(6560).29.

D'Souza, D.: The End of Racism. The Free Press. New York. 1995.

Duncan, K.: Hunting the 1918 Flu. University of Toronto Press. Toronto. 2003.

Easterly, W.: The White Man's Burden. The Penguin Press. New York. 2006.

Edwards, V.: The Aromatherapy Companion. Storey Books. North Adams, MA. 1999.

Fischer-Rizzi, S.: Complete Aromatherapy Handbook. Sterling Publishing Co., Inc. New York. 1990.

Gattefosse', Rene'-Maurice. Aromatherapy. Saffron Walden. UK. C.W. Daniel & Co. 1993.

Goodwin, D. K.: Team of Rivals. Simon & Schuster. New York. 2005

Guenther, Ernest. The Essential Oils. Malabar. Florida. 1950.

Halioua, B and Ziskind, B.: Medicine in the Days of the Pharaohs. The Belknap Press of Harvard University Press. Cambridge, Massachusetts and London, England. 2005.

Huddleston-Mattai, B.: The Sambo Mentality and the Stockholm Syndrome Revisited: Another Dimension to an Examination of the Plight of the African American. J. Black Studies. Vol. 23. No. 3. pp 344-357.

Isaacson, W.: Benjamin Franklin. Simon & Schuster Paperbacks. New York. 2003.

Keville, K.: Aromatherapy for Dummies. IDG Books Worldwide, Inc. Dummies Press. Indianapolis. 1999.

Keville, K. and Green, M.: Aromatherapy. The Crossing Press.

Freedom, CA. 1995.

King, jr., M. L.: Martin Luther King, Jr. Warner Books. New York. 1998.

Kurlansky, M.: Salt. Walker Publishing Company Inc. USA. 2002.

Mann, C.C.: 1491: New Revelations of the Americas Before Columbus. Alfred A. Knopf. New York. 2005.

McFeely, W.S.: Frederick Douglass. W. W. Norton & Company. New York. 1991.

McGlivery, C. and Reed, J.: Essential Aromatherapy. Acropolis Books, Enderby, England. 1993.

McGuffin, M. et al: Botanical Safety Handbook, CRC Press. Boca Raton, FL. 1997.

Murray, M: How to Prevent and Treat Diabetes with Natural Medicine. Riverhead Books. New York. 2003.

Niazi, H.: The Egyptian Prescription. Cairo, Egypt. Elias Modern Press. 1988.

Penoel, Daniel. Natural Home Health Care Using Essential Oils. . Essential Science Publishing. Salem, UT. 1998.

Ryman, D.: Aromatherapy: The Complete Guide to Plant and Flower Essences for Health and Beauty. New York. Bantam Books. 1993.

Sanday, P. R.: Divine Hunger. Cambridge University Press. Cambridge. 1986.

Simone, C.B.: Cancer & Nutrition. Princeton Institute. Princeton, New Jersey. 2005

Simone, C.B.: Prostate Health: Prostate Cancer. Pinceton Institute. Princeton, New Jersey. 2005.

Simone, C.B.: The Truth About Breast Health: Breast Cancer. Princeton Institute. Princeton, New Jersey. 2002.

Stetter, C.: The Secret Medicine of the Pharaohs. Quintessence Publishing Co, Inc. Carol Stream, Illinois. 1993.

Swanson, J. L.: Manhunt. William Morrow/HarperCollins. New York. 2006.

Theodosakis, J., Adderly, B. and Fox, B.: The Arthritis Cure. Wheeler Publishing, Inc. Rockland, Massachusettes. 1997.

Tisserand, R. and Balacs, T. (Ed.): Essential Oil Safety. Churchill Livingston. New York. 1995.

Valnet, J. and Tisserand, R. (ed): The Practice of Aromatherapy. Healing Arts Press. Rochester, VT. 1990.

Wallach, J. D. and Middleton, C. C.: Atherosclerosis in Aoudads. Acta Pathologica. 1971.

Wallach, J.D. and Boever, W.: The Diseases of Exotic Animals. W.B.Saunders and Co. Philadelphia. 1983.

Wallach, J.D. and Ma, L.: Let's Play Doctor. Wellness Publications, LLC. Bonita, CA. 1989.

Wallach, J.D. and Ma, L.: Let's Play Herbal Doctor. Wellness Publications, LLC. Bonita, CA. 2000.

Wallach, J.D. and Ma, L.: Rare Earths: forbidden cures. Wellness Publications, LLC. Bonita, CA. 1994.

Wallach, J.D. and Ma, L.: Dead Doctors Don't Lie. Wellness Publications, LLC. Bonita, CA. 1998.

Wallach, J. D. and Ma, L.: God Bless America. Wellness Publications, LLC. Bonita, CA. 2001.

Wallach, J.D. and Ma, L.: Hell's Kitchen. Wellness Publications, LLC. Bonita, CA. 2005.

Wallach, J.D. and Ma, L.: Passport to Aromatherapy. Wellness Publications, LLC. Bonita, CA. 2005.

Wildwood, C.: The Bloomsbury Encyclopedia of Aromatherapy. Bloomsbury Publishing Plc. London. 1996.

Worwood, V. A.: The Complete Book of Essential Oils and Aromatherapy. New World Library. Novato, CA. 1991.

Worwood, S. and Worwood, V.A.: Essential Aromatherapy. New World Library. Novato, California. 2003.

Young, A.: An Easy Burden. Harper Collins Books. New York. 2004.

Index

A

Abbott, Anderson R. 99
Abernathy, Ralph 67
Abolition 18, 26
Abolition Petition 28
Achilles 245
Acne 198
ACS 177
Adams, John 19
Adams, John Quincy 32
AEC 102
Aedes mosquito 84
African American 78
African Blacks 15
African folk medicine 97
Afro-Indians 20
Age of Exploration 82
Age of Jackson 93
AIDS 78, 114
Alabama 13
Alaska 94
Albany Herald 66
Alexander the Great 201
Allantoin 203
Allergies 199
American Cancer Society 177, 102
American Heart Assoc. 137
American Medical College 39, 96
American Medical Assoc. 92
American Missionary Assoc. 32
Amish 159
Amistad 32
Amphiarthroidal 168
An Easy Burden 75
Anacostia 59
Analgesic 203
Anaximander 121

Anaximenes 121
Anderson, Dr. Wm. 66
Andes 26
Aneurysm 137, 146
Angelica 190
Angiogenesis 183
Angiostatin 183
Anise 191
Annan, Kofi 73
Anopheles mosquito 85
Anorexia 218
Antebellum Period 93
Anthony, Susan B. 33
Anthrax 128
Antibacterial 201, 221
Antibiotic 239
Antifungal 221, 241
Anti-infectious 202, 239
Anti-inflammatory 203
Antimicrobial 203
Antioxidant 203
Antiparasitic 228
Antiseptic 202, 206, 214
Anti-slavery Society 34
Anti-spasmodic 202, 211
Antisudorific 202
Antiviral 207
Anus 120
Anxiety 218
Aphrodisiac 196, 2340
Arabia 207
Archaic medicine 118
Aristotle 121
Arkansas 14
Army Air Corps 108
Army of Northern Virginia 39
Arthritis 16

Asafetida herb 185
Asafetida pouch 185, 186
Asafizzit 185
Asthma 221
Astringent 205, 214
Atahuallpa 6
Atherosclerosis 211
Athlete's foot 239
Atlanta Compromise 60, 89
Atlanta Constitution 89
Atlantic Slave Trade 84, 127
Atzerodt, George 41
Augusta, Alexander T. 99
Autumnal fever 85
Aztec 6

B

Baby boomer 165
Bad Check speech 71
Bailey, Frederick 29
Baker, Luther 45
Bakken, Jill 79
Balkan 82
Baltimore Plot 34
Baptize 15
Barracoons 126
Basil 191
Battle of New Orleans 94
Bay 192
Bay of Benin Fever 84
Bay laurel 192
Bay rum 192
Bear Flag Republic 94
Beckwith, S. H. 48
Benzoin 192
Bergamot 193
Berry, Chuck 64
Bible 9

Biddle, Eli 34
Big Man 24
Bilharzias 125
Bilios remittent 84
Billups, Rev. Charles 68
Birch 194
Bitter orange 225
Black African 18, 81, 126
Black Freedman 14
Black genes 20
Black healers 95, 131
Black is Beautiful 39, 97
Black pepper 194
Black physician 92
Black Problem 88
Black Sea 82
Black skin 20
Black slave 13, 16, 82
Black State 33
Black suffrage 88
Black vomit 84
Blackamoor 18
Black Union Soldier 35
Blood flukes 125
Blow, Taylor 34
Blue tansy 240
BMC Medicine 138
Boils 216
Bondage 1, 23, 80
Bone (Bruised, broken, spurs) 239
Bone ache 239
Bongoism 188
Bonney, Rev. Isaac 32
Booth, John Wilkes 39
Boston 37, 16
Boston Celtics 142
Boston Tea Party 209
Bowling Green 45
Bows and arrows 2

Boynton v. Virginia 65
Branding 14
Breaking-in-Period 83
Breast cancer 179
Breeden, J. O. 88
Breeding farms 128
Brewer's yeast 129
Bronchitis 193
Brown v. Board of Ed/Topeka 64
Brown, John 32
Brucellosis 128
Bunch, Ralph J. 64
Bureau of Indian Affairs 102
Burns 208, 215
Bursae 168
Bus Boycott 64
Bush, Pres. George 79
Butler Island Plantation 98

C

Cachexia Africana 129
Caesar 131
Cajamarca 6
Cajeput 195
Calamus 196
Calcium 139
Caldwell, Dr. Charles 133
Calmative 197
Campeche 11
Cancer 173
Candida 210
Candle maker 16
Cannibalism 2
Capac, Huayna 11
Cape of Good Hope 125
Car sicknsess 209
Cardamom 196
Cardiomyopathy 145

Cardiotonic 229
Cardiovascular disease 141
Carnation 197
Cartilage 168
Castor oil 189
Catarrh 239
Catechins 183
CDC 78, 106
Cedarwood 198
Celsus 123
Center for the Biology of
    Natural Systems 86
Center for Disease Control 78, 106
Chai tea 196
Challcochima 13
Chamberlin, Wilt 113
Chamomile, German 199
Chamomile, Roman 199
Charles, Ray 129
Charles V 13
Charleston Harbor 35
Chase, Chief Justice Salmon P. 38
Chaste tree 244
Chatham Islands 21
Chattel slavery 21
Cherokee 19
Chester, Samuel Knapp 39
Chiefdoms 25
Chilblains 199
Cholesterol (high) 142
Chondroitin sulfate 169
Christ 9, 207, 76
Christian soldier 99
Christians 9, 82
Chromium 145
Cinnamon 200
Cinque 32
Citronella 201
Citrus 217

Civil Rights Act (1957) 65
Civil Rights Bill 74
Civil Rights Movement 116
Civil War 34, 88
Clans 24
Clary sage 201
Clay beds 2
Cleansing 189
Clove 202
Cnidus 122
Cobb, W. Montague 120
Cobo Hall 70
Cocoliztli 12
Code of Hammurabi 118
Coffee 161
Colitis 240
Collagen 168
Colon cancer 182
Colonial Wars 18
Columbus, Christopher 6
Comfrey 203
Committee on Civil Rights 64
Confederate 34
Confederate Congress 36
Confederate Cross 75
Confederate soldier 34
Conger, Everton 45
Conjure men 97
Connor, Bull 68
Conquistadores 26
Continental Army 19
Cook, Captain 219
Cooper, Dr. Richard S. 139
Corbett, Sgt. Boston 57
CORE 65
Coriander 204
Coronary artery disease 145
Correction Law 15
Cortes 11

Cos 122
Cosby Show 77
Coughs 200
Cow pox 132
Cox-2 inhibitor 170
Creek Confederation 19
Cribbing 160
Crispus Attacks Day 97
Cro-Magnon 2, 3
Cross 9
Crow, Jim 31
Cuba 11
Cuitlahuac 11
Culinary ashes 129
Culpepper, Nicholas 203
Cuyuchi, Ninan 11
Cypress 204
Cystitis 237

D

D-Day 69
Dandruff 198, 215
Daniels, Dr. Jennifer 116
Dark Continent 125
Darrow, Ann 108
Davidson, Basil 126
Dead Doctors Don't Lie 174
Declaration of Independence 19, 132
DeGrasse, J. V. 99
Delany, Dr. M. R. 96
Demolay 35
Deodorant 238
Derham, Dr. James 132
De Soto, Hernando 13
De Valverde, Fr. Vincente 9
Deringer 41
Devil's dung 185

Diabetes (type II) 148
Diabetes Care 153
Diabetes mellitus 148
Diamond, Jared 2, 7
Diet drinks 162
Digestive disorders 204
Digitalis 132
Diphtheria 128
Diuretic 210
Divan of Algiers 29
Dizziness 209
Dogwood, Silence 28
Doherty, Edward 45
Doisy, Dr. Richard J. 153
Douglas, Stephan A. 23
Douglas, Dr. Wm. 83
Douglass, Frederick 29
Douglass, Sgt. Maj. Lewis 36
Dove, Dr. Robert 132
Dove, Rita 78
Down's syndrome 129
Dream team 142
Dred Scott v. Sanford 33
Drugs 120, 210
Duke University 19
Dutch 14
Dutch West Indies Co. 14
Duffy antigen 86
Dysentery 84
Dysmenorrhea 120, 190

E

Earl Grey Tea 193
Ebers, Georg 120
Ebers papyrus 120
Eclectics 95
Eczema 198
Egalitarian 24

EGCG 183
Egypt 4
Ehrenreich, Barbara 101
Ehrenreich, John 101
Eisenhower, Pres. Dwight D. 65
Electoral College 88
Elite-rule 94
Elixir of Life 222
Ellis, William 99
Emancipation 100
Embalmers 191
Empire State Building 108
Empiricism 121
Emmenagogue 202
Endostatin 182
Erasistratus 123
Essential oil 189
Ethiopian regiment 19
Eucalyptus citriodora 205
Eucalyptus dives 205
Eucalyptus globulus 205
Eucalyptus oil 172, 205
Eucalyptus polybractea 205
Eucalyptus radiate 205
Eugenic Laws 104
Eugenical News 104
Eugenical sterilization 104
Eugenics 91, 104
Eugenics Record Office 104
Euphrates River 117
European Renaissance 124
Everlast 211
Evers, Medgar 70
Exodus 224
Expectorant 195

F

Family bands 24

Faneuil Hall 97
Farakhan, Minister Louis 78
Fatigue 137
FDA 102
Feces 127
Federilism 94
Fenn, Elizabeth 19
Fennel 206
Ferguson, James 42
Fertile Crescent 25
Fertility 125
Fertilizer 3
Fever 88
Fever and chills 86
Fever tree 205
Finley, M. I. 123
15th Amendment 87
54th Volunteer Infantry 34, 97
Fish hooks 2
Flatulence 230
Flexner/Johns Hopkins 91
Flowers, Vonetta 76
Flu 12, 128
Food poisoning 127
Forbes, Charles 42
Ford Theater 40, 52
Fort Sumter 34
Fort Wagner 35
Four Food Groups 117
Four Thieves Vinegar 234
Foxglove 132
14th Amendment 87
Frankfurter, Felix 34
Frankincense 207
Franklin, Benjamin 16
Frazier, E. Franklin 91
Freedmen 14
Freedmen's Bureau 87, 88, 89
Freedom 43

Freedom Riders 65, 66
Freemont, Capt. John C. 94
Free radicals 145
Frigidity 226
Fungal Infections 220, 221, 222

G

G-6-PD deficiency 86
Galactagogue 207
Gallbladder 218
Galeano, Eduardo 7
Galen 124
Galton, Sir Francis 104
Garbage dumps 2
Gardner, Alexander 39
Gargle 210
Garrett, John 43
Garrett, Richard 49
Garrett, William 44
Genetics 138
Genetically transmitted 138
Geophagia 129, 161
Geranium 208
Gettysburg 37
Gettysburg Address 37
Gilded Age 88
Gillum, Richard F. 136
Gin 186
Ginger 209
Ginger ale 209
Ginger beer 209
Gitt, George 36
Glory 34
Glucosamine sulfate 169
Glucose 153
God 9
god 119
Gold 6

Golden Age 121
Goldenrod 209
Gonorrhea 128
Gooch, Lt. Gov. 130
Good slave 20
Goose grease 186
Gouldman, Jesse 46
Gout 204
Governor Pizarro 7
Grady, Henry W. 88
Graham, Dee 110
Granada 82
Grant, Gen. Ulysses S. 39
Grapefruit 210
Great Awakening 16
Great Depression 90, 108
Great House 29
Great Leap Forward 2
Greeks 118
Green tea 172, 183
Guinea pig 92
Gunn's Domestic Medicine 97

H

Haley, Alex 77
Hamilton, Alexander 94
Hampton Institute 60
Hanta-virus 12
Harlem 90
Harlem Hospital Center 90
Harper's Ferry 34
Harpoons 2
Harvard School P.H. 106
Harvey, William 124
Hatcher, Richard 74
Haudenosaunee 19
Hawk, Harry 42
Hayes-Tilden Compromise 88

HDL 145
Hearst, Patty 110
Hearst, Wm. Randolph 110
Heart attack 141
Heart attack, stroke and
    Cancer belt 141
Heart burn 230
Heart disease 142
Hebrews 3
Helichrysum 211
Hemlock 243
Hemorrhoids 205
Herbs 187
Herb of Happiness 219
Herodotus 120
Herold, David 40
Herophilus 123
Hiccups 240
Hill-Burton Act 92
Hippocrates 122
Hippocratic Corpus 122
Hippocratic Oath 122
Hitler 90
HMS Seahorse 82
Hobbes, Thomas 15
Holy Law 9
Holy spirit root 190
Homeopathic 95
Homer 120
Homocysteine 162
Homo sapiens 2
Hood, James 69
Hoodoo 188
Hook worms 125
Howard, Gen. Oliver 89, 99
Howard School of Divinity 65
Howard University 58, 89
Hudson Valley 14
Hunger strikes 127

Hunza Land 187
Hyacinth 219
Hypertension 135, 138, 240
Hypnotic 212
Hyssop 212

I

I Have a Dream 71
Iberian Peninsula 82
ICC 66
Ideal slave 20
Idolatry 6
Imhotep 119
Immortelle 211
Inca 5
Inca Empire 7
Incest 6
Individualism 94
Indian slaves 20
Indians 9
Indigestion 209, 231
Infection 232
Infectious diseases 232
Infertility 120
Insect bites 217
Insecticides 217
Insect repellent 217
Insomnia 225
Insulin resistence 151
Interstate Commerce Com. 66
Iroquois League 19
Irrigation 25
Ishmaelites 4

J

Jackson, Pres. Andrew 32, 93
Jackson, Rev. Jesse L. 77
Jamestown 14
Jasmine 213
Jenner, Dr. Edward 132
Jet Magazine 64
Jett, Willie 45
Jews 83
Jim Crow Laws 32, 88
Johnson, Pres. Lyndon B. 74
Johnson, Vice Pres. Andrew 41
Johnson, Shoshana 79
Joint capsule 168
Jones, James H. 100
Joseph 3
Juice 162
Juniper 213
Junto 16
Justnian Code 15

K

Kahun papyrus 120
Kansas-Nebraska Act 33
Kardee, Allan 188
Kearny, Gen. Stephen 94
Keckly, Elizabeth 40
Kemble, Fanny 98
Kennedy, Pres. John F. 66
Kenny, Dr. John A. 92
Kerner Commission 74
Kerosene 116
Kerr-Mills Program 103
Kesso root 243
Kidney disorders 137
Kidney stones 120
King, Jr, Rev. Martin Luther 64, 74, 75
King Charles I 6
King, Coretta Scott 79
King/Drew Hospital 106

King of England 15
King Kong 107
King of Prussia 28
King, Rodney G. 78
King Solomon 223
King of Spain 10
Kinnamon 200
Kipling, Rudyard 242
Kleptocracies 25
Koran 29
Kuwait 117

L

Labrador tea 214
Laryngitis 195
Lavender 215
Laxative 212
LDL 145
Ledum 214
Lee, Gen. Robert E. 34
Lemon 216
Lemon balm 222
Lemongrass 216
Lemon-scented 217
Leptospirosis 128
Leukemia 182
Lewis, Reggie 113, 142
Licorice 206
Liberty Tea 209
Ligaments 168
Lincoln, Abraham 34
Lincoln's Inaugural Address 39
Lincoln, Mary 40
Lind, Dr. James 132
Litsea cubeba 217
Lloyd, Col. 30
Long, Jefferson Franklin 59
Lord of Cajamarca 11

Louis, Joe 61
Louisiana 14
Louisiana Purchase 94
Lucas, William 43
Lung cancer 175
Lynch Law 92

M

Macumba 188
Madagascan nutmeg 232
Maddox, Lester 75
Ma, Lan 81, 86
Malaria 83, 85
Malcom X 74
Malone, Vivian 69
Malta fever 128
Mandarin 218
Mandela, Pres. Nelson 78
Manuka 219
Manumitted 19
Maori 21
March on Washington 70
Marijuana 175
Marjoram 219
Maroon dance 188
Marsh fever 84
Marshall, Thurgood 74
Materia medica 185
Mather, Cotton 82
Matrilineal 20
McFeely, William 32, 132
McKenzie, Rev. V. M. 78
Measles 12, 127
Medicaid 103
Medicare 103
Mediterranean slave trade 82
Meharry University Medical
    School 89

Melaleuca alternifolia 220
Melaleuca ericifolia 221
Melaleuca quienquenervia 222
Melissa 222
Mertz, Dr. Walter 151
Mesoamerica 26
Mexican War 94
Mexico 11
Migraine headaches 243
Milk 162
Milliken's Bend 36
Million Man March 78
Mississippi appendectomies 106
Mississippian Chiefdoms 13
Missouri Compromise 34
Mitchell, Clarence 70
MLK, Jr. Day 75
Modern skeletons 3
Model Eugenical Sterilization 104
Montgomery Buss Boycott 64
Montgomery, Col. James 35
Moorish Moslem 82
Morgan v. Virginia 64
Moriori 21
Moslem Turkish 82
Motion sickness 209
Motley, Marion 64
Mountain savory 223
Mucolytic 211, 237
Mud fever 128
Mudd, Dr. Samuel 59
Mulattos 20
Munchies 160
Murine typhus 130
Murray, Anna 30
Muscles 213
Muscle cramps 213
Muscle pain 2213
Musket Wars 21

My Bondage My Freedom 32
Mycoplasma synoviae 169
Myocardial infarction 142
Myrrh 223
Myrtle 224

N

NAACP 63
Nail fungus 220, 221, 222
Name magic 188
Narcotic dropsy 84
Nard 201
Nashville VA Hospital 101
Nation of Islam 78
National Medical Assoc. 92
Native Americans 6, 93, 214
Natural Law 116, 121
Nausea 204
Nazi Germany 90
NCI 102
Neanderthals 2, 3
Negro car 31
Negro house 45
Negro servants 17
Negroes 17, 97
Neroli 225
Nervine 231
Nessa, Dr. W. Thomas 143
Neuralgia 247
New African Free School 95
New Amsterdam 14
New South 89
New World 5
New York Manumission Society 95
New Zealand 21
Nieman-Pick Disease 83
Nigerian 138
NIH 86

Nile River 118
Nippur 118
NMA 92
Nomads 24
North Star newspaper 32
Northwest Ordinance 33
Nutmeg 226
Nyannego 188

O

Obesity 155, 207
Observations 18
Ochberg, Frank 110
Oil of Angels 190
Old Confederacy 90
Old Hickory 94
Old Order Amish 159
Old South 141
Old Testament 3, 212
Old World 5
Oliver, Phil 86
Olsson, Jan-Erik 108
Omega-3 EFA 142
Operation PUSH 77
Orange 227
ORAC 183
Oregano 227
Oregon Territory 94
Osler, Sir William 119
Osteoarthritis 169
Osteoporosis 165, 170
Ottoman Empire 81
Our American Cousin 40
Owens, Jesse 63

P

Pain 211

Palmarosa 22
Pangaea 117
Parasites (intestinal) 201
Parasitic infestations 130
Parks, Rosa 64
Parsley 229
Patchouli 229
Peanut, John 41
Pearl ashes 187
Peck, Dr. David John 96
Pellagra 128
Peppermint 230
Peppermint oil 172
Pequots 18
Perfect storm 93, 166
Pernicious anemia 83
Perpetual servitude 28
Persian Gulf 82
Petitgrain 231
Pharaoh 4
Pharaoh Zoser 119
Phenotype 83
Phlebitis 211
Phillips, Gov. Wendell 34
Phytoestrogens 180
Pica 160
Pierce, Ronelda 113, 146
Pine 232
Pine oil 232
Pinel, Phillipe 132
Pinkerton, Allan 34
Pithom 5
Pizarro, Francisco 7
Pizarro, Hernando 6
Pizarro, Pedro 7
Pizarro, Juan 7
Plague 12, 214
Plant minerals 186
Plantation 97

Plasmodium spp. 85
Plato 121
Plessy v. Ferguson 63
Pliny 124, 206
PMS 190
Pneumonia 84
Point Coupee 17
Political pork 38
Polygamy 6
Poor Man's Friend 97
Porphyria 83
Porphyria cutania 83
Porphyria tarda 83
Port Royal 46
Potash 129, 187
Potash fever 187
Potiphar 3
Powell, Gen. Colin L. 78
Powell, Lewis 41
Powell, William 99
Pox Americana 19
Pre-Columbian 13
Prehypertension 137
Price, T. Douglas 12
Priest 25
Prisoner of Shark Island 59
Progressive Era 89, 92
Prosser, Gabriel 17
Prostate 181
Prostate cancer 181
Prostate Specific Antigen 181
Prostatitis 181
Proteoglycans 168
Protestant Reformation 82
Providence of God 35
PSA 181
Pu-We 247
Puritan 16, 82
Purvis, C. B. 99

Pythagoras 118

Q

Quakers 18
Quaker School 34
Queen of Sheba 223

R

Raamses 5
Race riots 74
Rapier, John 99
Retardation Centers 128
Ravensara 232
Rebel States 35
Reconstruction Era 87
Red-Black 20
Regan, Prews. Ronald 75
Remittent fever 85
Repel the devil 229
Republican Party 34
Rheumatoid arthritis 169, 171, 190
Riboflavin 129
Ringworm 220
Rio Grand Camp Knife 41
Robinson, Jackie 63
Rock, Dr. John Sweat 38, 96
Rogers, J. A. 120
Roman Code 15
Roman chamomile 199
Roman Empire 81
Root doctor 97
Roots 77
Rose 233
Rosemary 234
Rosmarinus officinalis 234
Rosemary verbenon 234
Rosewood 235

Royal African Co. 15
Rudolph, Welma 65, 113
Runaway "R" 14
Rush, Dr. Benjamin 132
Rush Medical College 96

S

Sage 236
Salt 128, 137
Sandalwood 236
Santeria 188
Santiago 10
Santomee, Lucas 131
Satcher, Sur. Gen. Dr. David 106
Savitt, Todd 83
Scar tissue 218
Scarlet fever 128
Sciatica 240
SCLC 70
Scrub typhus 130
Scurvy 132, 214
Seasickness 209
Second Revolution 75
Sedative 197
Selenium 142
Self examination 179
Seven Food Group Pyramid 117
Seward, Sec. Wm. H. 41
Shaddoc fruit 210
Shango 188
Shaw, Col. Robert Gould 35
Shingles 216, 220
Shock 226
Sick role 119
Sickle cell anemia 86
Sickle cell disease 86
Sickle Cell Foundation of
    Georgia 86

Sickle cell trait 86
SIDS 129
Sinusitis 221
Sixteenth New York 47
Skeletal remains 2
Skull Island 108
Slave 126
Slave barracoons 126
Slave castles 126
Slave coffles 126
Slave hospitals 98
Slave labor 12
Slave masters 20
Slave quarter cures 185, 190
Slave quarters 127
Slave trade 127
Slave uprising 17
Slaver 127
Sleeping distemper 84
Sleeping sickness 83
Smallpox 11, 12, 82
Smalls, Rep. Robert 59
Smart, Elizabeth 110
Smith, (Edwin) papyrus 120
Smith, Edwin 120
Smith, James McCune 95
Smith, William M. 39
SNCC 66
Social stigma 155
Sockdologizing 42
Sodium Task Force 137
Sodom and Gomorrah 106
Soft drinks 150, 162
Soporific 197
Sore eye 129
Sore throat 193
Spanish flu 186
Spearmint 237
Spear-throwers 2

Spider veins 205
Spikenard 238
Spruce 238
Stamey, Dr. Thomas A. 181
State Motto of Virginia 43
Stevens Committee 87
Stockholm syndrome 108, 109
Stockton, Com. Robert F. 94
Stokes, Carl 74
Stone tools 2
Storage ships 126
Stowe, Harriet Beecher 33
Stress 202
Stretch marks 218
Stringer, Cory 113
Strode, Woody 64
Stroke 144
Strontium-87 12
Sunburn 215
Swanson, James L. 43
Synarthroidal 168
Symbianese Liberation Army 110
Synovium 168
Syphilis 91
Syphilis experiment 91

T

Tagetes 239
Tampa Bay 13
Taney, Chief Justice Roger 33
Tansy, Blue 240
Tappan, Lewis 32
Tarragon 240
Tawneys 18
Taxation 25
Tea 161
Tea tree 172, 219, 220, 241
Tendons 168

Tendonitis 245
Tennessee 13
Texas 14
Thales 121
13th Amendment 38, 87
Thomas, Clarence 78
Thomsonians 95
Thrombosis 246
Thyme 242
Tiering 118
Tigris River 117
Tobacco 14, 196
Toe nail chromium 153
Tonic 200
Toothache 200
Torture 2, 3
Toxemia of pregnancy 137
Tribute 25
Triglycerides 142
Truman, Pres. Harry S. 64
Trypanosoma spp. 84
Tsalagi 19
Tsetse fly 84, 220, 241
Tsuga 243
Tuberculosis 88, 97
Tucker, Alpheus 99
Tuke, William 132
Turkish coffee 196
Turkish geranium oil 228
Tumors 208
Turner, Nat 17
Turpentine 189
Turpentine and Sugar 189, 238
Turpentine oils 189, 238
Tuscarora 18
Tuskegee experiment 91
Tuskegee Normal 60
Type setter 16

U

Ulcers (leg) 199
Uncle Tom's Cabin 15, 33
Underground Railroad 97
Undulant fever 128
United Auto Workers 69
University of Alabama 69
University of BC 151
University College of London 117
University of Glasgow 96
University of Mississippi 69
University of Pennsylvania 133
University of Wisconsin 12
Up from Slavery 81
Urban League 70
Urinary tract infection 194
U.S. Paternt (No. 1) 187

V

VA 102
Vaccination 82
Vaginal infection 242
Vaginal yeast 242
Valerian 243
Valnet, Dr. Jean 203
Valley Forge 19
Vanadium 145, 151
Vanderbilt Medical School 101
Vanderbilt University 101
Varicose veins (spider veins) 205
Venereal disease 120
Vesalius 124
Vetiver 244
Violet leaf tea 186
Vioxx 170
Viral hepatitis 127
Viral infection 127
Vitamin A 129
Vitamin B1 129
Vitamin B2 129
Vitamin B3 129
Vitex 244
Voodoo 188
Voodoo doctors 97, 186
Voting Rights Bill 74
Voudoun 186

W

Wallace, Gov. George 69
Wallach, Dr. Joel D. 81, 86, 142
War on Cancer 173
War of 1812 94
War on Poverty 74
Warriors 2
Warts 221
Washington, Booker T. 60
Washington, George 19
Washington, Kenny 63
Washington University 86
Water 161
Waterhouse, Dr. Benjamin 132
Watts Riot 74
Weaver, Robert 74
West African Blacks 12
Whipping 14
White Flight 101
White, Howard Ashley 99
Whites only 65
WHO 107
Wilder, L. Douglas 78
Williams, Ken 79
Williams, Serena 132
Willis, Ben 64
Wintergreen 245
Withering, William 132

WNBA 146
Women's Loyal League 38
Wood ashes 3, 116, 129, 186, 187
World Health Organization 107
World War II 90, 101
Wye House 29

Y

Yah, Dr. Yah 186
Yamasees 18
Yarrow 245
Yaws 127
Yeast 242
Yeast infections 242
Yellow Fever 83
Yellow Jack 84
Ylang-ylang 246
Young, Amb. Andrew 24, 75
Yuzu 247

Z

Zoser, Pharaoh 119

Dr. Joel D. Wallach, BS, DVM, ND
Dr. Ma Lan, MD, MS, LAc
Dr. Gerhard N. Schrauzer, PhD, MS, FACN, CNS

EPIGENETICS

THE DEATH OF THE GENETIC THEORY OF DISEASE TRANSMISSION

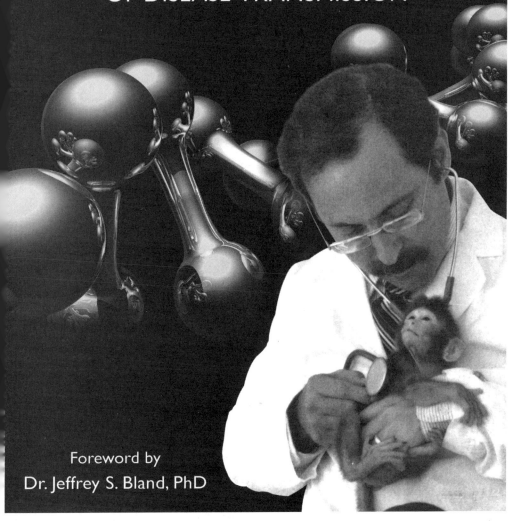

Foreword by
Dr. Jeffrey S. Bland, PhD

IMMORTALITY

The Age Beaters and Their Universal Currency for IMMORTALITY

We all have the genetic equipment to live healthfully well beyond 100. This book will guide you through with Calorie Restriction diet, Mineral supplementation, and the importance of Antioxidants. From the authors of "Dead Doctors Don't Lie"

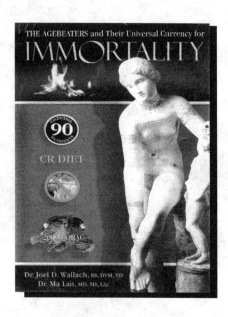

$19.95 - 10 or more $12.00 each

1-800-755-4656
www.drjwallach.com

Let's Play Doctor

The Book That "Orthodox" Doctors Couldn't Kill - "How to" maximize your genetic potential for health and longevity.

- Become your own primary health care provider
- Learn The Alternative Healing Arts
- Establish your own Health Clinic
- Establish a Home Pharmacy
- Home Surgery

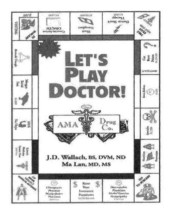

$14.95 - 10 or more $8.00 each

Rare Earths Forbidden Cures
Their Secrets of Health and Longevity

The definitive home reference on minerals, mineral deficiencies and their relationship to:

* Degenerative Diseases
* Learning Disabilities
* Criminal Behavior
* Birth Defects
* Addition
* Food Binges
* Depression
* Infertility and More!

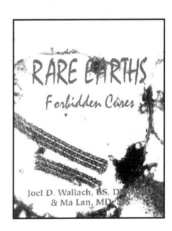

$19.95 - 10 or more $12.00 each

1-800-755-4656
www.drjwallach.com

Hell's Kitchen

What are the real cause of obesity?

Obesity is not a disease, obesity is but a symptom of a deeper nutritional deficiency. Dr.Wallach and Dr.Ma Lan looked beyond written history and looked for clues that would show what events, technology, and what people set us on the terrible path of the would pandemic of obesity. People can simply eliminate obesity and other degenerative diseases if only we would all adhere simple principals and supplement properly and cut cut back on most forms of dietary sugars and carbohydrates.

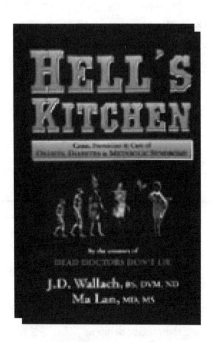

$19.95 - 10 or more $12.00 each

1-800-755-4656
www.drjwallach.com

LET'S PLAY HERBAL DOCTOR

- Learn about the pharmacologilcal properties of plan herbs.
- The history of herbal medicine
- Learn how herbs work
- Active constituents of medicinal herbs
- Growing, harvesting, selecting, storage and processing of herbs

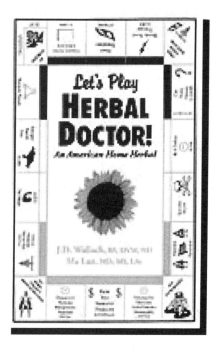

$19.95 - 10 or more $12.00 each

1-800-755-4656
www.drjwallach.com

PASSPORT TO AROMATHERAPY

Essential oils or "essences" are highly concentrated volatile oils extracted from aromatic plants

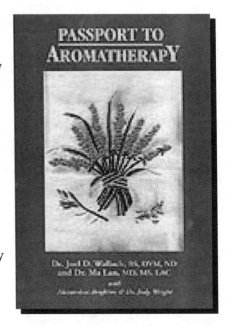

- Essential oils are legendary for their anti-microbial properties

- Essential oils are legendary for uplifting the emotions

$14.95 - 10 or more $8.00 each

Learn more about essential oils from this book

1-800-755-4656
www.drjwallach.com

GOD BLESS AMERICA!

- The epiphany
- American centenarians
- Medical dogmas/lies
- Health and longevity
- Weight loss
- Home defense and
- anti-terrorism plan
  Cash flow and tax plan
- Longevity recipes

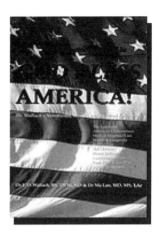

$14.95 - 10 or more $8.00 each

WALLach $Treet for kids

This book is about entrepreneurship, money and business for the purpose of educating entrepreneurial kids, teens and young adults opportunities to find a "good jobs" in a changing global economy, the obvious direction for entrepreneurs is to own their business. Ownership is the true measure of power of business

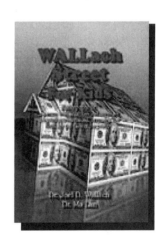

$19.95 - 10 or more $12.00 each

1-800-755-4656
www.drjwallach.com

Audio CDs

CD001	Dead Doctors Don't Lie	The origiinal tape that started it all
CD002	DDDL in Chinese, Korean, Spanish, Japanese	
CD003	Trust me, I am a Doctor	Dr.Wallach's 1996 health lecture series
CD004	Good Doctor, Bad Doctor	Dr.Wallach's 1997 health lecture series
CD005	Live Doctors Do Lie	
CD006	Medical Dogmas & Lies	Dr.Wallach's 2000 health lecture series
CD007	Medical Milking Machine	Dr.Wallach's 2000 health lecture series
CD008	What's Up Doc II	Health Products Information
CD009	Women, Athletes and Children	Menopause, ADHD and Athletes, 2003
CD010	Medical Mouse Trap	Dr.Wallach's lecture on Doctor's continue eduction
CD011	The Best of Dead Doctors Don't Lie	combination of DDDL I,II and III
CD012	Lucky Mo	Children's musical story
CD013	Hell's Kitchen	Dr.Wallach's 2004 health lecture series
CD014	God's Recipe	Health alternative to Ritalin
CD015	$10 Path to Financial Freedom	How to get your Youngevity products for free
CD016	Ferret Fat Pak 101	Weight loss product
CD017	Live Free or Die	Jonathan Emord
CD018	Healthier and Longer Life	
CD020	Dial MD for Murder	Dr.Wallach's 2004 health lecture series
CD030	Truth is Forever	Christian Songs by Dee Stocks
CD031	HE Has the Power to Heal	Christian Songs by Dee Stocks
CD033	WBA and Youngevity Opportunity	Dr.Wallach interviewed by Leroy MacMath -Athlete physical and financial health
CD034	Black Gene Lies I	interviewed by Herbalist Dirk Twine - the top killer diseases of African American
CD035	Black Gene Lies II	Dr.Wallach's lecture at World Changers Men's fellowship in Atlanta, GA
CD037	Tomato Warning	narration by Richard Dennis
CD046	Dead Athletes Don't Lie	
CD047	H5N1 Bird Flu	Dr.Ma Lan
CD048	Deadly Recipe	
CD056	Until Death Do Us Part	Outline information of Dr.Wallach's lectures
CD057	Energy Crisis	History on energy boost
CD058	Get your ACT together	Steve Wallach
CD059	New Best of DDDL	With 25 questions and answers
CD060	Tru Chocolate	Dr.Wallach , Sandy Elsberg and Elaine Lagatta
CD067	From Here To Immortality	Dr. Wallach
CD069	Aroma Therapy Oil	Dr. Wallach
CD070	Cerial Killer	Dr. Wallach
CD071	What Kills Billionaires	Dr.Wallach

order 1-10: $3.00/each, 11-20: $2.00/each, 50 and more: $1.00/each
personalized CD label is available for minimum of 50 CD order.